D1577393

Neonatology Questions and Controversies

ELSEVIER

Neonatology Questions and Controversies

Series Editor

Richard A. Polin, MD
William T. Speck Professor of Pediatrics
College of Physicians and Surgeons
Columbia University;
Director Division of Neonatology
New York Presbyterian
Morgan Stanley Children's Hospital
New York, New York

Other Volumes in the Neonatology Questions and Controversies Series

Neonatology Questions and Controversies

Third Edition

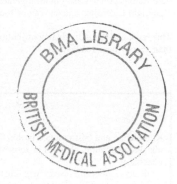

Jeffrey M. Perlman, MB, ChB

Professor of Pediatrics
Division of Newborn Medicine
Department of Pediatrics
New York Presbyterian Hospital
Komansky Children's Hospital
Weill Cornell Medicine
New York, New York

Maria Roberta Cilio, MD, PhD

Professor, Neurology and Pediatrics
Director of Pediatric Epilepsy Research
Director of Neonatal Neuromonitoring and Epilepsy Program
University of California, San Francisco
San Francisco, California

Consulting Editor

Richard A. Polin, MD
William T. Speck Professor of Pediatrics
College of Physicians and Surgeons
Columbia University;
Director Division of Neonatology
New York Presbyterian
Morgan Stanley Children's Hospital
New York, New York

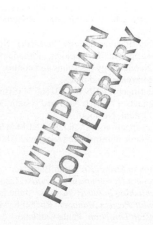

ELSEVIER

ELSEVIER

1600 John F. Kennedy Blvd.
Ste 1800
Philadelphia, PA 19103-2899

NEUROLOGY: NEONATOLOGY QUESTIONS AND CONTROVERSIES,
THIRD EDITION   ISBN: 978-0-323-54392-7

Notices

Knowledge and best practice in this field are constantly changing. As new research and experience broaden
our understanding, changes in research methods, professional practices, or medical treatment may become
necessary.

Practitioners and researchers must always rely on their own experience and knowledge in evaluating and
using any information, methods, compounds, or experiments described herein. In using such information or
methods they should be mindful of their own safety and the safety of others, including parties for whom they
have a professional responsibility.

With respect to any drug or pharmaceutical products identified, readers are advised to check the most
current information provided (i) on procedures featured or (ii) by the manufacturer of each product to be
administered, to verify the recommended dose or formula, the method and duration of administration, and
contraindications. It is the responsibility of practitioners, relying on their own experience and knowledge of
their patients, to make diagnoses, to determine dosages and the best treatment for each individual patient, and
to take all appropriate safety precautions.

To the fullest extent of the law, neither the Publisher nor the authors, contributors, or editors, assume
any liability for any injury and/or damage to persons or property as a matter of products liability, negligence
or otherwise, or from any use or operation of any methods, products, instructions, or ideas contained in the
material herein.

Previous editions copyrighted 2012 and 2008.

Library of Congress Cataloging-in-Publication Data

Names: Perlman, Jeffrey M., editor. | Cilio, Maria Roberta, editor. | Polin,
    Richard A. (Richard Alan), 1945- editor.
Title: Neurology: neonatology questions and controversies / [edited by]
    Jeffrey M. Perlman, Maria Roberta Cilio; consulting editor, Richard A.
Polin.
Other titles: Neurology (Perlman) | Neonatology questions and controversies.
Description: Third edition. | Philadelphia, PA: Elsevier, [2019] | Series:
    Neonatology questions and controversies | Includes bibliographical
    references and index.
Identifiers: LCCN 2018011667 | ISBN 9780323543927 (hardcover: alk. paper)
Subjects: | MESH: Nervous System Diseases | Infant, Newborn, Diseases
    | Infant, Newborn
Classification: LCC RJ290 | NLM WS 340 | DDC 618.92/8--dc23 LC record
available at https://lccn.loc.gov/2018011667

Content Strategist: Sarah Barth
Content Development Specialist: Lisa M. Barnes
Publishing Services Manager: Julie Eddy
Senior Project Manager: Rachel E. McMullen
Design Direction: Paula Catalano

Printed in China

Last digit is the print number: 9   8   7   6   5   4   3   2   1

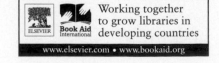

Contributors

Enrico Bertini, MD
Department of Neurosciences
Unit of Neuromuscular Disorders
Laboratory of Molecular Medicine
Bambino Gesù Children's Research
  Hospital
Rome, Italy
  Neonatal Hypotonia

Adrienne Bingham, MD
Teaching Fellow in Neonatal-Perinatal
  Medicine
Women and Infants Hospital of Rhode
  Island;
Department of Pediatrics
Warren Alpert Medical School
Brown University
Providence, Rhode Island
  Hypothermia for Neonatal Hypoxic-
  Ischemic Encephalopathy: Different
  Cooling Regimens and Infants Not
  Included in Prior Trials

Vann Chau, MD, FRCPC
Pediatric Neurologist
Department of Pediatrics
Division of Neurology
The Hospital for Sick Children;
Assistant Professor of Pediatrics
University of Toronto
Toronto, Ontario, Canada
  Congenital Heart Disease: An
  Important Cause of Brain Injury
  and Dysmaturation

Maria Roberta Cilio, MD, PhD
Professor of Neurology and Pediatrics
Department of Neurology
University of California, San Francisco
San Francisco, California
  Neonatal-Onset Epilepsies: Early
  Diagnosis and Targeted Treatment

Adele D'Amico, MD
Department of Neurosciences
Unit of Neuromuscular Disorders
Laboratory of Molecular Medicine
Bambino Gesù Children's Research
  Hospital
Rome, Italy
  Neonatal Hypotonia

Linda S. de Vries, MD, PhD
Professor
Department of Neonatology
Brain Center Rudolf Magnus
Wilhelmina Children's Hospital
University Medical Center Utrecht
Utrecht University
Utrecht, The Netherlands
  Amplitude-Integrated EEG and
  Its Potential Role in Augmenting
  Management Within the NICU

Donna M. Ferriero, MD, MS
Distinguished Professor
Departments of Pediatrics and
  Neurology
University of California, San Francisco
San Francisco, California
  Focal Cerebral Infarction

Dawn Gano, MD, MAS
Assistant Professor
Department of Neurology & Pediatrics
University of California, San Francisco
San Francisco, California
  Focal Cerebral Infarction

Torin J.A. Glass, BMBCh
Fellow
Department of Pediatrics
The Hospital for Sick Children
Toronto, Ontario, Canada
*Congenital Heart Disease: An
Important Cause of Brain Injury
and Dysmaturation*

Nazia Kabani, MD, BS
Fellow
Pediatric Infectious Diseases and
Neonatal-Perinatal Medicine
Department of Pediatrics
University of Alabama
Birmingham, Alabama
*Neonatal Herpes Simplex Virus,
Congenital Cytomegalovirus, and
Congenital Zika Virus Infections*

Ericalyn Kasdorf, MD
Assistant Professor
Department of Pediatrics
New York Presbyterian Hospital
Komansky Children's Hospital
Weill Cornell Medicine
New York, New York
*General Supportive Management
of the Term Infant With Neonatal
Encephalopathy Following
Intrapartum Hypoxia-Ischemia*

David Kaufman, MD
Department of Pediatrics
University of Virginia Medical School
Charlottesville, Virginia
*Neonatal Meningitis: Current
Treatment Options*

David W. Kimberlin, MD
Professor of Pediatrics,
Sergio Stagno Endowed Chair in
Pediatric Infectious Diseases
Co-Director, Division of Pediatric
Infectious Diseases
University of Alabama at Birmingham
Birmingham, Alabama
*Neonatal Herpes Simplex Virus,
Congenital Cytomegalovirus, and
Congenital Zika Virus Infections*

Abbot R. Laptook, MD
Professor of Pediatrics
Department of Pediatrics
Warren Alpert School of Medicine at
Brown University;
Medical Director
Neonatal Intensive Care Unit
Department of Pediatrics
Women and Infants Hospital of Rhode
Island
Providence, Rhode Island
*Hypothermia for Neonatal Hypoxic-
Ischemic Encephalopathy: Different
Cooling Regimens and Infants Not
Included in Prior Trials*

Jean-Baptiste Le Pichon, MD, PhD
Child Neurologist
Child Neurology Residency Program
Director
Associate Professor of Pediatrics
University of Missouri-Kansas City
School of Medicine;
Adjunct Assistant Professor of
Neurology
University of Kansas Medical School
Kansas City, Missouri
*Hyperbilirubinemia and the Risk for
Brain Injury*

**Neil Marlow, BA (Hons), MBBS, DM,
FMedSci**
Professor of Neonatal Medicine
Institute for Women's Health
University College London
London, Great Britain
*Long-Term Follow-Up of the Very
Preterm Graduate*

Claire McLean, MD
Attending Neonatologist
Kaiser Permanente Health System
Los Angeles, California
*Cerebral Circulation and
Hypotension in the Premature Infant:
Diagnosis and Treatment*

Shahab Noori, MD
Associate Professor of Clinical Pediatrics
Keck School of Medicine
University of Southern California
Los Angeles, California
*Cerebral Circulation and
Hypotension in the Premature Infant:
Diagnosis and Treatment*

Jeffrey M. Perlman, MB, ChB
Professor of Pediatrics
Division of Newborn Medicine
Department of Pediatrics
New York Presbyterian Hospital
Komansky Children's Hospital
Weill Cornell Medicine
New York, New York
*Intraventricular Hemorrhage and
White Matter Injury in the Preterm
Infant; General Supportive Man-
agement of the Term Infant With
Neonatal Encephalopathy Following
Intrapartum Hypoxia-Ischemia*

Francesco Pisani, MD
Child Neuropsychiatry Unit
Department of Neuroscience
University of Parma
Parma, Italy
*Diagnosis and Management of Acute
Seizures in Neonates*

Sean M. Riordan, PhD
Research Assistant Professor
Division of Child Neurology
Department of Pediatrics
Children's Mercy Kansas City
University of Missouri-Kansas City
School of Medicine
*Hyperbilirubinemia and the Risk for
Brain Injury*

Pablo J. Sánchez, MD
Professor of Pediatrics
Department of Pediatrics
Divisions of Neonatal-Perinatal
Medicine and Pediatric Infectious
Diseases
Center for Perinatal Research
Nationwide Children's Hospital
The Ohio State University College of
Medicine
Columbus, Ohio
*Neonatal Meningitis: Current
Treatment Options*

Tristan T. Sands, MD, PhD
Assistant Professor
Department of Neurology
Columbia University Medical Center
New York, New York
*Neonatal-Onset Epilepsies: Early
Diagnosis and Targeted Treatment*

Michael Seed, MBBS
Staff Cardiologist/Staff Cardiac
Radiologist
Department of Pediatrics
Division of Cardiology/Department of
Radiology
The Hospital for Sick Children
Toronto, Canada
*Congenital Heart Disease: An
Important Cause of Brain Injury and
Dysmaturation*

Istvan Seri, MD, PhD, HonD
Honorary Member
Hungarian Academy of Sciences;
First Department of Pediatrics
Semmelweis University
Faculty of Medicine
Budapest, Hungary;
Professor of Pediatrics (Adjunct)
Children's Hospital Los Angeles
USC Keck School of Medicine
Los Angeles, California
*Cerebral Circulation and
Hypotension in the Premature Infant:
Diagnosis and Treatment*

Steven M. Shapiro, MD, MSHA
Director, Kernicterus Center of
Excellence
Division of Neurology
Department of Pediatrics
Children's Mercy Hospital;
Professor
Department of Pediatrics
University of Missouri-Kansas City;
Professor
Department of Neurology and Pediatrics
University of Kansas Medical Center
Kansas City, Missouri
*Hyperbilirubinemia and the Risk for
Brain Injury*

Carlotta Spagnoli, MD
Child Neurology Unit
Department of Pediatrics
IRCCS Santa Maria Nuova Hospital
Reggio Emilia, Italy
*Diagnosis and Management of
Acute Seizures in Neonates*

Mona C. Toet, MD, PhD
Department of Neonatology
Brain Center Rudolf Magnus
Wilhelmina Children's Hospital
University Medical Center Utrecht
Utrecht University
Utrecht, The Netherlands
  *Amplitude-Integrated EEG and
  Its Potential Role in Augmenting
  Management Within the NICU*

Lauren C. Weeke, MD, PhD
Department of Neonatology
Brain Center Rudolf Magnus
Wilhelmina Children's Hospital
University Medical Center Utrecht
Utrecht University
Utrecht, The Netherlands
  *Amplitude-Integrated EEG and
  Its Potential Role in Augmenting
  Management Within the NICU*

Tai Wei-Wu, MD
Attending Neonatologist
Newborn and Infant Critical Care Unit
Children's Hospital, Los Angeles;
Assistant Professor of Clinical Pediatrics
Division of Neonatology
Keck School of Medicine of USC at
  Neonatology
Los Angeles, California
  *Cerebral Circulation and
  Hypotension in the Premature
  Infant: Diagnosis and Treatment*

Andrew Whitelaw, MD, FRCPCH
Professor of Neonatal Medicine
School of Clinical Science
University of Bristol
Bristol, Great Britain
  *Posthemorrhagic Hydrocephalus
  Management Strategies*

Jerome Y. Yager, MD, FRCP(C)
Professor
Department of Pediatrics
Stollery Children's Hospital;
Pediatric Neurosciences
Department of Pediatrics
University of Alberta
Edmonton, Alberta, Canada
  *Glucose and Perinatal Brain
  Injury—Questions and Controversies*

Vivien Yap, MD
Assistant Professor of Pediatrics
Division of Newborn Medicine
Department of Pediatrics
New York Presbyterian
Weill Cornell Medicine
New York, New York
  *Intraventricular Hemorrhage and
  White Matter Injury in the Preterm
  Infant*

Santina Zanelli, MD
Department of Pediatrics
University of Virginia Medical School
Charlottesville, Virginia
  *Neonatal Meningitis: Current
  Treatment Options*

Preface

Our understanding of the basic mechanisms contributing to perinatal brain injury continues to advance as a consequence of ongoing research, which has facilitated the introduction of targeted strategies in certain instances. The third edition of this book again addresses some of the prominent factors/events contributing to brain injury as well as describing some of the novel treatment options that have been introduced over the past decade. Two new chapters have been added related to neonatal-onset epilepsies (see Chapter 8) and the impact of congenital heart disease (CHD) on brain development (see Chapter 15). In Chapter 4, emergent data indicate that a longer duration of cooling or a lower temperature for cooling when treating neonates with hypoxic-ischemic encephalopathy can in fact be harmful. In addition, there is little data to indicate benefit from hypothermia for hypoxic-ischemic encephalopathy among infants with a mild encephalopathy, preterm infants, or infants in low- or middle-income countries. The new Chapter 8 on neonatal-onset epilepsies highlights the advances in the early diagnosis and treatment of these rare disorders made possible by the increasing use of neurodiagnostic testing in the neonatal intensive care unit (NICU), including neuro-imaging and video-EEG, coupled with readily available genetic and metabolic analysis, allowing for the recognition and personalized treatment of new electroclinical phenotypes, that is, KCNQ2 encephalopathy. In Chapter 10 on hyperbilirubinemia, the authors propose a new term "Kernicterus Spectrum Disorders (KSDs)" to clinically define and categorize kernicterus subtypes and severity.

In Chapter 12 on viral meningoencephalitis, the authors discuss the emerging Zika virus and its devastating consequences on developing brain. In Chapter 16 on long-term follow-up of the very premature graduate, the author stresses the point that these children are at risk of key executive functional deficits that may predispose to poor performance in the classroom. Chapter 15 focuses on the understanding of the specific pathophysiology of acquired brain injury in infants with CHD to optimize treatment and brain protection strategies.

The remaining chapter updates are all outstanding in their depth and comprehensive reviews and make for compelling reading.

The primary goal of this third edition is to provide the reader with a clearer management strategy of common and rare neurologic disorders of the neonate based on the most updated comprehension of their underlying pathophysiology. A desired secondary goal is that the highlighted gaps in knowledge will serve as a strong stimulus for future research.

Jeffrey M. Perlman, MB, ChB
Maria Roberta Cilio, MD, PhD

Series Foreword

Richard A. Polin, MD

"To study the phenomena of disease without books is to sail an uncharted sea, while to study books without patients is not to go to sea at all."

—William Osler

Physicians in training generally rely on the spoken word and clinical experiences to bolster their medical knowledge. There is probably no better way to learn how to care for an infant than to receive teaching at the bedside. Of course, that assumes that the "clinician" doing the teaching is knowledgeable about the disease, wants to teach, and can teach effectively. For a student or intern, this style of learning is efficient because the clinical service demands preclude much time for other reading. Over the course of one's career, it becomes clear that this form of education has limitations because of the fairly limited number of disease conditions one encounters even in a lifetime of clinical rotations and the diminishing opportunities for teaching moments.

The next educational phase generally includes reading textbooks and qualitative review articles. Unfortunately, both of those sources are often outdated by the time they are published and represent one author's opinions about management. Systematic analyses (meta-analyses) can be more informative, but more often than not the conclusion of the systematic analysis is that "more studies are needed" to answer the clinical question. Furthermore, it has been estimated that if a subsequent large randomized clinical trial had not been performed, the meta-analysis would have reached an erroneous conclusion more than one-third of the time.

For practicing clinicians, clearly the best way to keep abreast of recent advances in a field is to read the medical literature on a regular basis. However, that approach is problematic given the multitude of journals, unless one reads only the two or three major pediatric journals published in the United States. That approach however, will miss many of the outstanding articles that appear in more general medical journals (e.g., *Journal of the American Medical Association, New England Journal of Medicine, Lancet*, and the *British Medical Journal*), subspecialty journals, and the many pediatric journals published in other countries.

Whereas there is no substitute to reading journal articles on a regular basis, the "Questions and Controversies" series of books provides an excellent alternative. This third edition of the series was developed to highlight the clinical problems of most concern to practitioners. The series has been increased from six to seven volumes and includes new sections on genetics and pharmacology. In total, there are 70 new chapters not included previously. The editors of each volume (Drs. Bancalari, Davis, Keszler, Oh, Baum, Seri, Ohls, Christensen, Maheshwari, Neu, Benitz, Smith, Poindexter, Cilio, and Perlman) have done an extraordinary job in selecting topics of clinical importance to everyday practice. Unlike traditional review articles, the chapters not only highlight the most significant controversies, but when possible, have incorporated basic science and physiological concepts with a rigorous analysis of the current literature.

As with the first edition, I am indebted to the exceptional group of editors who chose the content and edited each of the volumes. I also wish to thank Lisa Barnes (Content Development Specialist at Elsevier) and Judy Fletcher (VP, Content Development at Elsevier) who provided incredible assistance in bringing this project to fruition.

Contents

Corresponding color figures for select images are available on Expert Consult.

CHAPTER 1

Cerebral Circulation and Hypotension in the Premature Infant: Diagnosis and Treatment

Shahab Noori, Claire McLean, Tai Wei-Wu, and Istvan Seri

- Neonatal hypotension can be defined by *population-based normative data*, by the *principles of developmental cardiovascular physiology* (autoregulatory, functional and ischemic blood pressure thresholds) or by the *pathophysiology* (morbidity and/or mortality).

- During the immediate transitional period, a given blood pressure value at a given point in time in a given patient may be associated with normal systemic and organ blood flow. However, depending on the underlying cardiovascular pathology and the patient's ability to compensate, the same blood pressure value in the same patient at a different time point may be associated with impaired systemic and organ blood flow and thus oxygen delivery.

- *Only an association* but *not causation* has been documented between hypotension and brain injury/poor neurodevelopmental outcome. Therefore at present, one cannot infer that long-term neurodevelopmental outcomes will improve if hypotension is rigorously avoided.

- Treatment of neonatal hypotension improves the major hemodynamic variables (blood pressure, cardiac output, organ blood flow and oxygen delivery) but improvement in neurodevelopmental outcomes has not yet been documented.

With the evolution of neonatology over the past few decades, improved methods of monitoring and more effective interventions have been developed to identify and manage the respiratory, fluid and electrolyte, and nutritional abnormalities frequently encountered in very low-birth-weight (VLBW) infants. However, the ability to effectively and continuously monitor the *hemodynamic changes* at the level of systemic and organ blood flow and tissue perfusion is still limited. Yet the advances achieved with the use of targeted neonatal echocardiography and other bedside monitoring devices providing noninvasive, continuous systemic, organ and tissue perfusion and cerebral function monitoring have started to usher in a new era in developmental hemodynamics. The novel monitoring modalities include but are not restricted to electrical impedance velocimetry, continuous wave Doppler ultrasonography, near-infrared spectroscopy (NIRS), visible light spectroscopy, laser Doppler technology, and amplitude-integrated electroencephalography (EEG, aEEG). Yet with the improvements in hemodynamic monitoring and a better understanding of the principles of developmental cardiovascular physiology have come the realization that little is known about circulatory compromise and its effects on organ function, especially brain blood flow, blood flow–metabolism coupling, and long-term outcomes. Although we can continuously and reliably monitor systemic blood pressure in absolute numbers and a great number of proposed interventions exist for "normalizing" it, blood pressure is only the dependent component among the three hemodynamic parameters regulating systemic perfusion. Accordingly, blood pressure is determined by changes in the two independent variables, cardiac output and systemic vascular resistance (SVR). Therefore in addition to monitoring and maintaining perfusion pressure (blood pressure), the goal is to preserve normal systemic and organ blood flow and thus tissue oxygenation especially in the vital organs—the brain, heart, and adrenal glands. In this regard, when it comes to the brain, medicine is at an even greater disadvantage. For instance, measuring cerebral blood flow (CBF) is more complex than continuously measuring systemic blood flow (left ventricular output), which itself has remained a significant challenge. Assessment of systemic blood flow becomes even more complicated when shunting through the fetal channels (ductus arteriosus and foramen ovale) occurs during the first few postnatal days in the preterm neonate. Unfortunately, it is more complicated to detect clinical evidence of ischemia in the brain in a timely manner in the neonate. In addition, distinct regions of the brain have different sensitivity to decreased oxygen delivery. Accordingly, injury to the normally less well-perfused white matter might occur before other regions suffer damage. Alterations in normal brain activity and seizures are clear signs of a pathologic process, but they can be difficult to recognize, especially in the VLBW neonate; although the use of aEEG might be helpful in this regard. As for seizures, by the time they are present, irreversible injury may have already occurred. Most importantly, the clinician faces the formidable task of effectively supporting and protecting the enormously complex developmental processes that take place in the brain of the preterm infant during the postnatal transitional period and beyond. In addition, the understanding of how to manage hemodynamic disturbances that affect CBF, flow-metabolism coupling, brain function and structure, and ultimately neurodevelopmental outcome is limited.

The intent of this chapter is to review the information available related to the definition of systemic hypotension as well as the pathogenesis, diagnosis, and treatment of early cerebral perfusion abnormalities that have been shown to precede intracranial hemorrhage and periventricular white matter injury (PWMI) in the VLBW infant. Because CBF flow-metabolism coupling and cerebral oxygenation in this population is complex, the discussion is focused on the first postnatal days, during which the cardiorespiratory transition from fetal to extrauterine life occurs and most pathologic processes take place. The discussion focuses on some bedside modalities potentially useful for identifying changes in CBF and cerebral oxygenation. In addition, a paradigm is presented for the treatment of the pathologic processes underlying clinically evident brain injury in the VLBW infant based on the most up-to-date monitoring and clinical evidence. Unfortunately, there is sparse evidence related to the appropriateness and effectiveness of current approaches to treatment of neonatal hypotension and cardiovascular compromise. The goal is to provide the practitioner with guidelines for establishing the diagnosis and treatment of neonatal hypotension. Finally, although the understanding of both the normal and pathologic processes in the developing preterm brain is improving, a definitive, safe, and effective clinical approach remains elusive.

Definition of Hypotension

Hypotension, defined by *population-based normative data*, is present in up to 50% of VLBW infants admitted to the neonatal intensive care unit. Hypotension in the immediate postnatal period has historically been thought to be one of the major factors contributing to central nervous system injury and poor long-term neurologic outcome, including cerebral palsy in VLBW neonates. Indeed, an *association* between hypotension and brain injury and poor neurodevelopmental outcome is well documented[1-9] and forms the basis of therapeutic efforts to normalize blood pressure. However, *causation* has not been demonstrated between hypotension and poor neurodevelopment and thus one cannot infer that long-term neurodevelopmental outcomes will improve if hypotension is rigorously avoided.[10] Therein lies the conundrum often faced by the neonatologist: when to treat early cardiovascular compromise in the VLBW neonate, what medication to use, and how quickly to normalize blood pressure and CBF. Thus a prospective observational study of more than 1000 infants less than 28 weeks' gestation showed that early postnatal hypotension was not associated with poorer outcomes.[11] Furthermore retrospective studies have raised additional concerns by demonstrating an association between "treated hypotension" and poor neurodevelopmental outcomes.[12–15] Of note, the use of the definition "treated hypotension" in these studies has introduced an additional bias by implying that, in addition to or independent of hypotension, the treatment might be a factor contributing to the described association. Although the implication of the potential negative effects of treatment of hypotension is plausible and thus needs to be prospectively studied, at present no conclusion can be drawn, especially because other investigators have reported essentially the opposite finding.[16] Unfortunately, all prior studies were uncontrolled, either retrospective or observational in nature, and hypotension was treated. There is only one randomized controlled trial published to date that had a no-treatment arm.[17] Owing to difficulties in obtaining informed consent in a timely fashion or refusal of enrollment by the attending neonatologist, these trials are not feasible to perform. Interestingly, a follow-up study[15] to a randomized prospective trial[18] comparing the effectiveness of dopamine and epinephrine in increasing blood pressure and CBF in hypotensive VLBW neonates during the first postnatal day found that neonates who responded to dopamine or epinephrine had long-term neurodevelopment outcomes comparable to those of age-matched normotensive controls. However, infants who did not respond to vasopressor-inotrope treatment had worse long-term outcome. However, as the primary outcome measure of the original study[18] was not long-term neurodevelopmental outcome, the follow-up study[15] was not appropriately powered to put this concern to rest.

It is clear that the relationship between a given mean blood pressure and associated brain oxygen delivery below which the risk for injury is increased remains unclear. Moreover, there is no clear evidence that increasing blood pressure to the normal range will normalize oxygen delivery. Mean arterial pressure (MAP) is considered by some to be less important than other indirect clinical indicators of decreased perfusion, such as capillary refill time (CRT), urine output, and lactic acidosis. This approach ignores the physiologic principle that a pressure gradient is necessary to drive flow (Poiseuille's law). Simplistically, to provide blood flow to the brain, the systolic arterial pressure has to be higher than the intracranial pressure. Obviously, the dependent variables of systemic hemodynamics (cardiac output and SVR) determine blood pressure and thus tissue oxygen delivery. However, ignoring MAP itself, as implied by some, may not be prudent and even feasible.[17] In summary, *blood pressure should be considered as one of the markers* of adequacy of circulatory function but *not the only or primary marker*. Indeed, low blood pressure implies impairment of vasomotor tone, low cardiac output, or both. Conversely, a normal blood pressure indicates either normal cardiac output and vasomotor tone or a compensated state, in which either cardiac output is increased to compensate for the low vasomotor tone or the vasomotor tone is elevated to compensate for the low cardiac output (Fig. 1.1).[19] In older children and adults, vital organs are relatively protected in the compensated phase of shock. Unfortunately, this may not be the situation in the preterm infant—hence the limitation of primarily relying on blood pressure monitoring in an effort to assess the adequacy of circulation.

In clinical practice, hypotension is usually defined as the blood pressure value below the 5th or 10th percentile for the gestational and postnatal age–dependent normative blood pressure values (Fig. 1.2).[20,21] Interestingly, findings of a recent study suggest that the normative values may actually be low; that is, physiologically normal blood pressure in VLBW infants may actually be higher than has been commonly accepted.[22] Moreover, owing to the compensatory mechanisms, a certain blood pressure value in a given patient might be associated with normal oxygen delivery at one point in time while the same value may indicate true hypotension (abnormal tissue oxygen delivery) at another time.[19] Accordingly, there is no consensus among neonatologists about the acceptable lower limit of systemic mean or systolic arterial blood pressure, and most units have different guidelines for the initiation of treatment of hypotension. From a pathophysiological standpoint, three levels of functional

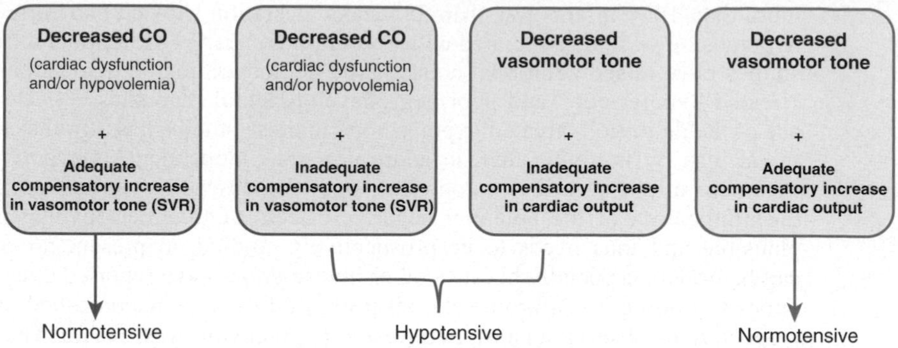

1

Decreased CO

(cardiac dysfunction and/or hypovolemia)

+

Adequate compensatory increase in vasomotor tone (SVR)

↓

Normotensive

Decreased CO

(cardiac dysfunction and/or hypovolemia)

+

Inadequate compensatory increase in vasomotor tone (SVR)

Decreased vasomotor tone

+

Inadequate compensatory increase in cardiac output

Hypotensive

Decreased vasomotor tone

+

Adequate compensatory increase in cardiac output

↓

Normotensive

Fig. 1.1 Pathophysiology of neonatal cardiovascular compromise in primary myocardial dysfunction and primary abnormal vascular tone regulation with or without compensation by the unaffected other variable. This figure illustrates why blood pressure can be considered normal when there is appropriate compensatory increase in either vasomotor tone or cardiac output. In the hypotensive scenarios, there is inadequate compensatory increase in these variables. *CO,* Cardiac output; *SVR,* systemic vascular resistance. (From Wu T, Noori S, Seri I. Neonatal hypotension. In: Polin R, Yoder M, eds. *Workbook in Practical Neonatology.* 5th ed. Philadelphia, PA: Elsevier; 2014.)

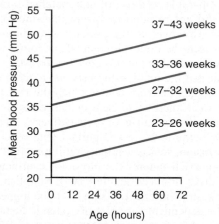

Fig. 1.2 Gestational age– and postnatal age–dependent nomogram for mean blood pressure values in preterm and term neonates during the first 3 postnatal days. The nomogram is derived from continuous arterial blood pressure measurements obtained from 103 neonates with gestational ages between 23 and 43 weeks. As each line represents the lower limit of 80% confidence interval of mean blood pressure for each gestational age group, 90% of infants for each gestational age group will have a mean blood pressure equal or greater than the value indicated by the corresponding line (the lower limit of confidence interval). (From Nuntnarumit P, Yang W, Bada-Ellzey HS. Blood pressure measurements in the newborn. *Clin Perinatol.* 1999;26(4):981–996. Used with permission.)

alterations of increasing severity can be used to guide the definition of hypotension (Fig. 1.3). Findings of a small study[23] underscore this point. However, it is important to keep in mind that no prospectively collected information is available on mortality and morbidity associated with the different proposed blood pressure thresholds.

First, the mean blood pressure associated with the loss of CBF autoregulation is the generally accepted definition of hypotension (*autoregulatory blood pressure threshold*).[24] Indeed, there is considerable information in the literature indicating that CBF autoregulation is functional, albeit within a narrow range, in normotensive but not in hypotensive VLBW neonates in the immediate postnatal period (Fig. 1.4).[5,25,26] Also of interest is that CBF velocity increases in a pressure-passive fashion as systolic blood pressure is increased with dopamine during the first postnatal day.[27] A study found that cerebral pressure passivity in the VLBW neonatal population was associated with an increased risk for periventricular/intraventricular hemorrhage (P/IVH).[28] These findings implicate blood pressure and pressure passivity as risk factors for intracranial pathology.

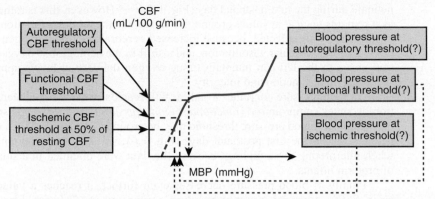

Fig. 1.3 Definition of hypotension by three pathophysiologic phenomena of increasing severity: autoregulatory, functional, and ischemic thresholds of hypotension. *CBF,* Cerebral blood flow; *MBP,* mean blood pressure.

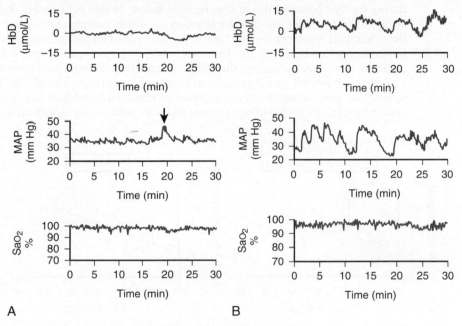

Fig. 1.4 Intact and compromised cerebral blood flow (CBF) autoregulation in very low-birth-weight neonates in the immediate postnatal period. Changes in cerebral intravascular oxygenation (hemoglobin D *[HbD]* = oxyhemoglobin *[HbO₂]* – hemoglobin [Hb]) correlate with changes in CBF. A, Changes in *HbD* (i.e., CBF), mean arterial pressure *(MAP),* and oxygen saturation *(Sao₂)* in a 1-day-old 28-week gestation preterm infant whose subsequent head ultrasound findings remained normal. No change occurs in CBF in relation to the sudden increase in MAP associated with endotracheal tube suctioning *(arrow).* B, Changes in HbD (CBF), MAP, and Sao₂ in a 1-day-old, 27-week–gestational age preterm infant whose subsequent head ultrasound revealed the presence of periventricular white matter injury. Changes in blood pressure are clearly associated with changes in CBF. (From Tsuji M, Saul PJ, duPlessis A, et al. Cerebral intravascular oxygenation correlates with mean arterial pressure in critically ill premature infants. *Pediatrics.* 2000;106(4):625–632. Used with permission.)

Autoregulation is the ability of the arteries to constrict or dilate in response to an increase or decrease, respectively, in the transmural pressure to maintain blood flow relatively constant within a range of arterial blood pressure changes (see Fig. 1.4). However, in the neonate the vascular response has a limited capacity. In addition, and as mentioned previously, the autoregulatory blood pressure range is narrow in the neonatal patient population, with the 50th percentile of the mean blood pressure being relatively close to the lower autoregulatory blood pressure threshold. In other words, small decreases in blood pressure may result in loss of CBF autoregulation, especially in the VLBW infant.[25] Available data suggest that the autoregulatory blood pressure threshold is around 28 to 29 mm Hg even in the extremely LBW (ELBW) neonate during the first postnatal day (Fig. 1.5).[25,26] However, this is rather arbitrary as it remains unclear at values around this range whether cellular function and structural integrity are affected, because increased cerebral fractional oxygen extraction (CFOE), microvascular vasodilation, and a shift in the hemoglobin-oxygen dissociation curve to the left can maintain tissue oxygen delivery at levels appropriate to sustain cellular function and integrity.[29,30]

If blood pressure continues to fall, it will reach a value at which cerebral function becomes compromised (*functional blood pressure threshold*). Data suggest that the functional blood pressure threshold may be around 22 to 24 mm Hg in the VLBW neonate during the first postnatal days (Fig. 1.6).[31,32] However, caution is needed when interpreting these findings because the data were obtained in a small number of preterm infants.

Finally, if blood pressure decreases even further, it reaches a value at which brain tissue structural integrity becomes compromised (*ischemic blood pressure threshold*). On the basis of findings in immature animals, it is assumed that the ischemic CBF threshold is around 50% of resting CBF.[25] Although it is unclear which blood pressure value represents the ischemic CBF threshold in the VLBW neonate during the first postnatal day, it may be at or below 20 mm Hg (see Fig. 1.3).[31,32] It is important to emphasize that the situation is further complicated by the fact that these numbers represent moving targets for the individual patient influenced by his or her ability to compensate for decreases in blood pressure and oxygen delivery. In addition, other factors, such as the different sensitivity of brain structures to perfusion changes, arterial partial pressure of carbon dioxide ($Paco_2$) levels, the presence of acidosis, preexisting insults (interruption of placental blood flow [i.e., asphyxia]), and underlying pathophysiology (sepsis, anemia), all have an impact on the critical

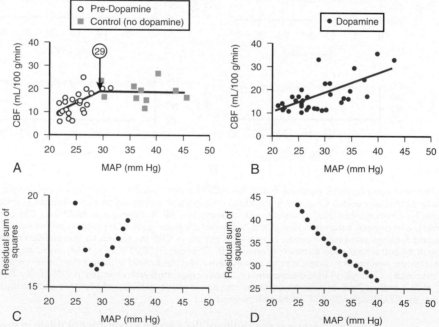

Fig. 1.5 Relationship between cerebral blood flow (*CBF*) and mean arterial pressure (*MAP*) in hypotensive and normotensive extremely low-birth-weight (ELBW) neonates during the first postnatal day and the effect of dopamine on this relationship. A and B, MAP (mm Hg) and CBF (mL/100 g/min) assessed by near-infrared spectroscopy in normotensive ELBW neonates not requiring dopamine (Control [*solid squares*]; n = 5) and hypotensive ELBW neonates before dopamine administration (pre-dopamine [*open circles*]; n = 12). The lower threshold of the CBF autoregulatory blood pressure limit (29 mm Hg; A) is identified as the minimum of the residual sum of squares of the bilinear regression analysis (B). C and D, MAP (mm Hg) and CBF (mL/100 g/min) in previously hypotensive ELBW neonates after dopamine treatment (*solid circles*). No breakpoint is evident in the CBF-MAP curve in ELBW neonates receiving dopamine (C), because there is no minimum identified by the bilinear regression analysis (D). (From Munro MJ, Walker AM, Barfield CP. Hypotensive extremely low birth weight infants have reduced cerebral blood flow. *Pediatrics.* 2004;114(6):1591–1596. Used with permission.)

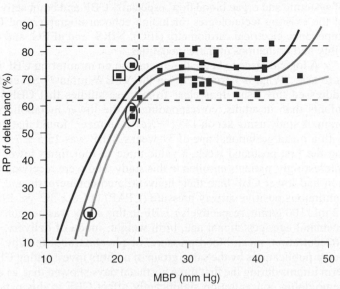

Fig. 1.6 Relationship between mean blood pressure *(MBP)* and cerebral electrical activity in very low-birth-weight neonates during the first 4 postnatal days. The relationship between MBP and the relative power *(RP)* of the delta band of the electroencephalogram (EEG) is shown as the line of best fit with 95% confidence interval ($n = 35$; $R^2 =$ 0.627; $P < .001$). The horizontal dotted lines represent the normal range of the relative power of the delta band (10th–90th percentile), while the vertical dotted line identifies the point of intercept. The open square identifies the infant with abnormal cerebral fractional oxygen extraction and the abnormal EEG records are circled. (From Victor S, Marson AG, Appleton RE, et al. Relationship between blood pressure, cerebral electrical activity, cerebral fractional oxygen extraction and peripheral blood flow in very low birth weight newborn infants. *Pediatr Res.* 2006;59(2):314–319. Used with permission.)

blood pressure value at which perfusion pressure and cerebral oxygen delivery cannot satisfy cellular oxygen demand to sustain autoregulation, then cellular function, and finally structural integrity.

In most units, continuous monitoring of blood pressure and assessment of indirect signs of tissue perfusion (urine output, CRT, and lactic acidosis) still form the basis for identifying the presence of cardiovascular compromise. As discussed earlier, though, "adequate" blood pressure may not always guarantee adequate organ perfusion in VLBW neonates, especially during the first postnatal day.[33] Indeed, blood pressure only weakly correlates with superior vena cava (SVC) flow in VLBW neonates during the period of immediate postnatal adaptation.[34] Of note, SVC flow has increasingly been used in the clinical practice as a surrogate for systemic blood flow in the VLBW neonate during the immediate postnatal period, when shunting through the fetal channels prohibits the use of left ventricular output to assess systemic blood flow.[35] The finding that adequate blood pressure may not always guarantee adequate systemic blood flow in these patients may be explained, at least in part, by the notion that the cerebral vascular bed, especially of the 1-day-old ELBW neonate, may not be of high priority assignment yet and thus it will constrict, as do the vessels do in the nonvital organs, rather than dilate in response to a decrease in the perfusion pressure (see later text).[36,37]

Pathogenesis and Diagnosis of Pathologic Cerebral Blood Flow

Fluctuations in CBF are implicated in the pathogenesis of P/IVH and PWMI in the VLBW infant.[1,5,28,37] Both systemic and local (intracerebral) factors play a role in the pathogenesis of these central nervous system injuries and therefore are important to establish the underlying pathogenesis. In addition, the level of maturity, postnatal age, and intercurrent clinical factors (e.g., infection/inflammation, vasopressor-resistant hypotension) also need to be considered.[38] In this section, we briefly discuss the monitoring parameters currently in clinical use (systemic arterial pressure and arterial blood gas sampling) and then delve into the emerging field of bedside monitoring of systemic and organ blood flow, especially CBF and brain activity. We review most of the existing technologies, including echocardiography and Doppler ultrasound, impedance electrical cardiometry (IEC), NIRS, and aEEG, and discuss the applicability and limitations of these modalities.

A logical place to begin the discussion on monitoring CBF in the VLBW infant is to ask, "What is normal CBF in the VLBW infant?" Several investigators have addressed this issue. It is clear from these studies that CBF is lower in preterm infants than in adults, corresponding to the lower metabolic rate of the preterm brain. A study using xenon 133 (^{133}Xe) clearance[39] found that in 42 preterm infants with a mean gestational age of 31 weeks, CBF was 15.5 ± 7.2 mL/100 g/min during the first postnatal week, a value three to four times lower than that in adults. Interestingly, patients enrolled in this study who were receiving mechanical ventilation had lower CBF than their nonventilated counterparts and those supported by continuous positive airway pressure (CPAP) (11.8 ± 3.2 vs. 19.8 ± 5.3 and 21.3 ± 12 mL/100 g/min, respectively). CBF in this study was not consistently affected by postnatal age, gestational age, birth weight, mode of delivery, Pa_{CO_2}, hemoglobin concentration, mean blood pressure, or phenobarbital therapy. In contrast, subsequent publications by the same group of authors investigating CBF reactivity in preterm infants during the first three postnatal days showed that, as expected, Pa_{CO_2} and hemoglobin concentration significantly affect CBF in this patient population.[40–42] However, the relationship between Pa_{CO_2} and CBF appears to be also affected by postnatal age during the immediate postnatal period (see later text). Using positron emission tomography (PET) to measure CBF, a study found[43] lower values for CBF in preterm and term neonates compared with those obtained by the use of ^{133}Xe clearance. More importantly, the authors reported that, in 1 term and 5 preterm infants with CBF between 4.9 and 10 mL/100 g/min, the term neonate and 3 of the preterm infants had normal neurodevelopmental outcome at 24 months.[43] These data suggest that the "neurodevelopmentally safe" lower limit of CBF in the neonate is lower than predicted and may be between 5 and 10 mL/100 g/min. Finally, as mentioned earlier, because CBF is affected by many factors other than blood pressure, it is not possible to define the blood pressure value consistently associated with a decrease of CBF below the safe limit that results in ischemic brain injury.

Kluckow and Evans, using SVC flow as a surrogate for CBF, established normal values of SVC flow during the first 48 postnatal hours in well preterm neonates younger than 30 weeks' gestation who were receiving minimal ventilatory support.[35] However, it must be stated that the extent to which SVC flow is representative of systemic or CBF in preterm neonates during the first postnatal days is not understood. In a subsequent study that included sick preterm infants younger than 30 weeks' gestation, the same group found that 38% of infants had a period of low SVC in the first 24 postnatal hours.[33] The incidence of low SVC flow was significantly related to the level of immaturity, and more than 70% of low SVC flow occurred in very preterm neonates (< 27 weeks' gestation). The sudden increase in the peripheral vascular resistance caused by the loss of the low-resistance placental circulation when the cord is clamped immediately after delivery, the complex process of cardiorespiratory transition to the postnatal circulatory pattern, and myocardial and autonomic central nervous system immaturity have all been proposed to contribute to these findings. Indeed, these factors may explain why many of these very preterm neonates struggle to maintain normal systemic blood flow during the first 12 to 24 postnatal hours. Of note is that using "physiologic" (delayed) rather than immediate cord clamping, immediate postnatal hemodynamic transition, and the incidence of associated cerebral pathologies have changed.[44,45] Importantly, a proportion of the very preterm infants with extremely low SVC flow were found to have systemic blood pressures in the "normal" range (i.e., greater than or equal to their gestational age in weeks), a finding supported by subsequent studies of this group of researchers.[34,36,37] Because normal blood pressure and decreased organ blood flow to nonvital organs are the hallmarks of the compensated phase of shock and because a portion of SVC flow represents blood returning from the brain, a vital organ, it is conceivable that that the proposed low-priority vessel (nonvital organ) assignment of the vascular beds of the forebrain (cerebral cortex and white matter) in the very preterm neonate during the immediate postnatal period explain these findings. This hypothesis, which is supported by studies in different animal models[46,47] and, indirectly, in the human neonate,[36,37,48] may explain, at least in part, why SVC blood flow may be decreased in some very preterm neonates who have normal systemic blood pressure. Most preterm neonates with documented low SVC flow in the first 24 to 48 hours who do not go on to have P/IVH or PWMI are more mature (28 weeks' and beyond vs. 25–26 weeks' gestation). Thus for preterm infants of less than 30 weeks' gestation, preexisting low systemic blood flow (and CBF) may be necessary but not sufficient to cause intracranial pathology. Importantly, all patients studied had an increase in SVC flow by 24 to 36 hours, and all P/IVHs occurred after the SVC flow had increased. Findings of a later prospective observational study by our group using echocardiography and NIRS confirm and expand these observations.[49] In this study, very preterm neonates who presented with lower systemic blood flow and higher cerebral vascular resistance during the first 12 postnatal hours were at a higher risk for the development of P/IVH. Importantly, the bleeding occurred only after cardiac output and brain blood flow had increased. In addition, lower cerebral tissue oxygenation levels detected by NIRS during the first 12 postnatal hours might identify the patients who will subsequently develop P/IVH.[49] Taken together, these findings implicate an ischemia-reperfusion cycle in the pathogenesis of P/IVH in very preterm neonates during the immediate transitional period.

It is important to note that the methods used to assess systemic and CBF in VLBW neonates in the immediate transitional period have significant limitations. When SVC flow is used to assess systemic and CBF, the measurements are operator dependent owing to the uncertainties associated with the accurate measurement of vessel diameter and flow velocity. The fluctuations in vessel size during the cardiac cycle and the flow velocity pattern in the SVC are important factors contributing to these technical difficulties. In addition, the shape of the SVC, the lack of data on the magnitude of the contribution of CBF to SVC flow in the human neonate, and the lack of a documented association between $Paco_2$ and SVC flow in this patient population call for caution in the interpretation of these findings.

Yet an association has been found between SVC flow and aEEG indices of oxygen utilization (continuity and amplitude) in the first 48 postnatal hours.[50] A finding of this study also demonstrated that hypotension, either treated or untreated, was associated with decreased levels of brain activity as assessed by aEEG.[50] This finding supports the previously referenced data[18,23,29] indicating that blood pressure and brain oxygen utilization are inextricably linked.

In another study, CBF was measured in both the internal carotid and vertebral arteries and the sum of the flow in the four arteries supplying the brain was used to assess the changes in CBF volume in preterm infants of 28 to 35 weeks' gestation over the first 2 postnatal weeks.[51] Although the technique, again, has significant limitations, the findings suggest that a steep rise in CBF occurs from the first to the second postnatal day and that this pattern is independent of gestational age. Thereafter CBF continues to rise gradually (Fig. 1.7). Because brain weight does not significantly increase during the first 48 postnatal hours, the investigators inferred that the observed increase in CBF during that period was secondary to increased cerebral perfusion per unit weight of tissue. On the other hand, the more gradual increase over the ensuing 2 weeks is likely due to a combination of both increased brain weight and increased perfusion.[51] This study enrolled only healthy preterm infants with normal brains, whereas investigations in other studies[33,34,52,53] included a group of preterm infants who were sicker and had a higher incidence of significant intracranial pathology. Nevertheless, the results in the two groups of patients are complementary as they provide evidence for a decreased CBF in the first postnatal day, followed by a significant increase by the second postnatal day. Although low CBF in the first postnatal day and the ensuing "reperfusion" appears to be a physiologic phenomenon likely occurring in all very preterm neonates, CBF is even lower in those who later develop P/IVH.[49] Therefore the phenomenon of low CBF is also a

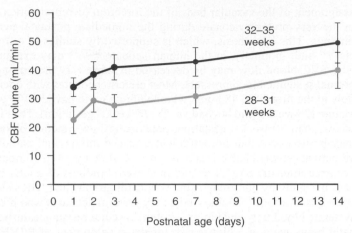

Fig. 1.7 Changes in cerebral blood flow *(CBF)* volume in preterm neonates during the first 14 days after delivery. Development of CBF volume with increasing postnatal age in two different gestational age groups (28–31 and 32–35 weeks' gestation). Mean and 95% confidence interval are shown (analysis of variance; n = 29, P < .0001). (From Kehrer M, Blumenstock G, Ehehalt S, et al. Development of cerebral blood flow volume in preterm neonates during the first two weeks of life. *Pediatr Res.* 2005;58(5):927–930. Used with permission.)

necessary but not sufficient cause of intracranial pathology (P/IVH or PWMI) in this patient population. Although the vast majority of studies found low CBF on the first examination performed during the first few hours after birth, some have described a decrease in CBF at 12 hours compared with 3 to 6 hours after delivery.[54] The reason for the discrepancy in the findings is unclear at present.

The ultimate goal is to improve neurodevelopmental outcome in preterm infants. In addition to the association between low SVC flow in the early postnatal period and P/IVH, low SVC flow in the early postnatal period is also independently associated with impaired neurologic outcome at 3 years of age.[6] Therefore, infants most at risk must be identified in the immediate postnatal period. In addition to ultrasonography, NIRS and other monitoring modalities may be helpful in this regard. Indeed, and as mentioned earlier, preterm infants who develop P/IVH have a pattern of changes in cerebral regional tissue oxygen saturation and oxygen extraction that is different from those without risk for P/IVH.[49] Thus combining different systemic and organ blood flow and tissue oxygenation monitoring technologies may be helpful in the early identification of infants at greater risk for the development of intracerebral pathologies.[55]

It is clear from the large number of epidemiologic and hemodynamic studies, though, that the level of immaturity is one of the most important predisposing factors for the occurrence of more abrupt changes in CBF and the increased vulnerability during postnatal adaptation and for poor neurologic outcome. Therefore assessment of CBF during the first 24 to 48 postnatal hours in the most immature and vulnerable patients is important. However, owing to the technical difficulties associated with reliable and continuous assessment of CBF, clinical practice currently relies on indirect measures for diagnosis of changes in cerebral perfusion, especially because the sole reliance on blood pressure in the indirect assessment of CBF in this patient population during the first postnatal day is not appropriate.

In addition to blood pressure, monitoring of the indirect clinical indicators of tissue perfusion such as urine output, CRT, and acid-base status in the routine clinical practice remain important. Although these indirect clinical indicators by themselves are fairly nonspecific for evaluating systemic flow, using CRT and blood pressure together results in greater sensitivity. Indeed, when blood pressure and CRT are less than 30 mm Hg and 3 seconds or less, respectively, the sensitivity for identifying low systemic blood flow is 86%.[56] In addition, avoidance of both hypocapnia and hypercapnia is of utmost importance because of their effect on CBF. However, and as mentioned earlier, the manifestation of the effect of $Paco_2$ on CBF appears to be dependent on postnatal age. A recent study reported a gradual change in the relationship between Pa_{CO_2} and middle cerebral artery mean velocity, a surrogate for CBF, from none on the first day to the expected positive linear pattern by the third postnatal day.[57] Others have also described an attenuated relationship on the first postnatal day with an increase in the reactivity of CBF to carbon dioxide (CO_2) during the following days.[58,59]

Monitoring of Blood Pressure, Systemic and Organ Blood Flow, and Cerebral Function

Blood pressure is invasively and continuously monitored in most critically ill neonates using an indwelling arterial catheter and a calibrated pressure transducer. Available techniques more likely to be used for systemic blood flow and CBF monitoring are ultrasound (echocardiography and Doppler ultrasound), electrical impedance, and NIRS. As for continuous monitoring of cerebral function in neonates, aEEG has also been increasingly used at the bedside. We briefly discuss these modalities used for systemic and organ blood flow monitoring in the following sections with a primary focus on those that can be performed noninvasively at the bedside.

Doppler Ultrasound

Velocity of blood flow can be measured through the use of the Doppler principle, which states that the change in frequency of reflected sound is proportional to the velocity of the passing object (in this case, blood). The calculated velocity needs to be corrected for the angle between the vessel and the emitted sound beam (angle of insonation), and the straightforward idea is complicated by the fact that arterial blood is pulsatile and its speed varies within the vessel (i.e., it is faster in the center of the vessel). It is important to recognize that speed of blood (distance traveled per unit time) in a vessel means little by itself; we are interested in the absolute blood flow (volume per unit time). Thus volumetric measurements are crucial and can be obtained by the product of velocity time integral (VTI) and cross-sectional area of the vessel that the blood travels in. Investigators have used several different volumetric indices, including SVC, internal carotid artery, and vertebral artery flow, as previously discussed.[35,51] The limitations of SVC flow measurements were discussed earlier. In general, major technical problems with volumetric measurements include but are not restricted to the small size of the vessels, the motion of vessel wall, and whether or not an angle of insonation of less than 20 degrees can be achieved. In addition to volumetric measurements of vessel blood flow, right ventricular and left ventricular outflow measurements have excessively been studied. However, both are fraught with pitfalls in the very preterm neonate in the immediate postnatal period, because the patent foramen ovale (PFO) and patent ductus arteriosus (PDA) represent shunts that confound measurements of the right ventricular and left ventricular flows, respectively. It is believed that right ventricular output may be a more reliable indicator of systemic blood flow during the immediate postnatal period with the fetal channels open, because shunting through the PFO is less significant than PDA shunting during the first 24 postnatal hours.[60] Indeed, right ventricular output and systemic blood pressure have been correlated with EEG parameters (brain function) in VLBW infants in the immediate postnatal period.[61] Ultrasound techniques are noninvasive and widely accessible in the intensive care setting and can be done at the bedside. The procedure itself minimally affects hemodynamic and physiological variables of the infant.[62] However, all ultrasound measurements are noncontinuous, operator dependent, and have their significant limitations. As for the issues related to operator skills, centers using these methods to diagnose pathologic CBF in neonates must have a rigorous quality control system in place with neonatologists trained in functional echocardiography and available at the bedside at any time.[63]

   With regard to the limitations to the use of vascular Doppler ultrasonography in assessing organ blood flow, the most important limitation is the small size of the artery of interest (e.g., middle or anterior cerebral artery), which precludes accurate measurement of its diameter. As previously mentioned, the estimation of blood flow (Q) depends on assessment of mean velocity of the blood (V) and the vessel diameter (D)

$(Q = V[\pi D^2/4] \times 60)$; any small error in measuring the diameter will translate into a significant error in estimating the actual blood flow. Therefore instead of directly measuring blood flow, investigators often use changes in various Doppler-derived indices, such as mean blood flow velocity or the pulsatility or resistance index, as surrogates for changes in blood flow. This approach is based on the premise that the vessel diameter remains constant despite the changes in blood flow. However, this concept in not universally accepted.[63] Nevertheless, both animal and human studies have shown an acceptable correlation between these indices and other measures of blood flow.[64–67]

Finally, although normative data for the Doppler ultrasonography–derived indices for various vessels are available, the previously described limitations require caution in the interpretation of a single measurement. Rather, repeated measurements and the use of trends over time are thought to be more informative of the hemodynamic status and the changes in organ blood flow.

Impedance Electrical Cardiometry

IEC is a noninvasive and continuous bedside method of measuring beat-to-beat left ventricular output on the basis of detection of changes in thoracic electrical bioimpedance (Aesculon, Cardiotronic; La Jolla, CA) caused by the changes in the orientation of the red blood cells in the ascending aorta during systole and diastole normalized for the body mass of the patient.[68] The method has been validated against thermodilution and other direct methods of cardiac output measurement and has shown good correlation in adults and children.[68,69] Although its clinical utility in neonates is still untested, data from our group show a clinically acceptable precision and quantitation of left ventricular output comparable to echocardiography in term neonates.[70] However, a recent study comparing magnetic resonance imaging (MRI) and IEC in adults found poor agreement between the two methods in estimating left ventricular output.[71] In addition to the inherent limitations of MRI, in this study the IEC measurements were done before and after MRI and not simultaneously. Another recent study by our group, however, also found poorer correlation with MRI-derived values of cardiac output and its changes with those obtained by simultaneous IEC monitoring in adults during rest and exercise.[72] These findings suggest that the absolute values obtained using IEC may not appropriately represent cardiac output. Yet because of its reproducibility, continuous beat-to-beat cardiac output measurements, and ease of application, IEC appears to possess clinical applicability when the measurements are trended over time. The recent publication of reference values for cardiac output measured by IEC in premature infants of different gestational age[73] may be helpful if one considers IEC as a screening tool for the detection of infants at risk for low cardiac output. Further validation of this technique is needed, especially in the premature infant population, before the routine use of IEC can be recommended in the neonatal patient population. In conclusion, IEC remains an interesting approach with the ability to obtain continuous, beat-to-beat and noninvasively collected data in absolute numbers on stroke volume and cardiac output at the bedside in neonates, especially when trending changes in cardiac output and assessing the efficacy of therapeutic interventions.

Near-Infrared Spectroscopy

NIRS has received much attention since its first use in newborns in 1985,[74] and numerous papers have been published describing its use and clinical relevance in neonatology. As absorption of light in the near-infrared range (600–900 nm) depends on the oxygenation status of chromophores such as hemoglobin and cytochrome aa3, the absorption during passage through brain tissue can be measured and oxygenation indices calculated. Different wavelengths of light can be used to assess different parameters, such as oxyhemoglobin, deoxyhemoglobin, and cytochrome aa3 oxidase. Through induction of a small but rapid change in arterial oxygen saturation in the subject, CBF can even be calculated using the Fick principle. This method assumes that during the measurement period, cerebral blood volume (CBV) and cerebral oxygen extraction remain constant. However, the technique may not be feasible in infants with severe lung disease, in whom no or very little change in oxygen saturation occurs with an increased fraction of inspired oxygen (F_{IO_2}), and in infants with normal lungs in whom oxygen saturation is 100% when they breathe room air. To circumvent this problem, an injected tracer dye such as indocyanine green has been used instead of oxygen with comparable results.[75] Some instruments use the tissue oxygenation index (TOI), which is the weighted average of arterial, capillary, and venous oxygenation and theoretically allows the measurement of regional cerebral hemoglobin oxygen saturation (rScO$_2$) without manipulation of F$_{IO_2}$ or use of dye. However, this index also has significant potential for inaccuracy, with an intrameasurement agreement in a single subject as large as -17% to $+17\%$.[76] Indeed, reproducibility of NIRS measurements in general has been an ongoing issue for investigators, especially in the detection of focal changes in cerebral hemodynamics. This is a significant problem because focal hemodynamic changes are at least as likely as global changes to contribute to neuropathology. Despite these limitations, NIRS has been validated through comparison with ^{133}Xe clearance in human newborns.[77] As the penetration depth of NIRS is around 2.5 cm, unless the patient is a very preterm neonate, rScO$_2$ is primarily assessed in the frontal lobes when the optodes are placed on the forehead.

For clinical use, an algorithm allowing for continuous monitoring of regional tissue oxygen saturation (rSO$_2$) in absolute numbers has been developed for adult, pediatric, and neonatal use.[78] More recently, newly developed MRI techniques that do not require respiratory calibration have allowed comparison of cerebral oxygen saturation measurements by NIRS and MRI in neonates. The agreement is reasonable with strong linear relation between the two methods.[79,80] Although NIRS represents a practical solution and information on its use in neonates has been encouraging,[81] accumulation of more data and prospective studies looking at both short- and long-term outcomes are needed to provide an evidence-based utilization of NIRS in neonatal medicine. A multicenter randomized clinical trial (SafeBoosC II [Safeguarding the Brain of Our Smallest Children II]) proposes a treatment guideline to reduce the burden of cerebral hypoxia or hyperoxia of extremely preterm infants by targeting a hypothesized "acceptable" rScO$_2$ range of 55% to 85% by use of NIRS monitoring during the first 3 postnatal days.[82] Short-term outcomes have shown an overall 58% (95% confidence interval [CI] 35%–73%) reduction of hypoxia or hyperoxia burden in the NIRS group versus the control group (36.1% vs. 81.3% hours) using a preset treatment guideline.[83] However, despite the decrease in cerebral hypoxia/hyperoxia burden, no significant differences in incidence of severe brain injury detected by cranial ultrasound and MRI,[84] EEG (burst rates), or certain biomarkers of brain injury[85] were found between the NIRS and control groups. Data collection for long-term neurodevelopmental outcomes is still underway. Limited animal data suggest that cerebral rSO$_2$ of 45% to 55% may be an important threshold below which ischemic brain injury likely occurs.[86,87]

A recent case-control study comparing hypotensive preterm infants receiving moderate-high doses of dopamine with normotensive control subjects found no difference in the percentage time spent with cerebral saturation less than 50% in the first 3 postnatal days. However, patients who spent more than 10% of the time with saturation less than 50% had worse neurodevelopmental outcomes.[88] In addition to the interest in absolute rScO$_2$ values, assessment of cerebral autoregulation in premature infants using NIRS has also become a focus of active research. Assuming a constant arterial oxygen saturation (SaO$_2$), hematocrit, metabolic rate, CBV, and arterial and venous blood distribution in the tissue, alteration in cerebral rSO$_2$ reflects changes in CBF. When coupled with mean arterial blood pressure measurement, cerebral autoregulation can be characterized. However, this is a challenging approach because maintaining a constant oxygen saturation in extremely premature infants is difficult in the clinical setting.[89,90] In summary, before NIRS monitoring can be recommended to guide routine clinical care, well-designed, large, multicenter randomized control trials need to be completed.

Amplitude-Integrated EEG (Cerebral Function Monitoring)

Amplitude integrated EEG is one of the most accurate bedside methods to establish a neurologic prognosis[91] in asphyxiated infants during the first several hours after birth. Accordingly, aEEG has been used to select candidates for enrollment in head-cooling neuroprotection trials. This technology uses either a single-channel EEG recording with biparietal electrodes or duo-channel EEG with four electrodes. Frequencies lower than 2 Hz and higher than 15 Hz are selectively filtered out, and the amplitude of the signal is integrated. The signal is then recorded semilogarithmically with slow speed, effectively compressing hours of EEG recording into shorter segments that reflect global background activity and major deviations from baseline (e.g., seizures). Studies have shown that aEEG correlates with conventional EEG[92] and has the distinct advantage of being easily applied and interpreted by non-neurologists. In an earlier study, normal aEEG findings in the first 72 postnatal hours in asphyxiated term neonates have been found to be prognostic of normal neurologic outcome at 2 years of age.[93] Coupled with early neurologic examination, simultaneous aEEG improved specificity and positive predictive value of abnormal results for abnormal neurologic outcome at 18 months of age.[94] A growing interest for the utilization of aEEG in the preterm population has enabled gathering of normative data. Typical patterns of background activity for preterm infants have been established, and a number of studies exist that point to its applicability in this group. West and colleagues[61] examined the relationships among echocardiographic blood flow findings, mean arterial blood pressure, and aEEG findings in preterm infants (<30 weeks' gestation) during the first 48 hours after birth. They found that low right ventricle output, used as a surrogate for systemic blood flow owing to the shunting across the fetal channels at 12 hours of postnatal age, correlated with low aEEG amplitude, whereas low mean blood pressure (<31 mm Hg) correlated with low EEG continuity. However, there was no relationship between aEEG amplitude and SVC flow. Although preliminary in nature, this study at least succeeded in drawing attention to an association between a hemodynamic parameter in wide clinical use (blood pressure) and two more experimental modes of CBF monitoring (echocardiography and aEEG). Taken together with evidence that early aEEG in preterm infants can be helpful in predicting long-term neurodevelopmental outcome, it is reasonable to suggest that aEEG merits further study in the VLBW population, especially along with the use of NIRS, as a means of identifying infants at risk for low CBF and oxygen delivery and/or for pathologic fluctuations in CBF.

Summary of the Monitoring Methods Discussed

Methods capable of diagnosing altered CBF and the associated changes in brain function in the VLBW population in the first hours to days after delivery are still largely in the experimental arena. It is extremely unlikely that one monitoring parameter will be sufficient to encapsulate the status of CBF and oxygen delivery. Instead, and in addition to clinical assessment, a combination of a variety of technologies will likely prove helpful; these technologies range from conventional (heart rate, blood pressure, oxygen saturation, transcutaneous CO_2) to advanced (Doppler ultrasonography, IEC, NIRS, aEEG) methods. Both systemic and CBF, as well as cerebral oxygen delivery and extraction, have to be evaluated simultaneously and continuously to enable the collection of in-depth information allowing for more informed, minute-to minute decisions about how, when, and what to treat. This goal has not been achieved, but it is likely that a number of these modalities will be incorporated into routine clinical use in the not too distant future.

Fig. 1.8 illustrates an example of a comprehensive, real-time, hemodynamic bedside monitoring and data acquisition system developed by our group.[95]

Treatment Strategies

In the previous section we discussed the available noninvasive bedside techniques with the potential to monitor CBF in the VLBW neonate. However, these techniques are not yet currently appropriate for widespread routine clinical use for CBF monitoring, as their application and interpretation require specialized technology and further confirmation. By extension, application of these methods in clinical practice must eventually be shown to improve long-term neurologic outcome. However, results of studies using these experimental strategies can at least be useful for tailoring routine

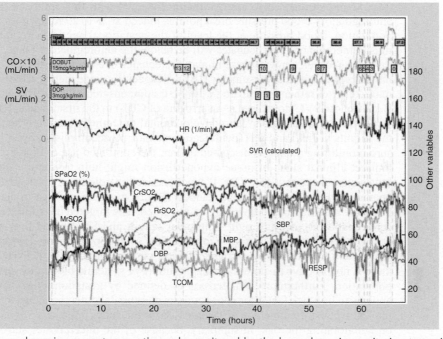

Fig. 1.8 Hemodynamic parameters continuously monitored by the hemodynamic monitoring tower in a term, 3-day-old neonate with hypoxic-ischemic encephalopathy undergoing rewarming from therapeutic whole-body hypothermia. Parameters continuously monitored included arterial oxygen saturation ($SPao_2$; %), heart rate (HR; 1/min), respiratory rate ($RESP$; L/min), systolic (SBP, mm Hg), diastolic (DBP; mm Hg) and mean (MBP; mm Hg) blood pressure, beat-to-beat cardiac output (CO; mL/min); and stroke volume (SV; mL/min) using impedance electrical cardiometry, cerebral ($CrSo_2$), renal ($RrSo_2$), and muscle ($MrSo_2$) mixed venous tissue oxygen saturation using near-infrared spectroscopy, and transcutaneous carbon dioxide ($TCOM$, mm Hg). These parameters are depicted on the y-axis, and age after delivery in hours is shown on the x-axis. Rewarming started at 30 hours of monitoring. Core temperature ($TEMP$) is shown in small boxes and dopamine (DOP) and dobutamine ($DOBUT$) doses are depicted over the cardiac output and stroke volume data. Automatically calculated systemic vascular resistance (SVR, mm Hg × min/mL) is also depicted. See text for details.

care because they provide some insight of how MAP and systemic blood flow interact and affect CBF. This section focuses on how routinely monitored indices such as arterial blood pressure (hypotension), acid-base status, and arterial oxygenation, the commonly used medications, presence of a PDA, and intercurrent infection may affect CBF. We discuss management options, including evidence for when and how to treat systemic hypotension and clinical signs of systemic and organ hypoperfusion. Ultimately we propose a treatment strategy for maintaining brain perfusion and oxygenation in the VLBW infant during the first few postnatal days.

Systemic Hypotension

There are several clinical approaches to the diagnosis and treatment of neonatal hypotension. First, as mentioned earlier, two groups of researchers independently identified a MAP of 28 to 29 mm Hg as a breakpoint below which autoregulation was absent in preterm neonates.[23,29] Use of dopamine to raise the mean blood pressure resulted in a normalization of CBF in these hypotensive infants. Although treatment of hypotension with dopamine quickly restored normal blood pressure and CBF,[29] CBF autoregulation was not immediately restored. Findings of an earlier study suggested that it may take up to an hour or more for CBF autoregulation to be restored after treatment of systemic hypotension.[96] If a mean blood pressure higher than 28 to 29 mm Hg were considered normal in VLBW infants, this would result in an over-treatment of many preterm infants for a mean blood pressure less than 28 mm Hg who would not need an intervention. Instead, the most widespread approach to the definition of hypotension in the VLBW neonate during the immediate transitional period is use of a mean blood pressure value that equals the gestational age in numerals (e.g.,

23, 25, and so on). There are two major concerns with this approach. First, if the autoregulatory blood pressure breakpoint is indeed at 28 to 29 mm Hg for this patient population, blood pressure at the level of the gestational age in more immature and thus vulnerable preterm neonates will be below the autoregulatory range. Second, as discussed earlier, some of these immature neonates even with normal blood pressure have low systemic and presumably CBFs,[30] especially since their cerebral vasculature may constrict rather than dilate in the first, compensated phase of shock.[36,37,46,47,97] Because low SVC flow (used as a surrogate of CBF) in the first postnatal day is a risk factor for P/IVH and poor neurodevelopmental outcome,[6] it is important to identify the infants at risk, and this identification cannot be accomplished with blood pressure monitoring alone. As discussed earlier, the combined use of blood pressure and indirect clinical signs of tissue hypoperfusion might help to identify patients with low systemic and thus low CBF. If functional echocardiography is available, VLBW neonates who are normotensive (blood pressure ≥ gestational age in numerals) but have low systemic blood flow may be identified. The targeted use of functional echocardiography to measure right ventricular output and SVC blood flow may be the best approach currently available to detect low systemic perfusion. However, even if low systemic blood flow is recognized during the first hours after delivery, at present there is no effective treatment strategy to improve systemic blood flow in this patient population. Furthermore, hypotension as defined by gestational age–based criteria appears to be a risk factor for poor neurodevelopmental outcome; however, it remains unclear whether treatment with vasopressors or inotropes improves[15] or has no effect[9] on ameliorating the risk. In summary, because of the uncertainties surrounding the definition of hypotension as well as the potential side effects of vasopressors coupled with a lack of evidence that treatment of hypotension improves neurodevelopmental outcome, some advocate that early hypotension in the VLBW neonate be treated only if there is clear evidence of organ hypoperfusion (i.e., lactic acidosis). This strategy may result in delay in treatment and carries the theoretical risk of allowing significant cerebral hypoperfusion to occur. Therefore an individualized approach based on early (direct or indirect) evidence of decreases in systemic and/or brain blood flow in hypotensive preterm neonates is the most prudent choice at present.

There is general consensus that once the fetal channels are closed and the blood pressure–CBF relationship is restored after the first few days following delivery, blood pressure becomes a more reliable indicator of cerebral perfusion even in the most immature neonates. In this scenario, it can be more stringently advocated that hypotension should be treated promptly with cautious volume administration and careful titration of the most appropriate vasoactive medication (vasopressor/inotrope or inotrope) to avoid sustained changes in systemic blood pressure and blood flow.

Treatment of Hypotension Associated With PDA

PDA is a common presentation in VLBW infants in the immediate postnatal period, with significant left-to-right shunting often manifesting as hypotension.[60,98] It has been demonstrated that the direction of shunting through a nonrestrictive PDA is already primarily left to right in the first 6 hours after delivery and is highly associated with a low SVC flow state.[35,99] Treatment of a PDA before 6 hours of postnatal life with indomethacin induces ductal constriction within 2 hours, but this effect is not associated with simultaneous improvement in systemic blood flow.[100] Indomethacin decreases CBF via a direct cerebrovascular vasoconstrictive effect that is independent of the drug's inhibitory action on prostaglandin synthesis.[101] It is possible that the documented decrease in severe P/IVH with early indomethacin use may be due to this selective cerebral vasoconstrictive effect during the first 2 to 3 days after delivery when reperfusion occurs[100] and has less to do with improving the low systemic blood flow state by closing the ductus arteriosus.

Although treatment of a hemodynamically insignificant PDA has become more controversial in the past few years, there is general consensus that a symptomatic, hemodynamically significant PDA should be treated. Cardiovascular management of the VLBW neonate with a large PDA should focus on measures that induce stepwise and reversible increases in pulmonary vascular resistance until pharmacologic or, if this fails, surgical closure of the PDA takes place. Such measures may include the avoidance of respiratory (and/or metabolic) alkalosis and maintenance of the oxygen saturation value at the lower end of the acceptable range. It is not known how vasopressors affect ductal shunting. Limited data suggest that dopamine may not worsen ductal shunting and might actually improve systemic blood flow along with increases in blood pressure in preterm infants.[102] However, if used the hemodynamic effects of dopamine or epinephrine need to be closely monitored in these patients with the use of functional echocardiography.

Treatment of Hypotension Associated With Other Causes Such as Sepsis, Adrenal Insufficiency, and Hypovolemia

In the treatment of hypotension in preterm infants with sepsis, adrenal insufficiency, and hypovolemia, every effort should be made to specifically treat the underlying primary cause. Although there are few experimental data regarding the response of CBF to vasopressor/inotropes or inotropes in the hypotensive VLBW infant, some evidence is accumulating.

Dopamine is the first-line medication because of its beneficial cardiovascular and renal effects.[103] It effectively increases blood pressure in the preterm infant, but its effect on organ blood flow is less well described. Evidence indicates that despite its effect on increasing blood pressure and renal perfusion, dopamine does not have a selective vasoactive action on the cerebral circulation in normotensive VLBW neonates.[104,105] However, in hypotensive VLBW infants, the dopamine-induced increase in blood pressure is associated with an increase in CBF.[27,29,96] This finding suggests strongly that cerebrovascular autoregulation is impaired in hypotensive VLBW infants and that effective treatment of hypotension is associated with an increase in CBF but with a delay in the restoration of CBF autoregulation (see earlier text).

Are other vasopressors more effective in restoring normal CBF in this population than dopamine? A randomized controlled trial compared the cerebrovascular, hemodynamic, and metabolic effects of dopamine and epinephrine using careful, stepwise titration of the two medications to achieve optimum blood pressure in VLBW neonates in the first 24 postnatal hours.[15] Both medications were effective in increasing cerebral perfusion in the medium dose range, with epinephrine being slightly more effective in infants of less than 28 weeks' gestation and dopamine being more effective in those of greater than 28 weeks' gestation. Because both medications were effective at increasing blood pressure and CBF, there is no reason to choose one vasopressor over the other for this particular application. Vasopressin has also been proposed for the treatment of hypotension in this context and was found to be a viable candidate in a small pilot study.[106] However, more data are needed before vasopressin can be considered a first-line medication for the treatment of hypotension. There has been growing interest in the potential use of milrinone, a selective phosphodiesterase III inhibitor, in neonates and infants who have undergone cardiac surgery and in VLBW neonates with low systemic blood flow during the first postnatal day. Indeed, milrinone effectively decreases the incidence of low cardiac output in infants after cardiac surgery.[107,108] Because the low-flow state in preterm infants immediately after birth is in many ways similar to the low cardiac output syndrome in postoperative cardiac patients, this drug has the potential as both treatment for and prophylaxis of low systemic blood flow (and presumably low CBF) in the VLBW patient population. A pilot study examined the safety, efficacy, and optimal dosing of milrinone in infants of less than 29 weeks' gestation during the first hours of postnatal life.[109] At the applied dose, milrinone appeared to be relatively safe in the 1-day-old VLBW neonate. However, findings of a likely somewhat underpowered randomized controlled trial by the same group of researchers indicate that milrinone is likely *ineffective to prevent* the occurrence of low SVC flow (a surrogate of systemic blood flow) in the 1-day-old VLBW neonate.[110] Therefore, at present, routine use of milrinone in this population cannot be recommended. Dobutamine, another sympathomimetic amine with direct positive inotropic and mild vasodilatory effects, effectively increases cardiac output and blood pressure in the VLBW neonate, especially when the cardiovascular compromise is caused by myocardial dysfunction.[111] Virtually no data are available on the cerebrovascular effects of dobutamine in the VLBW neonate. Beyond the presentation of different forms of neonatal shock treated with vasopressors/inotropes, inotropes, and lusitropes, there has been increasing recognition that vasopressor-resistant hypotension frequently develops in the VLBW population. This presentation is thought to be due to cardiovascular adrenergic receptor downregulation and the higher incidence of relative adrenal insufficiency in the VLBW neonate.[112–115] A prospective observational study examining the hemodynamic effects of low-dose hydrocortisone administration in preterm neonates with vasopressor resistance and borderline hypotension found no independent effect of this treatment modality on CBF.[115]

The Impact of Provision of Intensive Care on Systemic and Cerebral Hemodynamics

In addition to the impact of the hemodynamic changes on CBF during postnatal transition, the effects of all interventions must be considered at all times. They include ventilatory maneuvers, the use of medications other than vasopressors/inotropes or inotropes, and invasive procedures. Premature infants with a median gestational age of 31 weeks have been reported to have a decrease in CBF velocity (and presumably in CBF) in response to *transient hyperoxia*.[116] This occurred without a decrease in $Paco_2$, implicating hyperoxia directly in the decrease in CBF. *Hypocapnia* is a well-described cause of cerebral vasoconstriction; a direct association between $Paco_2$ and CBF, and an inverse association between $Paco_2$ and cerebral oxygen extraction, have been demonstrated in VLBW infants during the first postnatal days.[36,117,118] Lower levels of $Paco_2$ are also associated with slowing of the EEG, likely induced by decreased cerebral oxygen delivery.[118] Interestingly, the effects on aEEG are most significant in the first 24 hours, less evident on the second day, and gone by the third postnatal day. These findings support the notion that the first hours of postnatal life represent a period of heightened vulnerability to CBF fluctuations. Not surprisingly, severe hypocapnia in VLBW neonates during the immediate transition period is associated with PWMI and cerebral palsy.[119] *Hypercapnia* affects cerebral hemodynamics by increasing CBF and attenuating CBF autoregulation. The increase in CBF appears to be more prominent after the first postnatal day[57,58] and with a $Paco_2$ greater than 51 to 53 mm Hg.[57] $Paco_2$ values higher than 45 mm Hg during the first 2 postnatal days have been shown to progressively attenuate CBF autoregulation (Fig. 1.9).[120] It is tempting to speculate that these effects may explain the findings of retrospective studies, revealing a strong independent association between hypercapnia and P/IVH in very preterm neonates.[121–123] Interestingly, a recent randomized controlled trial comparing the impact of mild versus high permissive hypercapnia on the rate of bronchopulmonary dysplasia found no pulmonary benefits of the high CO_2 strategy, and there was also no difference in the incidence of severe P/IVH between the mild and high permissive hypercapnia groups.[124] The follow-up study of this trial also

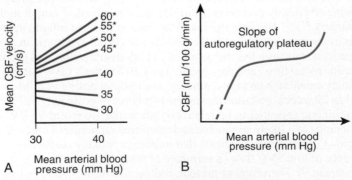

Fig. 1.9 Effect of hypercapnia on cerebral blood flow *(CBF)* autoregulation in 43 ventilated very low-birth-weight neonates during the first 2 postnatal days. A, Lines represent the estimated mean slopes of the autoregulatory plateau from 30 to 60 mm Hg arterial partial pressure of carbon dioxide *(Paco₂)* with mean blood pressure values between 30 and 40 mm Hg. The horizontal line at slope zero indicates intact autoregulation with lines at 30, 35, and 40 mm Hg being not significantly different from zero. B, The estimated means of the slope of the autoregulatory plateau (cm/s/mm Hg) increased as $Paco_2$ increased from 40 mm Hg (P = .004).

found no independent effects (positive or negative) of the high CO_2 strategy on neurodevelopment.[125] However, secondary exploratory data analysis of another randomized controlled trial on the subject found that higher CO_2 is an independent risk factor for severe P/IVH or death, neurodevelopmental impairment or death, and bronchopulmonary dysplasia or death,[126] thereby supporting the findings of the earlier retrospective studies.[120–122] Accordingly, the use of permissive hypercapnia during the immediate postnatal period may put the VLBW neonate at higher risk for cerebral injury.[127] Finally, high mean airway pressures in the immediate postnatal period have also been implicated in low systemic and CBF and a predilection for P/IVH.[34] Beyond ventilatory maneuvers and interventions, commonly used medications such as midazolam and morphine have also been associated with potentially harmful changes in CBF.[128] and even umbilical arterial blood sampling could have an effect on cerebral hemodynamics in these tiny infants.[129] The clinical relevance of the latter finding is unclear.

Summary and Recommendations

As discussed in this chapter, the management of hypotension and low systemic and CBF in the VLBW infant during the first postnatal days presents a significant challenge because immaturity, the physiologic changes during transition, and the underlying pathology all affect the hemodynamic response to pathologic processes and interventions.

Because of these factors and the lack of evidence on how treatment affects mortality and short- and long-term morbidity, straightforward recommendations on the treatment of cardiovascular compromise in the VLBW neonate during the period of transition to postnatal life cannot be given. Therefore the following approach to diagnosis and treatment represents our view and should be considered only as such, especially because evidence on the effectiveness and impact of treatment of shock, particularly on long-term neurodevelopmental outcomes, in the VLBW neonate during the first postnatal days is not available.

Diagnosis of Hypotension

1. We use the 5th or 10th percentile of the gestational and postnatal age–dependent population-based blood pressure values as a crude definition of hypotension. However, treatment at this point is initiated only if signs of tissue hypoperfusion or echocardiographic evidence of decreased systemic perfusion and/or poor myocardial contractility are present. However, we attempt to maintain mean blood pressure at 23 to 24 mm Hg even if signs of tissue hypoperfusion are not present in the most immature ELBW neonates during the first postnatal day, because cerebral electrical activity appears to be depressed at blood pressure values below this level.
2. Irrespective of the blood pressure value, whenever there is indirect or direct evidence of poor tissue perfusion, both systemic blood flow and blood pressure are monitored closely and attempt to maintain appropriate systemic blood flow without much fluctuation in the blood pressure. Because a blood pressure breakpoint of the CBF autoregulatory curve may exist at 28 to 29 mm Hg and because more than 90% of even ELBW neonates not receiving vasopressor support maintain their mean blood pressure at 30 mm Hg or higher by the third postnatal day, we carefully attempt to slowly increase mean blood pressure during the first 3 postnatal days and maintain it in the 28- to 30-mm Hg range by the third postnatal day. However, it must be kept in mind that an increase in blood pressure during this period does not necessarily ensure normalization of systemic and CBF and that there are no data that this approach improves long-term neurodevelopmental outcomes. Finally, the presence of a hemodynamically significant PDA affects our approach to maintaining and focusing primarily on mean arterial blood pressure; in these cases we carefully consider diastolic blood pressure and interrogate the cardiovascular system for evidence of systemic steal during diastole.
3. Although some neonatologists may agree with the approach described here, there is another, less frequently practiced approach that is worthy of discussion. Neonatologists using this approach initiate cardiovascular support only if there is

clear evidence of poor systemic perfusion as long as mean blood pressure is at or higher than 20 mm Hg in the ELBW neonate during the first postnatal day. Because it is difficult to define poor perfusion within the first 24 hours, especially without the use of functional echocardiography, and because lactic acidosis heralds the presence of (ongoing or previously present) tissue ischemia, we do not practice this diagnostic and treatment philosophy and do not allow mean arterial blood pressure to be maintained around 20 mm Hg during the first postnatal day. However, there is no direct evidence at present that the use of permissive hypotension as an approach to diagnosis and management of cardiovascular compromise in VLBW neonates during the immediate postnatal period (positively or negatively) affects outcomes.

Treatment of Hypotension

With regard to the kind of treatment used, the most appropriate strategy requires identification of the underlying pathogenesis of hypotension. The most common etiologic factors are inappropriate peripheral vasoregulation and dysfunction of the myocardium complicated by the presence of a large PDA in VLBW neonates during the first postnatal days. However, recent data on physiologic (delayed) cord clamping also implicate a certain level of hypovolemia if the cord clamped immediately after delivery.[44,45]

1. In the case of hypotension, because low to moderate doses of dopamine (or epinephrine) improve both blood pressure and CBF, we carefully titrate dopamine in a stepwise manner using 3- to 5-minute cycles and make every effort to avoid inducing significant rapid changes in blood pressure. If there is evidence of hypovolemia, we carefully administer volume (usually isotonic saline solution). If low systemic blood flow is detected with low-normal to normal blood pressure during the first postnatal day, we use dobutamine (with or without low-dose dopamine) and monitor for indirect (CRT, urine output, base deficit) and direct (functional echocardiography) signs of improvement in systemic perfusion.

2. In the presence of a hemodynamically significant PDA, we attempt to close the ductus arteriosus with a cyclooxygenase inhibitor (we use indomethacin) along with providing appropriate supportive care. If pharmacologic closure fails in the patient with a hemodynamically significant PDA and there is evidence of ongoing or worsening systemic tissue hypoperfusion, we surgically ligate the ductus arteriosus. During the wait for surgical closure to take place, our goal is to decrease the left-to-right shunting across the ductus. As briefly described earlier, we attempt to achieve this goal by carefully increasing pulmonary resistance in a stepwise manner. Using this approach, we frequently are successful at increasing pulmonary vascular resistance, and the associated decrease in left-to-right shunting usually results in improvement of systemic blood flow and blood pressure. We also use dopamine in infants with a hemodynamically significant PDA, because it has been shown that, in patients with increased pulmonary blood flow, dopamine increases pulmonary vascular resistance and systemic perfusion.[102] Interestingly, there is no evidence that dopamine preferentially increases pulmonary vascular resistance in neonates without preexisting pulmonary overcirculation. It is tempting to speculate that the increased pulmonary blood flow–associated protective upregulation of vasoconstrictive mechanisms (enhanced α-adrenergic and endothelin-1 receptor expression) and downregulation of the vasodilatory mechanisms (endogenous nitric oxide and vasodilatory prostaglandin production) in the pulmonary arteries are responsible for this observation. We add dobutamine only in the presence of impaired myocardial function, because most VLBW neonates with hemodynamically significant PDA after the first postnatal day usually have normal or hyperdynamic cardiac function. Indeed, the indiscriminate use of dobutamine in these patients may compromise diastolic function and thus cardiac filling. Finally, administration of fluids to increase blood volume must be restricted because excessive (or even liberal) use of volume is associated with greater mortality and morbidity (pulmonary hemorrhage) in this patient population. However, careful, small-volume transfusions might be used to increase viscosity and thus pulmonary vascular

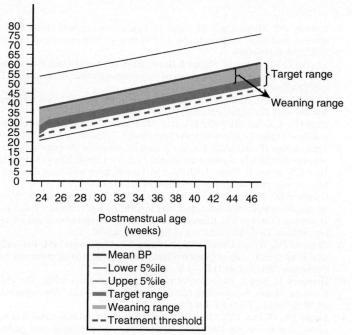

Fig. 1.10 Postmenstrual age–dependent definition of hypotension and the target and weaning blood pressure *(BP)* ranges. Hypotension is defined as the treatment threshold, which is 1 to 3 points above the 5th percentile *(5%ile)* for postmenstrual age (14–16 weeks). Below the treatment threshold, the authors usually initiate treatment for hypotension. The target range is defined as the mean BP that is intended to be maintained. The target range is between 2 and 3 mm Hg above the treatment threshold and the 50th percentile of the mean BP (14–16 weeks). Finally, the weaning range is defined as the mean BP range where careful weaning of vasopressor/inotropes and/or inotropes is commenced. This range is between 5 mm Hg above the lower limits of the target range and the 50th percentile of the mean BP. Note that the upper limit of the target range does not exceed the 50th percentile of the mean BP to decrease the risk of achieving an increase in BP by causing significant increases in systemic vascular resistance and thus potentially decreases in cardiac output when vasopressor/inotropes are being administered. This graph was developed in collaboration with the Under Pressure hemodynamic group created as part of a Vermont-Oxford Network (VON) initiative for 2004–2006. One of the authors (I.S.) served as the VON expert on hemodynamics for this initiative.

resistance in patients not responding to maneuvers aimed to decrease pH and keep oxygenation in the lower end of the accepted range.

3. Finally, because Pa_{CO_2} is a more potent mediator of cerebral vascular tone than blood pressure, we make every effort to keep Pa_{CO_2} around 45 to 50 mm Hg during the first 3 postnatal days. We hope that by keeping a Pa_{CO_2} relatively constant we minimize the risk for the hypocapnia-associated white matter injury and cerebral palsy and the hypercapnia-associated increased risk of P/IVH. In addition, in the presence of constant Pa_{CO_2} levels, the integrity of CBF autoregulation is likely to be optimized.

Fig. 1.10 illustrates our postmenstrual age–dependent approach to the diagnosis and treatment of hypotension in preterm and term neonates. It is important to note that our definition of hypotension (*dotted line*) and the target and weaning ranges have all been arbitrarily defined with the use of epidemiologic data, extrapolation of hemodynamic findings, and the data on the association between blood pressure and systemic and CBF. As this approach, just like any other approach to managing cardiovascular compromise in the neonatal patient population, is not evidenced based, therefore it cannot be recommended for routine use and illustrates only one of the many approaches to the diagnosis and treatment of neonatal hypotension.

Finally, we use these numbers only as guidance, carefully assess the indirect clinical signs of tissue perfusion, and perform targeted echocardiographic evaluations when more information is needed. In the future and after completion of the ongoing investigations, we plan to use the real-time information provided by our comprehensive cardiovascular monitoring and data acquisition system.

REFERENCES

1. Perlman JM, McMenamin JB, Volpe JJ. Fluctuating cerebral blood-flow velocity in respiratory-distress syndrome. Relation to the development of intraventricular hemorrhage. *N Engl J Med.* 1983;309(4):204–209.
2. Van Bel F, Van de Bor M, Stijnen T, Baan J, Ruys JH. Aetiological rôle of cerebral blood-flow alterations in development and extension of peri-intraventricular haemorrhage. *Dev Med Child Neurol.* 1987;29(5):601–614.
3. Miall-Allen VM, de Vries LS, Whitelaw AG. Mean arterial blood pressure and neonatal cerebral lesions. *Arch Dis Child.* 1987;62(10):1068–1069.
4. Bada HS, Korones SB, Perry EH, et al. Mean arterial blood pressure changes in premature infants and those at risk for intraventricular hemorrhage. *J Pediatr.* 1990;117(4):607–614.
5. Tsuji M, Saul JP, du Plessis A, et al. Cerebral intravascular oxygenation correlates with mean arterial pressure in critically ill premature infants. *Pediatrics.* 2000;106(4):625–632.
6. Hunt RW, Evans N, Rieger I, Kluckow M. Low superior vena cava flow and neurodevelopment at 3 years in very preterm infants. *J Pediatr.* 2004;145(5):588–592.
7. Goldstein RF, Thompson RJ, Oehler JM, Brazy JE. Influence of acidosis, hypoxemia, and hypotension on neurodevelopmental outcome in very low birth weight infants. *Pediatrics.* 1995;95(2):238–243.
8. Dammann O, Allred EN, Kuban KC, et al. Systemic hypotension and white-matter damage in preterm infants. *Dev Med Child Neurol.* 2002;44(2):82–90.
9. Fanaroff JM, Wilson-Costello DE, Newman NS, Montpetite MM, Fanaroff AA. Treated hypotension is associated with neonatal morbidity and hearing loss in extremely low birth weight infants. *Pediatrics.* 2006;117(4):1131–1135.
10. Dempsey E, Seri I. Definition of normal blood pressure range: the elusive target. In: Seri I, Kluckow M, eds. *Neonatology Questions and Controversies: Hemodynamics and Cardiology.* 3rd ed. Philadelphia, PA: Saunders Elsevier; 2017.
11. Logan JW, O'Shea TM, Allred EN, et al. Early postnatal hypotension is not associated with indicators of white matter damage or cerebral palsy in extremely low gestational age newborns. *J Perinatol.* 2011;31(8):524–534.
12. Batton B, Li L, Newman NS, et al. Early blood pressure, antihypotensive therapy and outcomes at 18–22 months' corrected age in extremely preterm infants. *Arch Dis Child Fetal Neonatal Ed.* 2016;101(3):F201–F206.
13. Batton B, Li L, Newman NS, et al. Use of antihypotensive therapies in extremely preterm infants. *Pediatrics.* 2013;131(6):e1865–e1873.
14. Dempsey EM, Al Hazzani F, Barrington KJ. Permissive hypotension in the extremely low birthweight infant with signs of good perfusion. *Arch Dis Child Fetal Neonatal Ed.* 2009;94(4):F241–F244.
15. Pellicer A, Bravo MC, Madero R, Salas S, Quero J, Cabañas F. Early systemic hypotension and vasopressor support in low birth weight infants: impact on neurodevelopment. *Pediatrics.* 2009;123(5):1369–1376.
16. Faust K, Härtel C, Preuß M, et al. Short-term outcome of very-low-birthweight infants with arterial hypotension in the first 24 h of life. *Arch Dis Child Fetal Neonatal Ed.* 2015;100(5):F388–F392.
17. Batton BJ, Li L, Newman NS, et al. Feasibility study of early blood pressure management in extremely preterm infants. *J Pediatr.* 2012;161(1):65–69.e61.
18. Pellicer A, Valverde E, Elorza MD, et al. Cardiovascular support for low birth weight infants and cerebral hemodynamics: a randomized, blinded, clinical trial. *Pediatrics.* 2005;115(6):1501–1512.
19. Wu T-W, Noori S, Seri I. *Neonatal Hypotension.* 5th ed. Philadelphia: Elsevier Health Sciences; 2014.
20. Nuntnarumit P, Yang W, Bada-Ellzey HS. Blood pressure measurements in the newborn. *Clin Perinatol.* 1999;26(4):981–996, x.
21. Development of audit measures and guidelines for good practice in the management of neonatal respiratory distress syndrome. Report of a joint working group of the british association of perinatal medicine and the research unit of the royal college of physicians. *Arch Dis Child.* 1992;67(10 Spec No):1221–1227.
22. Vesoulis ZA, El Ters NM, Wallendorf M, Mathur AM. Empirical estimation of the normative blood pressure in infants <28 weeks gestation using a massive data approach. *J Perinatol.* 2016;36(4):291–295.
23. Børch K, Lou HC, Greisen G. Cerebral white matter blood flow and arterial blood pressure in preterm infants. *Acta Paediatr.* 2010;99(10):1489–1492.
24. Seri I. Circulatory support of the sick preterm infant. *Semin Neonatol.* 2001;6(1):85–95.
25. Greisen G. Autoregulation of cerebral blood flow in newborn babies. *Early Hum Dev.* 2005;81(5):423–428.
26. Milligan DW. Failure of autoregulation and intraventricular haemorrhage in preterm infants. *Lancet.* 1980;1(8174):896–898.
27. Lightburn MH, Gauss CH, Williams DK, Kaiser JR. Observational study of cerebral hemodynamics during dopamine treatment in hypotensive ELBW infants on the first day of life. *J Perinatol.* 2013;33(9):698–702.
28. O'Leary H, Gregas MC, Limperopoulos C, et al. Elevated cerebral pressure passivity is associated with prematurity-related intracranial hemorrhage. *Pediatrics.* 2009;124(1):302–309.
29. Munro MJ, Walker AM, Barfield CP. Hypotensive extremely low birth weight infants have reduced cerebral blood flow. *Pediatrics.* 2004;114(6):1591–1596.
30. Kissack CM, Garr R, Wardle SP, Weindling AM. Cerebral fractional oxygen extraction is inversely correlated with oxygen delivery in the sick, newborn, preterm infant. *J Cereb Blood Flow Metab.* 2005;25(5):545–553.

31. Victor S, Marson AG, Appleton RE, Beirne M, Weindling AM. Relationship between blood pressure, cerebral electrical activity, cerebral fractional oxygen extraction, and peripheral blood flow in very low birth weight newborn infants. *Pediatr Res.* 2006;59(2):314–319.

32. Victor S, Appleton RE, Beirne M, Marson AG, Weindling AM. The relationship between cardiac output, cerebral electrical activity, cerebral fractional oxygen extraction and peripheral blood flow in premature newborn infants. *Pediatr Res.* 2006;60(4):456–460.

33. Kluckow M, Evans N. Low superior vena cava flow and intraventricular haemorrhage in preterm infants. *Arch Dis Child Fetal Neonatal Ed.* 2000;82(3):F188–F194.

34. Kluckow M, Evans N. Relationship between blood pressure and cardiac output in preterm infants requiring mechanical ventilation. *J Pediatr.* 1996;129(4):506–512.

35. Kluckow M, Evans N. Superior vena cava flow in newborn infants: a novel marker of systemic blood flow. *Arch Dis Child Fetal Neonatal Ed.* 2000;82(3):F182–F187.

36. Kissack CM, Garr R, Wardle SP, Weindling AM. Cerebral fractional oxygen extraction in very low birth weight infants is high when there is low left ventricular output and hypocarbia but is unaffected by hypotension. *Pediatr Res.* 2004;55(3):400–405.

37. Seri I. Low superior vena cava flow during the first postnatal day and neurodevelopment in preterm neonates. *J Pediatr.* 2004;145(5):573–575.

38. Strunk T, Inder T, Wang X, Burgner D, Mallard C, Levy O. Infection-induced inflammation and cerebral injury in preterm infants. *Lancet Infect Dis.* 2014;14(8):751–762.

39. Greisen G. Cerebral blood flow in preterm infants during the first week of life. *Acta Paediatr Scand.* 1986;75(1):43–51.

40. Pryds O, Andersen GE, Friis-Hansen B. Cerebral blood flow reactivity in spontaneously breathing, preterm infants shortly after birth. *Acta Paediatr Scand.* 1990;79(4):391–396.

41. Pryds O, Greisen G. Effect of PaCO2 and haemoglobin concentration on day to day variation of CBF in preterm neonates. *Acta Paediatr Scand Suppl.* 1989;360:33–36.

42. Greisen G, Trojaborg W. Cerebral blood flow, PaCO2 changes, and visual evoked potentials in mechanically ventilated, preterm infants. *Acta Paediatr Scand.* 1987;76(3):394–400.

43. Altman DI, Powers WJ, Perlman JM, Herscovitch P, Volpe SL, Volpe JJ. Cerebral blood flow requirement for brain viability in newborn infants is lower than in adults. *Ann Neurol.* 1988;24(2):218–226.

44. Backes CH, Rivera BK, Haque U, et al. Placental transfusion strategies in very preterm neonates: a systematic review and meta-analysis. *Obstet Gynecol.* 2014;124(1):47–56.

45. Katheria AC, Lakshminrusimha S, Rabe H, McAdams R, Mercer JS. Placental transfusion: a review. *J Perinatol.* 2017;37(2):105–111.

46. Hernandez M, Hawkins R, Brennan R. *Sympathetic Control of Regional Cerebral Blood Flow in the Asphyxiated Newborn Dog.* New York: Elsevier; 1982.

47. Ashwal S, Dale PS, Longo LD. Regional cerebral blood flow: studies in the fetal lamb during hypoxia, hypercapnia, acidosis, and hypotension. *Pediatr Res.* 1984;18(12):1309–1316.

48. Lightburn MH, Gauss CH, Williams DK, Kaiser JR. Cerebral blood flow velocities in extremely low birth weight infants with hypotension and infants with normal blood pressure. *J Pediatr.* 2009;154(6):824–828.

49. Noori S, McCoy M, Anderson MP, Ramji F, Seri I. Changes in cardiac function and cerebral blood flow in relation to peri/intraventricular hemorrhage in extremely preterm infants. *J Pediatr.* 2014;164(2):264–270.e261–e263.

50. Shah D, Paradisis M, Bowen JR. Relationship between systemic blood flow, blood pressure, inotropes, and aEEG in the first 48 h of life in extremely preterm infants. *Pediatr Res.* 2013;74(3):314–320.

51. Kehrer M, Blumenstock G, Ehehalt S, Goelz R, Poets C, Schöning M. Development of cerebral blood flow volume in preterm neonates during the first two weeks of life. *Pediatr Res.* 2005;58(5):927–930.

52. Kluckow M, Evans N. Low systemic blood flow and hyperkalemia in preterm infants. *J Pediatr.* 2001;139(2):227–232.

53. Osborn D, Evans N, Kluckow M. Randomized trial of dobutamine versus dopamine in preterm infants with low systemic blood flow. *J Pediatr.* 2002;140(2):183–191.

54. Takami T, Sunohara D, Kondo A, et al. Changes in cerebral perfusion in extremely LBW infants during the first 72 h after birth. *Pediatr Res.* 2010;68(5):435–439.

55. Seri I, Noori S. Fetal and neonatal hemodynamics. *Semin Fetal Neonatal Med.* 2015;20(4):209.

56. Osborn DA, Evans N, Kluckow M. Clinical detection of low upper body blood flow in very premature infants using blood pressure, capillary refill time, and central-peripheral temperature difference. *Arch Dis Child Fetal Neonatal Ed.* 2004;89(2):F168–F173.

57. Noori S, Anderson M, Soleymani S, Seri I. Effect of carbon dioxide on cerebral blood flow velocity in preterm infants during postnatal transition. *Acta Paediatr.* 2014;103(8):e334–e339.

58. Pryds O, Greisen G, Lou H, Friis-Hansen B. Heterogeneity of cerebral vasoreactivity in preterm infants supported by mechanical ventilation. *J Pediatr.* 1989;115(4):638–645.

59. Levene MI, Shortland D, Gibson N, Evans DH. Carbon dioxide reactivity of the cerebral circulation in extremely premature infants: effects of postnatal age and indomethacin. *Pediatr Res.* 1988;24(2):175–179.

60. Evans N, Iyer P. Longitudinal changes in the diameter of the ductus arteriosus in ventilated preterm infants: correlation with respiratory outcomes. *Arch Dis Child Fetal Neonatal Ed.* 1995;72(3):F156–F161.

61. West CR, Groves AM, Williams CE, et al. Early low cardiac output is associated with compromised electroencephalographic activity in very preterm infants. *Pediatr Res.* 2006;59(4 Pt 1):610–615.

62. Noori S, Seri I. Does targeted neonatal echocardiography affect hemodynamics and cerebral oxygenation in extremely preterm infants? *J Perinatol.* 2014;34(11):847–849.

63. Kluckow M, Seri I, Evans N. Functional echocardiography: an emerging clinical tool for the neonatologist. *J Pediatr*. 2007;150(2):125–130.
64. Gilbert RD, Pearce WJ, Ashwal S, Longo LD. Effects of hypoxia on contractility of isolated fetal lamb cerebral arteries. *J Dev Physiol*. 1990;13(4):199–203.
65. Hansen NB, Stonestreet BS, Rosenkrantz TS, Oh W. Validity of Doppler measurements of anterior cerebral artery blood flow velocity: correlation with brain blood flow in piglets. *Pediatrics*. 1983;72(4):526–531.
66. Greisen G, Johansen K, Ellison PH, Fredriksen PS, Mali J, Friis-Hansen B. Cerebral blood flow in the newborn infant: comparison of Doppler ultrasound and 133xenon clearance. *J Pediatr*. 1984;104(3):411–418.
67. Raju TN. Cerebral Doppler studies in the fetus and newborn infant. *J Pediatr*. 1991;119(2):165–174.
68. Suttner S, Schöllhorn T, Boldt J, et al. Noninvasive assessment of cardiac output using thoracic electrical bioimpedance in hemodynamically stable and unstable patients after cardiac surgery: a comparison with pulmonary artery thermodilution. *Intensive Care Med*. 2006;32(12):2053–2058.
69. Norozi K, Beck C, Osthaus WA, Wille I, Wessel A, Bertram H. Electrical velocimetry for measuring cardiac output in children with congenital heart disease. *Br J Anaesth*. 2008;100(1):88–94.
70. Noori S, Drabu B, Soleymani S, Seri I. Continuous non-invasive cardiac output measurements in the neonate by electrical velocimetry: a comparison with echocardiography. *Arch Dis Child Fetal Neonatal Ed*. 2012;97(5):F340–F343.
71. Trinkmann F, Berger M, Doesch C, et al. Comparison of electrical velocimetry and cardiac magnetic resonance imaging for the non-invasive determination of cardiac output. *J Clin Monit Comput*. 2016;30(4):399–408.
72. Borzage M, Heidari K. T C, I S, J W, S B. Phase contract MR imaging does not support the accuracy of impedance cardiography stroke volume determination. *American Journal of Critical Care*. 2017: in press.
73. Hsu K-H, Wu T-W, Wang Y-C, Lim W-H, Lee C-C, Lien R. Hemodynamic reference for neonates of different age and weight: a pilot study with electrical cardiometry. *J Perinatol*. 2016;36(6):481–485.
74. Brazy JE, Lewis DV, Mitnick MH, Jöbsis vander Vliet FF. Noninvasive monitoring of cerebral oxygenation in preterm infants: preliminary observations. *Pediatrics*. 1985;75(2):217–225.
75. Patel J, Marks K, Roberts I, Azzopardi D, Edwards AD. Measurement of cerebral blood flow in newborn infants using near infrared spectroscopy with indocyanine green. *Pediatr Res*. 1998;43(1):34–39.
76. Dullenkopf A, Kolarova A, Schulz G, Frey B, Baenziger O, Weiss M. Reproducibility of cerebral oxygenation measurement in neonates and infants in the clinical setting using the NIRO 300 oximeter. *Pediatr Crit Care Med*. 2005;6(3):344–347.
77. Bucher HU, Edwards AD, Lipp AE, Duc G. Comparison between near infrared spectroscopy and 133xenon clearance for estimation of cerebral blood flow in critically ill preterm infants. *Pediatr Res*. 1993;33(1):56–60.
78. Dujovny M, Ausman JI, Stoddart H, Slavin KV, Lewis GD, Widman R. Somanetics INVOS 3100 cerebral oximeter. *Neurosurgery*. 1995;37(1):160.
79. Alderliesten T, De Vis JB, Lemmers PM, et al. Brain oxygen saturation assessment in neonates using T2-prepared blood imaging of oxygen saturation and near-infrared spectroscopy. *J Cereb Blood Flow Metab*. 2017;37(3):902–913.
80. Alderliesten T, De Vis JB, Lemmers PM, et al. T2-prepared velocity selective labelling: a novel idea for full-brain mapping of oxygen saturation. *Neuroimage*. 2016;139:65–73.
81. Toet MC, Lemmers PM. Brain monitoring in neonates. *Early Hum Dev*. 2009;85(2):77–84.
82. Pellicer A, Greisen G, Benders M, et al. The SafeBoosC phase II randomised clinical trial: a treatment guideline for targeted near-infrared-derived cerebral tissue oxygenation versus standard treatment in extremely preterm infants. *Neonatology*. 2013;104(3):171–178.
83. Hyttel-Sorensen S, Pellicer A, Alderliesten T, et al. Cerebral near infrared spectroscopy oximetry in extremely preterm infants: phase II randomised clinical trial. *BMJ*. 2015;350. g7635.
84. Plomgaard AM, Hagmann C, Alderliesten T, et al. Brain injury in the international multicenter randomized SafeBoosC phase II feasibility trial: cranial ultrasound and magnetic resonance imaging assessments. *Pediatr Res*. 2016;79(3):466–472.
85. Plomgaard AM, van Oeveren W, Petersen TH, et al. The SafeBoosC II randomized trial: treatment guided by near-infrared spectroscopy reduces cerebral hypoxia without changing early biomarkers of brain injury. *Pediatr Res*. 2016;79(4):528–535.
86. Kurth CD, McCann JC, Wu J, Miles L, Loepke AW. Cerebral oxygen saturation-time threshold for hypoxic-ischemic injury in piglets. *Anesth Analg*. 2009;108(4):1268–1277.
87. Hagino I, Anttila V, Zurakowski D, Duebener LF, Lidov HG, Jonas RA. Tissue oxygenation index is a useful monitor of histologic and neurologic outcome after cardiopulmonary bypass in piglets. *J Thorac Cardiovasc Surg*. 2005;130(2):384–392.
88. Alderliesten T, Lemmers PM, van Haastert IC, et al. Hypotension in preterm neonates: low blood pressure alone does not affect neurodevelopmental outcome. *J Pediatr*. 2014;164(5):986–991.
89. Greisen G. Cerebral autoregulation in preterm infants. How to measure it—and why care? *J Pediatr*. 2014;165(5):885–886.
90. Eriksen VR, Hahn GH, Greisen G. Cerebral autoregulation in the preterm newborn using near-infrared spectroscopy: a comparison of time-domain and frequency-domain analyses. *J Biomed Opt*. 2015;20(3):037009.
91. Toet MC, Hellström-Westas L, Groenendaal F, Eken P, de Vries LS. Amplitude integrated EEG 3 and 6 hours after birth in full term neonates with hypoxic-ischaemic encephalopathy. *Arch Dis Child Fetal Neonatal Ed*. 1999;81(1):F19–F23.

92. Toet MC, van der Meij W, de Vries LS, Uiterwaal CS, van Huffelen KC. Comparison between simultaneously recorded amplitude integrated electroencephalogram (cerebral function monitor) and standard electroencephalogram in neonates. *Pediatrics.* 2002;109(5):772–779.

93. ter Horst HJ, Sommer C, Bergman KA, Fock JM, van Weerden TW, Bos AF. Prognostic significance of amplitude-integrated EEG during the first 72 hours after birth in severely asphyxiated neonates. *Pediatr Res.* 2004;55(6):1026–1033.

94. Shalak LF, Laptook AR, Velaphi SC, Perlman JM. Amplitude-integrated electroencephalography coupled with an early neurologic examination enhances prediction of term infants at risk for persistent encephalopathy. *Pediatrics.* 2003;111(2):351–357.

95. Azhibekov T, Soleymani S, Lee BH, Noori S, Seri I. Hemodynamic monitoring of the critically ill neonate: an eye on the future. *Semin Fetal Neonatal Med.* 2015;20(4):246–254.

96. Seri I, Rudas G, Bors Z, Kanyicska B, Tulassay T. Effects of low-dose dopamine infusion on cardiovascular and renal functions, cerebral blood flow, and plasma catecholamine levels in sick preterm neonates. *Pediatr Res.* 1993;34(6):742–749.

97. Noori S, Stavroudis TA, Seri I. Systemic and cerebral hemodynamics during the transitional period after premature birth. *Clin Perinatol.* 2009;36(4):723–736, v.

98. Evans N, Moorcraft J. Effect of patency of the ductus arteriosus on blood pressure in very preterm infants. *Arch Dis Child.* 1992;67(10 Spec No):1169–1173.

99. Kluckow M, Evans N. Early echocardiographic prediction of symptomatic patent ductus arteriosus in preterm infants undergoing mechanical ventilation. *J Pediatr.* 1995;127(5):774–779.

100. Osborn DA, Evans N, Kluckow M. Effect of early targeted indomethacin on the ductus arteriosus and blood flow to the upper body and brain in the preterm infant. *Arch Dis Child Fetal Neonatal Ed.* 2003;88(6):F477–F482.

101. Yanowitz TD, Yao AC, Werner JC, Pettigrew KD, Oh W, Stonestreet BS. Effects of prophylactic low-dose indomethacin on hemodynamics in very low birth weight infants. *J Pediatr.* 1998;132(1):28–34.

102. Bouissou A, Rakza T, Klosowski S, Tourneux P, Vanderborght M, Storme L. Hypotension in preterm infants with significant patent ductus arteriosus: effects of dopamine. *J Pediatr.* 2008;153(6):790–794.

103. Seri I. Cardiovascular, renal, and endocrine actions of dopamine in neonates and children. *J Pediatr.* 1995;126(3):333–344.

104. Seri I, Abbasi S, Wood DC, Gerdes JS. Regional hemodynamic effects of dopamine in the sick preterm neonate. *J Pediatr.* 1998;133(6):728–734.

105. Lundstrøm K, Pryds O, Greisen G. The haemodynamic effects of dopamine and volume expansion in sick preterm infants. *Early Hum Dev.* 2000;57(2):157–163.

106. Rios DR, Kaiser JR. Vasopressin versus dopamine for treatment of hypotension in extremely low birth weight infants: a randomized, blinded pilot study. *J Pediatr.* 2015;166(4):850–855.

107. Chang AC, Atz AM, Wernovsky G, Burke RP, Wessel DL. Milrinone: systemic and pulmonary hemodynamic effects in neonates after cardiac surgery. *Crit Care Med.* 1995;23(11):1907–1914.

108. Hoffman TM, Wernovsky G, Atz AM, et al. Efficacy and safety of milrinone in preventing low cardiac output syndrome in infants and children after corrective surgery for congenital heart disease. *Circulation.* 2003;107(7):996–1002.

109. Paradisis M, Evans N, Kluckow M, Osborn D, McLachlan AJ. Pilot study of milrinone for low systemic blood flow in very preterm infants. *J Pediatr.* 2006;148(3):306–313.

110. Paradisis M, Evans N, Kluckow M, Osborn D. Randomized trial of milrinone versus placebo for prevention of low systemic blood flow in very preterm infants. *J Pediatr.* 2009;154(2):189–195.

111. Noori S, Friedlich P, Seri I. Cardiovascular and renal effects of dobutamine in the neonate. *NeoReviews.* 2004;5:E22–E26.

112. Ng PC, Lee CH, Lam CW, et al. Transient adrenocortical insufficiency of prematurity and systemic hypotension in very low birthweight infants. *Arch Dis Child Fetal Neonatal Ed.* 2004;89(2):F119–F126.

113. Fernandez E, Schrader R, Watterberg K. Prevalence of low cortisol values in term and near-term infants with vasopressor-resistant hypotension. *J Perinatol.* 2005;25(2):114–118.

114. Seri I, Tan R, Evans J. Cardiovascular effects of hydrocortisone in preterm infants with pressor-resistant hypotension. *Pediatrics.* 2001;107(5):1070–1074.

115. Noori S, Friedlich P, Wong P, Ebrahimi M, Siassi B, Seri I. Hemodynamic changes after low-dosage hydrocortisone administration in vasopressor-treated preterm and term neonates. *Pediatrics.* 2006;118(4):1456–1466.

116. Niijima S, Shortland DB, Levene MI, Evans DH. Transient hyperoxia and cerebral blood flow velocity in infants born prematurely and at full term. *Arch Dis Child.* 1988;63(10 Spec No):1126–1130.

117. Tyszczuk L, Meek J, Elwell C, Wyatt JS. Cerebral blood flow is independent of mean arterial blood pressure in preterm infants undergoing intensive care. *Pediatrics.* 1998;102(2 Pt 1):337–341.

118. Victor S, Appleton RE, Beirne M, Marson AG, Weindling AM. Effect of carbon dioxide on background cerebral electrical activity and fractional oxygen extraction in very low birth weight infants just after birth. *Pediatr Res.* 2005;58(3):579–585.

119. Murase M, Ishida A. Early hypocarbia of preterm infants: its relationship to periventricular leukomalacia and cerebral palsy, and its perinatal risk factors. *Acta Paediatr.* 2005;94(1):85–91.

120. Kaiser JR, Gauss CH, Williams DK. The effects of hypercapnia on cerebral autoregulation in ventilated very low birth weight infants. *Pediatr Res.* 2005;58(5):931–935.

121. Kaiser JR, Gauss CH, Pont MM, Williams DK. Hypercapnia during the first 3 days of life is associated with severe intraventricular hemorrhage in very low birth weight infants. *J Perinatol.* 2006;26(5):279–285.

122. Kaiser JR. Both extremes of arterial carbon dioxide pressure and the magnitude of fluctuations in arterial carbon dioxide pressure are associated with severe intraventricular hemorrhage in preterm infants. *Pediatrics*. 2007;119(5):1039, author reply 1039–1040.
123. Vela-Huerta MM, Amador-Licona M, Medina-Ovando N, Aldana-Valenzuela C. Factors associated with early severe intraventricular haemorrhage in very low birth weight infants. *Neuropediatrics*. 2009;40(5):224–227.
124. Thome UH, Genzel-Boroviczeny O, Bohnhorst B, et al. Permissive hypercapnia in extremely low birthweight infants (PHELBI): a randomised controlled multicentre trial. *Lancet Respir Med*. 2015;3(7):534–543.
125. Thome UH, Genzel-Boroviczeny O, Bohnhorst B, et al. Neurodevelopmental outcomes of extremely low birthweight infants randomised to different PCO2 targets: the PHELBI follow-up study. *Arch Dis Child Fetal Neonatal Ed*. 2017. http://dx.doi.org/10.1136/archdischild-2016-311581. *[Epub ahead of print.]*
126. Ambalavanan N, Carlo WA, Wrage LA, et al. PaCO2 in surfactant, positive pressure, and oxygenation randomised trial (SUPPORT). *Arch Dis Child Fetal Neonatal Ed*. 2015;100(2):F145–F149.
127. McKee LA, Fabres J, Howard G, Peralta-Carcelen M, Carlo WA, Ambalavanan N. PaCO2 and neurodevelopment in extremely low birth weight infants. *J Pediatr*. 2009;155(2):217–221. e211.
128. van Alfen-van der Velden AA, Hopman JC, Klaessens JH, Feuth T, Sengers RC, Liem KD. Effects of midazolam and morphine on cerebral oxygenation and hemodynamics in ventilated premature infants. *Biol Neonate*. 2006;90(3):197–202.
129. Roll C, Hüning B, Käunicke M, Krug J, Horsch S. Umbilical artery catheter blood sampling volume and velocity: impact on cerebral blood volume and oxygenation in very-low-birthweight infants. *Acta Paediatr*. 2006;95(1):68–73.

CHAPTER 2

Intraventricular Hemorrhage and White Matter Injury in the Preterm Infant

Vivien Yap and Jeffrey M. Perlman

- Periventricular-intraventricular hemorrhage
- Periventricular white matter injury associated with IVH
- White matter injury in the absence of hemorrhage
- Outcome
- Gaps in knowledge

CASE HISTORY

HW was a 700-g 24-week premature twin B male infant born to a 29-year-old G1P0 (gravida 1, para 0) mother whose pregnancy was complicated by the onset of premature labor. The mother received a dose of betamethasone approximately 6 hours before a vaginal delivery. She also received antibiotics and was given magnesium sulfate. The infant was delivered with minimal respiratory effort and a heart rate of 70 beats/min. Resuscitation included bag-mask ventilation with room air and intubation, with a rapid improvement in heart rate. The infant was admitted to the intensive care unit and was given one dose of a surfactant for respiratory distress syndrome (RDS). The early course was complicated by a pneumothorax as well as a pulmonary hemorrhage, with associated hypoxic respiratory failure and significant metabolic acidosis. A head ultrasound scan showed a grade III intraventricular hemorrhage on the left with dilation of the ventricle and an associated ipsilateral intraparenchymal echodensity involving frontoparietal white matter. In addition, the infant developed a hemodynamically significant patent ductus arteriosus (PDA) that was initially treated with indomethacin. The infant was weaned to continuous positive airway pressure by day of life (DOL) 14, and was briefly reintubated for the surgical ligation of the PDA and on the second occasion for a late-onset sepsis. Other issues included recurrent apnea and bradycardia and frequent unprovoked desaturation episodes. He required supplemental oxygen through the 35th week of postmenstrual age. He required parenteral nutrition for 3 weeks and subsequently received enteral breast milk. Serial head ultrasound scans on DOLs 7, 14, 28, 42, and 56 revealed progressive communicating hydrocephalus involving the lateral third and fourth ventricles that peaked in dilation by DOL 28 and then gradually decreased in size by DOL 56. The parenchymal lesion evolved into a small left porencephalic cyst. The infant underwent a magnetic resonance imaging (MRI) evaluation on DOL 92 that revealed mild ventriculomegaly and the left cystic lesion and some periventricular white matter loss. The infant was discharged on DOL 100. He was seen and evaluated at 18 months. At that time the clinical findings indicated mild right hemiparesis. He recently started walking, was very active, and had minimal speech. Evaluation using the Bayley Scales of Infant and Toddler Development (BSID) found that he had a cognitive score of 75 and a motor score of 82.

Continued

CASE HISTORY—cont'd

> This case illustrates a typical course of an extremely premature infant who is at greatest risk for severe periventricular-intraventricular hemorrhage (PV-IVH) even when managed in the current era of neonatology. Although the overall incidence of PV-IVH in the premature infant has decreased, hemorrhage remains an important problem in the extremely low-birth-weight infant (ELBW, birth weight <1000 g), particularly in cases of rapid delivery when the potential for full dosing of glucocorticoids around the time of delivery is not possible.[1,2] This chapter focuses on a brief review of the pathogenesis of PV-IVH as well as white matter injury. Various approaches or strategies for the prevention, diagnosis, and treatment as well as outcomes are discussed, with gaps in knowledge highlighted.

Periventricular-Intraventricular Hemorrhage

Background

The overall occurrence of PV-IVH has declined with time, although severe intraventricular hemorrhage remains a significant clinical problem in the ELBW population.[3,4] For those born at or before 28 weeks' gestation, 15% still have the most severe forms of hemorrhage, occurring in 37% of those born at 23 weeks and 24% in infants born at 24 weeks.[4] This observation is highly relevant because survival of the infants born at the limits of viability continues to increase, and long-term neurocognitive deficits are more likely with severe hemorrhage.[5,6] However, evidence also points to neurodevelopmental deficits even with lesser grades of hemorrhage and even when the cranial sonogram is interpreted as being normal (see later discussion).[6–9] These observations are important because they point to the limitations of cranial sonography in identifying more subtle injury to the cortex, deep gray matter, or cerebellum. These are more readily identified by MRI studies performed closer to term.[10,11]

Neuropathology: Relevance to Clinical Findings

The primary lesion in PV-IVH is bleeding from small vessels in the subependymal germinal matrix (GM), a transitional gelatinous region that provides limited support for the luxurious but very immature capillary bed that courses through it.[12] With maturation, this matrix region becomes less prominent and is essentially absent by term gestation. The hemorrhage, when it evolves, may be confined to the GM region (grade I IVH), or it may extend and rupture into the adjacent ventricular system (grade II or III IVH, depending on the extent of hemorrhage), or extend into the white matter (termed a grade IV or intraparenchymal echogenicity [IPE]) (Fig. 2.1A).[1,13,14] IPE, which is invariably unilateral, represents an area of hemorrhagic necrosis of varying size within periventricular white matter, dorsal and lateral to the external angle of the lateral ventricle (Fig. 2.1B).[1,15,16]

Pathogenesis

The genesis of bleeding from capillaries within the GM is complex and includes a combination of intravascular, vascular, and extravascular influences. Intravascular factors, especially those that involve perturbations in cerebral blood flow (CBF), have a critical role in capillary rupture and hemorrhage. Thus it has been shown, through the use of different methods to assess CBF, including Doppler ultrasonography, near-infrared spectroscopy, and xenon-enhanced computed tomography (CT), that the cerebral circulation of the sick infant is pressure passive—that is, CBF varies directly with changes in systemic blood pressure.[17–20] This state would be expected to increase the vulnerability of the GM capillaries to periods of both hypotension and hypertension, and this is supported in experimental studies and clinical observations. In a beagle puppy model, GM hemorrhage can be produced by systemic hypertension with or without prior hypotension.[21,22] In addition, clinical temporal associations have been demonstrated between fluctuations in systemic blood pressure and

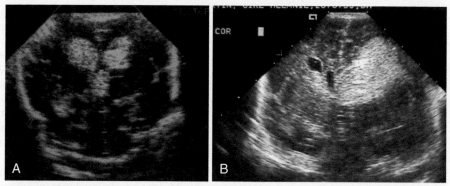

Fig. 2.1 Coronal ultrasound scans. A, Note a bilateral germinal matrix and intraventricular hemorrhage (grade III). B, Note the large left-sided germinal matrix and intraventricular hemorrhage. There is a large ipsilateral intraparenchymal echodensity involving periventricular white matter.

simultaneous fluctuations in CBF velocity as may occur in the ventilated premature infant with RDS, increases in CBF as may occur with rapid volume expansion or a pneumothorax, and the subsequent development of PV-IVH.[23–26] Conversely, decreases in CBF secondary to systemic hypotension, which may occur in utero or postnatally, may also play a prominent role in the genesis of PV-IVH in certain infants.[27] Hypercarbia produced by potential modulation of autoregulation increases the risk for severe IVH.[28,29] A presumed mechanism in this context is that of rupture upon reperfusion.[2,18] Finally, elevations in venous pressure may be an important additional intravascular mechanism of hemorrhage and may reflect the peculiarity of the anatomy of the venous drainage of GM and the white matter.[1] Thus at the level of the head of the caudate nucleus and the foramen of Monro, the terminal, choroidal, and thalamostriate veins course anteriorly to a point of confluence to form the internal cerebral vein. The blood flow then makes a U-turn at the usual site of hemorrhage, raising the possibility that an elevation in venous pressure increases the potential for venous distention with obstruction of the terminal and medullary veins and hemorrhagic infarction. Indeed, simultaneous increases in venous pressure have been observed in infants who exhibit variability in arterial blood pressure, such as when it occurs with RDS and associated complications, such as pneumothorax and pulmonary interstitial emphysema, or with mechanical or high-frequency ventilation.[30] To summarize, it is likely that both arterial and venous perturbations contribute to the genesis of IVH. Later evidence suggests that these intravascular responses may be modulated by inflammation or the administration of medications to the mother, such as glucocorticoids (see later discussion).[31–33] In one series, infants with fetal inflammation had a significantly higher incidence of severe IVH than infants with no fetal inflammation (49% vs. 17%) ($P = .04$). Infants with fetal inflammation had a significantly higher heart rate ($P = .005$), catecholamine index ($P = .02$), and volume load ($P = .02$) in the first 24 hours of life.[34]

In addition to the intravascular factors, vascular and extravascular influences—the poorly supported blood vessels, excessive fibrinolytic activity noted within the matrix region, and a prominent postnatal decrease in extravascular tissue pressure—may all contribute to hemorrhage.[1,35,36]

Periventricular White Matter Injury Associated With IVH

The pathogenesis of white matter injury associated with hemorrhage remains unclear but appears to be closely linked to the adjacent bleed. Two potential pathways have been proposed to explain this intricate relationship. The first suggests a direct relationship to the PV-IVH, on the basis of several clinical observations, as follows: (1) the white matter lesion is always noted concurrent with or following a large

GM and/or IVH and is rarely if ever observed before the hemorrhage; and (2) the white matter injury is always observed ipsilateral to the side of the larger hemorrhage when there is bilateral involvement of the ventricular system.[1,2,16] This consistent relationship between the GM and the white matter injury may in part be explained by the venous drainage of the deep white matter (see earlier discussion). A second explanation is a de novo evolution of white matter injury. Thus it is proposed that the PV-IVH and the white matter injury occur concurrently. Because both the GM and the periventricular white matter are border-zone regions, the risk for ischemic injury is increased during periods of systemic hypotension, particularly in the presence of a pressure-passive cerebral circulation.[1,2,18] Hemorrhage in these regions may then occur as a secondary phenomenon, or reperfusion injury. In support of this theory is the fairly consistent observation of the simultaneous detection of PV-IVH and white matter injury on cranial ultrasonography. Moreover, elevated hypoxanthine and uric acid levels (as markers of reperfusion injury) have been observed on the first postnatal day in infants in whom white matter injury subsequently developed.[37,38]

Identification of the mechanisms contributing to periventricular white matter injury is crucial to prevention of this lesion. If the white matter injury is directly related to PV-IVH, then prevention of the latter should reduce the occurrence of the white matter injury. However, if the PV-IVH and the white matter injury occur simultaneously as a result of a primary ischemic event with the hemorrhage occurring as a secondary phenomenon, then prevention of the secondary hemorrhage may not affect the primary ischemic lesion. Indeed, the two follow-up studies on indomethacin treatment to prevent IVH in the neonatal period are supportive of this latter concern. Thus, although the incidence of severe IVH was reduced in infants treated with indomethacin in both studies, neurodevelopmental outcomes at 18-month follow-up, including cerebral palsy, were comparable in the indomethacin-treated group controls.[39,40]

Clinical Features

In most cases (up to 70% of less severe IVH cases), the diagnosis is made with a screening sonogram. In the earlier descriptions of PV-IVH, the majority of cases, about 90%, evolved within the first 72 hours of postnatal life.[41] However, the time to initial diagnosis of hemorrhage has shifted to a later onset in recent years.[13] Thus for neonates weighing less than 1000 g, the IVH diagnosis is made early, within the first 24 hours in approximately 80% of infants. However, some cases are now noted after the 10th postnatal day. This changing pattern may reflect the complexity of disease in the tiniest infants and the extent of supportive medical care, especially the prolonged use of high-frequency ventilation. Infants with the more severe IVH frequently exhibit clinical signs such as a bulging fontanel, seizures, a drop in hematocrit, hyperglycemia, metabolic acidosis, and pulmonary hemorrhage.[2]

Complications

The two most significant complications of IVH are extension into adjacent white matter (see earlier discussion) and the development of posthemorrhagic hydrocephalus.

Prevention

Perinatal Strategies

Antenatal Steroids

Various perinatal and postnatal strategies have been investigated for the prevention of PV-IVH. The antenatal administration of glucocorticoids to augment pulmonary maturation has had the positive, unanticipated benefit of a significant reduction in the incidence of IVH and severe IVH.[32,42–47] A systematic review of 26 trials showed antenatal corticosteroid therapy to be associated with a reduction in the occurrence of PV-IVH (relative risk [RR] 0.54, 95% confidence interval [CI] 0.43–0.69; 13 studies, 2872 infants), and severe hemorrhage (RR 0.28, 95% CI 0.16–0.5; 5 studies, 572 infants).[32] The mechanisms whereby glucocorticoids reduce severe IVH remain unclear but may relate to less severe RDS, possibly minimizing fluctuation in cerebral blood flow and accelerated stabilization of the germinal matrix vasculature by modulating vascular growth factors.[25,36,48–50] Serial courses of antenatal corticosteroids are not recommended; a single rescue course is to be considered if preterm birth does not occur within a week to further decrease the risk of RDS but has no further impact on the rate of IVH or severe IVH.[51] There are concerns that multiple courses of antenatal corticosteroids may have adverse effects on the developing brain. Thus infants who were exposed to multiple courses (median of 4) of antenatal steroids had a higher incidence of cerebral palsy than a placebo group, although the difference was not statistically significant (6/206 vs. 1/195; $P = .12$).[52]

Pregnancy-Induced Hypertension

One maternal medical condition associated with a lower incidence of IVH is pregnancy-induced hypertension (PIH). In one report a lower incidence of severe PV-IVH was found in infants born to mothers with PIH (8.2%) than to those without PIH (14%), with an odds ratio (OR) estimate of 0.43 (95% CI 0.30–0.61),[53] a finding consistent with other reports.[54–57] The mechanisms through which the risk of IVH may be reduced by the presence of PIH remain unclear, but accelerated brain maturation in such infants is possible.[58,59]

Magnesium Sulfate

The use of magnesium sulfate in these women was initially suggested to be contributory to the reduction in IVH,[55,60] but subsequent studies have shown that it is not.[61–63] Tocolytic agents, in general, including magnesium sulfate, are associated with an increased risk for IVH.[64–66] However, a large prospective, randomized controlled trial of magnesium sulfate administered to mothers at 24 to 31 weeks' gestation demonstrated a reduced rate of cerebral palsy among infant survivors.[67] Subsequent randomized controlled trials showed similar neuroprotection. Thus a meta-analysis of antenatal magnesium sulfate therapy given to women at risk for preterm birth concluded that it substantially reduced the risk of cerebral palsy in the child (RR 0.68; 95% CI 0.54–0.87; in 5 trials involving 6145 infants).[68] The number of women needed to be treated to benefit one infant by avoiding cerebral palsy is 63 (95% CI 43–155).[69] The American Congress of Obstetricians and Gynecologists (ACOG) recommends intrapartum magnesium for women at less than 32 weeks' gestation who are at risk for delivery within 7 days.[70]

Route of Delivery

There are conflicting data regarding the route of delivery and subsequent IVH.[55,71–73] Interpretation of the data is difficult because most studies are retrospective, but this does not exclude the possibility that under certain circumstances, intrapartum events may contribute to the pathogenesis of severe IVH. Some studies show a higher risk for IVH with increasing duration of the active phase of labor, and a lower risk in infants delivered via cesarean section before active phase of labor.[55,71] Many of these studies were analyzed before the more frequent use of antenatal glucocorticoids.[74] In a study in infants born at less than 750 g whose mothers were given steroids, vaginal delivery was a predictor for severe IVH.[75] By contrast, in a retrospective cohort study of ELBW infants, the influence of labor on those born by cesarean delivery was examined and this analysis revealed that labor does not appear to play a significant role in the genesis of IVH.[76] Similarly, in a later retrospective analysis, severe IVH was not influenced by mode of delivery in vertex-presenting, singleton, very LBW infants after data were controlled for gestational age.[77] Any analysis that evaluates the impact of labor or route of delivery must account for an important role of placental inflammation, in particular fetal vasculitis, in the genesis of IVH, a role that may supersede the influence of the route of delivery. Thus in one study, although vaginal delivery was associated with an increased risk of IVH by univariate analysis, the risks attributable to vaginal delivery were no longer increased when adjustments were made in multivariate analysis for fetal vasculitis and other potential confounding factors.[78]

2

Delayed Cord Clamping

Several randomized controlled trials have shown improved neonatal outcomes, including a decreased rate of IVH, with delayed cord clamping.[79,80] A meta-analysis showed a reduction of all grades of IVH by ultrasound (RR 0.59, CI 0.41–0.85 in 10 trials involving 539 infants).[81] Other benefits seen include increases in the neonatal hematocrit, the need for fewer blood transfusions, and a lower risk for necrotizing enterocolitis.[81] One study in preterm infants born before 32 weeks showed that delayed cord clamping was protective against low motor scores at 18 to 22 months corrected age.[82] ACOG and the American Academy of Pediatrics (AAP) recommend a delay in cord clamping for vigorous preterm infants for at least 30 to 60 seconds.[83] Proposed mechanisms for the benefits associated with delayed cord clamping include an improved cardiovascular transition.[84,85] The optimal timing for infants requiring resuscitation is not yet clear, and further studies are currently under investigation to answer gaps in knowledge with this practice.

Postnatal Strategies

Any approach to intervention should at the least consider the following: (1) the target population should be those infants in whom severe IVH is most likely to develop—that is, with birth weights less than 1000 g[3]; and (2) the condition of the infant at delivery, which appears to be an important mediator of subsequent IVH (Box 2.1). The latter appears to be strongly influenced in part by perinatal events and, in particular, the administration of antenatal glucocorticoids[32] or the presence of fetal vasculitis.[78]

Postnatal Factors Associated With an Increased Risk

Postnatal factors associated with a higher risk for IVH include decreasing gestational age, lower birth weight (<1000 g), male sex, intubation, and RDS (see Box 2.1).[1,86,87] In contrast, the risk for severe IVH in the nonintubated infant is low(<10%).[88] For infants with RDS, the risk for IVH is even greater with associated perturbations in arterial and venous pressures as well as with hypercarbia.[23,24,28,29,89] These vascular perturbations are in part related to the infant's breathing patterns, which are usually out of synchrony with the ventilator breath.[90] The perturbations can be minimized with careful ventilator management, including the use of synchronized mechanical ventilation, assist/control ventilation, sedation, or, in more difficult cases, paralysis.[1,91] Interestingly enough, although surfactant administration improved respiratory

---

Box 2.1   FACTORS ASSOCIATED WITH RISK FOR THE DEVELOPMENT OF SEVERE INTRAVENTRICULAR HEMORRHAGE

High Risk
Minimal intrapartum care
No glucocorticoid exposure
Chorioamnionitis/funisitis
Fetal distress
Lower gestational age
Lower birth weight
Respiratory distress syndrome
Respiratory morbidity (i.e., pneumothorax)
Fluctuations or rapid elevations in systemic blood pressure and/or cerebral blood flow
Hypotension
Sudden and repeated increases in venous pressure

Lower Risk
Antenatal glucocorticoids (short course)
Medical condition (e.g., pregnancy-induced hypertension)
Intrauterine growth restriction
Higher gestational age
Higher birth weight
Postnatal medications (e.g., indomethacin)

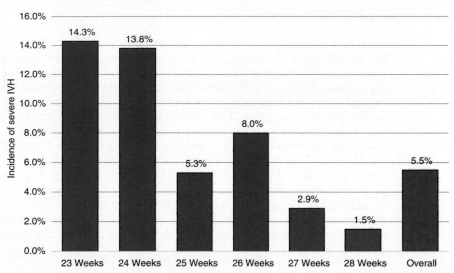

Fig. 2.2 Incidence of severe intraventricular hemorrhage (IVH) for infants of gestational age 23 5/7 through 28 6/7 weeks for the period of 2010 through 2015 at the Weill Cornell Neonatal Intensive Care Unit. Notably, indomethacin was introduced in 2011, administered to infants not exposed to antenatal glucocorticosteroids. *VLBW*, Very low birth weight.

ventilation, the improvement was not accompanied by a significant reduction in the incidence of IVH.[92]

Postnatal Administration of Medications to Reduce Severe IVH

Medications administered postnatally to reduce or prevent IVH have included phenobarbital,[93–95] vitamin E,[96] ethamsylate,[97] and indomethacin.[40,98–100] Although there was initial enthusiasm for the use of each of these medications in the prevention of IVH, the effect has not been borne out over time. In one noteworthy study, infants who received phenobarbital exhibited a higher incidence of severe IVH than controls.[95]

Indomethacin. Currently, the early postnatal administration of indomethacin is believed to be of benefit in the prevention of severe hemorrhage.[40,99] Two studies demonstrated a significant reduction in the incidence of severe IVH in infants who received indomethacin in comparison with control infants. However, at long-term follow-up, the incidence of cerebral palsy was comparable in the two groups.[40,99] This observation, coupled with the known reduction in CBF that accompanies indomethacin administration, warrants cautious use of this agent.[100,101] We administer indomethacin to those infants at greatest risk, such as those delivered precipitously without the benefit of antenatal steroids. Using this approach the overall incidence of severe IVH for infants between 23 5/7 weeks and 28 6/7 weeks was 5.5% for the years 2010–2015. (Fig. 2.2).

White Matter Injury in the Absence of Hemorrhage

CASE HISTORY

BS was a 28-week appropriate for gestational age (AGA) female infant born to a 42-year-old primigravida whose pregnancy was complicated by cervical shortening with funneling. The mother was started on bed rest, given a course of betamethasone, treated with antibiotics, and received magnesium sulfate. However, after 3 days fetal distress was noted and the infant was delivered vaginally. Delivery room resuscitation included brief bag-mask ventilation, and continuous positive airway pressure (CPAP) was started and the

Continued

CASE HISTORY—cont'd

infant was assigned to the neonatal intensive care unit. The Apgar scores were 6 (1 minute) and 8 (5 minutes). The infant was rapidly weaned to room air while receiving CPAP. She was treated with antibiotics for 7 days, in part because of the perinatal history as well as abnormal blood count indices (initial immature-to-total neutrophil ratio 0.39, which normalized within 24 hours). The culture results remained negative. The clinical course was characterized by recurrent apnea and bradycardia, for which caffeine was administered. A cranial sonogram performed on DOL 5 revealed increased bilateral periventricular echodensities (Fig. 2.3A). Sonograms performed on DOL 28 showed the evolution of bilateral diffuse cystic encephalomalacia (see Fig. 2.3B). An MRI performed at 36 weeks postmenstrual age revealed extensive cystic periventricular leukomalacia (PVL) with mild diffuse parenchymal volume loss and diffuse thinning of the corpus callosum (see Fig. 2.3C). Placental pathology demonstrated an immature placenta with evidence of acute chorioamnionitis and funisitis.

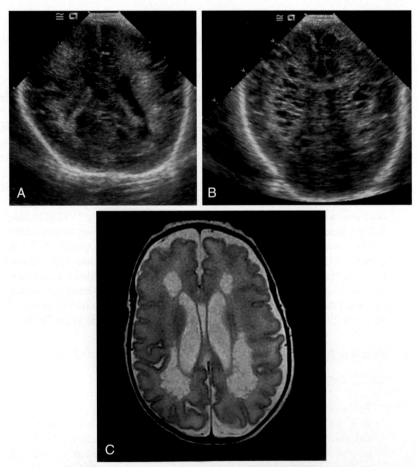

Fig. 2.3   A, Coronal ultrasound scan from an infant in the first week showing increased periventricular echogenicity. B, Coronal scan from the same infant at 4 weeks showing bilateral cystic formation in the areas of prior hyperechogenicity. C, Magnetic resonance image (axial view) before discharge showing T2-hyperintense periventricular signal abnormality bilaterally that is consistent with cystic periventricular leukomalacia.

This case illustrates the more typical ultrasonographic expression of white matter injury in the premature infant, characterized by hyperechogenicity, followed by the evolution of cystic changes in the absence of overt postnatal provocative clinical factors.[1,13,102,103] Although cysts usually became apparent within the first 2 to 3 weeks of life, data have now shown the evolution of cysts beyond the first month in an increasing numbers of cases.[13,104] Moreover, progressive dilation of the lateral ventricles, which in some cases is consistent with diffuse white matter injury, is also becoming more common.[105–107] However, MRI indicates that white matter injury is more prevalent than is apparent from cranial ultrasonography.[11,108]

Periventricular Leukomalacia

Periventricular leukomalacia refers to injury to the cerebral white matter and has long been regarded as the characteristic brain lesion of the premature infant.[1] PVL is characterized by a focal component of necrosis with loss of cellular elements and a diffuse component with astrogliosis, microglial gliosis, and maturational injury to the premyelinating oligodendrocytes.[102,109–112] The focal necrosis can be macroscopic in size and evolve over weeks into cystic lesions readily seen on serial ultrasounds, referred to as "cystic PVL" (see Fig. 2.2). The incidence of this pathology has declined over time, occurring in fewer than 5% of very low-birth-weight (VLBW) preterm infants. Focal necrosis can also be microscopic, and this type occurs more commonly and evolves into glial scars that are less readily seen on neuroimaging, referred to as "noncystic PVL." White matter injury may also occur beyond the focal necrosis and occurs as diffuse white matter injury. This is now the most frequent form of white matter injury in preterm infants. From the early necrotic lesions, there is a widespread initial degeneration of premyelinating oligodendrocytes, followed by a compensatory increase in dysmature oligodendroglial progenitors that are not able to fully differentiate into mature myelin-producing cells. This results in poorly myelinated axons with ventriculomegaly. This diffuse component is less well characterized on imaging, even on MRI, but does include diffuse signal abnormalities and disturbances in diffusion imaging of the white matter.[109,113,114]

Pathogenesis

Experimental and clinical observations suggest a complex interaction of vascular factors, inflammation, and the intrinsic vulnerability of the differentiating oligodendrocyte that leads to white matter injury in the preterm infant.[112,113,115,116]

Vascular Factors

Several features peculiar to the premature infant are important in the vascular mechanism of PVL. The first relates to the vascular development and supply. Specifically, the penetrating branches of the anterior, middle, and posterior cerebral arteries end in border zones, which are most vulnerable to decreases in CBF. It is within these border zones that the focal necrosis of PVL typically occurs.[116,117] Furthermore, the penetrating cerebral vessels, which include long branches that terminate in the deep periventricular white matter and short branches that terminate in the subcortical white matter, vary as a function of gestational age.[118] Thus early on, at approximately 24 to 30 weeks' gestation, the long penetrators have few side branches and limited intraparenchymal anastomosis with the short branches, resulting in border zones in white matter beyond the periventricular region. This feature may account for the more diffuse lesion noted in the smaller premature infant.[103] From 32 weeks on, there is a marked increase in vascular supply as a result of increase in vessel length and anastomoses. It is this vascular maturation that likely accounts for the uncommon presentation of this lesion in the larger infant. A second feature relates to the limited vasodilatory response of the blood vessels supplying the white matter to increases in the arterial partial pressure of carbon dioxide ($Paco_2$) in comparison with the vasodilatory responses of the blood vessels supplying other regions of brain, such as the medulla and gray matter,[119] as well as a persistent decrease in CBF to white matter during the phase of reperfusion following ischemia, despite recovery in all other brain areas.[120] Finally, impairment of CBF autoregulation, as may occur in the sick premature infant, increases the risk for ischemia to the border-zone regions of white matter during episodes of systemic hypotension.[18,111,121] Clinically, loss of CBF autoregulation and/or decreases in CBF may occur in the sick infant secondary to events such as hypotension, acidosis, septic shock, hypocarbia, PDA, recurrent apnea, and bradycardia, and may in part explain the association of such events with PVL.[122–130]

Intrinsic Vulnerability of the Differentiating Oligodendrocyte

It has been established that the premyelinating oligodendrocyte (pre-OL) is most vulnerable to injury secondary to release of numerous factors, including free radicals, excitotoxins, and cytokines. These cells undergo cell death via apoptosis,[131] as seen in newborn animal models subjected to hypoxia-ischemia and/or infection demonstrating apoptotic cell death in immature cerebral white matter.[132,133] After the initial depletion of these pre-OLs, early oligodendrocyte progenitors that are more resistant to the initial ischemic/inflammatory insult proliferate robustly in the setting of pre-OL depletion.[134] However, this new population of pre-OLs displays maturational arrest and the pre-OLs fail to develop into mature myelin-producing oligodendrocytes, leading to failed myelination of intact axons.[135–137] In a neuropathologic study, apoptosis of pre-OLs was observed significantly more often in infants dying of white matter injury than in infants without white matter injury.[138] In the diffuse white matter lesions, neuropathology has also shown a marked prominence of activated microglia and reactive astrocytosis, as identified by immunocytochemical markers for oxidative and nitrative attacks.[139] The presence of the activated microglia raises the possibility of a key role for these cells in the causation of the diffuse injury to the premyelinating oligodendrocyte (see later discussion).[109]

Free Radical Injury

The prominence of activated microglia in the diffuse component of PVL suggests that these cells may be involved in the generation of reactive oxygen species (ROS) and reactive nitrogen species (RNS) found in the human lesion.[139] Microglia have been shown to be activated by ischemia and inflammation and remain activated for weeks following the insult. Activation of microglia releases ROS and RNS, which then cause pre-OL cell death. Experimental studies have demonstrated vulnerability of the pre-OL to injury by free radicals.[109,140,141] This maturation-dependent vulnerability to injury by ROS and RNS appears to be related to deficient antioxidant defenses and acquisition of iron during development, which may result in hydroxyl radical formation. The role of free radical–induced damage in triggering the death of the early differentiating oligodendrocyte is supported by the cryoprotection provided by the Fenton reaction.[142,143] Human studies have shown a delay in the development of free radical scavengers, such as superoxide dismutase, desferrioxamine, and vitamin E, leaving tissues without the requisite antioxidant enzyme cascade following preterm birth to an oxygen-rich postnatal environment.[143] Neonatal rat models studied on postnatal day 3 (P3) and P6 showed bilateral reduction in myelin basic protein expression with 24 hours of exposure to 80% oxygen, an effect not noted when they were studied on P10. Hyperoxia caused oxidative stress and triggered maturation-dependent apoptosis in pre-OLs, which involved the generation of ROS and caspase activation, and led to white matter injury in the neonatal rat brain.[144] This effect could be blocked by estradiol, which produced significant dose-dependent protection by preventing hyperoxia-induced proapoptotic Fas upregulation and caspase-3 activation.[145]

Excitotoxic Injury (Glutamate)

Glutamate can lead to the death of oligodendroglial precursors via both receptor and nonreceptor-mediated mechanisms. The nonreceptor mechanism involves intracellular entry of glutamate in exchange for cystine via activation of a glutamine-cystine exchange transporter, resulting in a decrease in intracellular cystine and thereby glutathione synthesis.[109,140] The result is glutathione depletion and free radical–mediated cell death. The receptor-mediated injury appears to be mediated via activation of 2-amino-3-[5-methyl-3-oxo-1,2-oxazol-4-yl]propanoic acid (AMPA)/kainate–type glutamate receptors. Experimental data suggest that this form of cell death occurs only in developing and not mature oligodendroglia, related to upregulation of this receptor in oligodendrocyte precursors.[146] It has also been shown, in an immature animal model of diffuse white matter injury, that non–N-methyl-D-aspartate (NMDA) receptors are present on pre-OLs that cause free radical–mediated death of these cells when activated in vitro, and that in vivo cause death of pre-OLs when activated by hypoxia-ischemia.[147] The relevance of this mechanism to hypoxia-ischemia–induced white matter injury has been demonstrated in an immature rat model, in which such injury is prevented by the systemic administration of the non-NMDA receptor antagonist 6-nitro-7-sulfamoylbenzo[f]quinoxaline-2,3-dione (NBQX) following termination of the insult.[148] NMDA receptors have also been found in the processes of oligodendrocytes across its developmental lineage. Ischemia resulting in excess glutamate may result in loss of oligodendrocyte processes.[149]

Cytokines

Cytokines released by activated microglia also participate in an important mechanism for pre-OL cell death. The paradigm of ischemia-reperfusion accompanied by a rapid activation of microglia, secretion of cytokines, and migration of inflammatory cells has been well established in animal models.[150] Within the central nervous system, microglia release tumor necrosis factor α (TNF-α), interleukin-1 (IL-1), and IL-6. Cell culture studies suggest that TNF-α is toxic to oligodendroglia.[151] Interferon-γ is also toxic to oligodendroglia, an effect potentiated by TNF-α.[152] However, numerous additional cytokines, microglia, or white blood cells may be involved in this process.[153] Indeed, in one study, increased levels of circulating proinflammatory cytokines during the first 72 hours of life were associated with arterial hypotension and with the development of brain damage as detected by ultrasonography.[154] Increases in IL-6, IL-8, and IL-10 were associated with arterial hypotension, and increases in IL-6 and IL-8 with severe IVH. Prolonged rupture of membranes was associated with increased postnatal levels of interferon-γ, which in turn were associated with white matter injury.[154] The potential deleterious effects of cytokines may be mediated via other mechanisms, including increased permeability of the blood-brain barrier,[155] vascular endothelial damage,[156] and decreased CBF to white matter after endotoxin exposure.[157]

Maternal Fetal Infection and/or Inflammation and White Matter Injury

Both experimental and clinical evidence demonstrate an association between maternal infection/inflammation of the chorion and amnion with or without fetal vascular involvement (i.e., funisitis) and white matter injury. Thus intraperitoneal injection of lipopolysaccharides into kittens and exposing pregnant rabbits to intrauterine infection induce white matter injury similar to that observed in humans.[133,158] Several clinical studies have demonstrated an association between chorioamnionitis and PVL.[127,159] As in IVH, this association appears to be accentuated in the presence of funisitis.[160] The link between chorioamnionitis may be mediated via cytokines. High levels of cytokines (IL-6 and IL-1β) have been found in the amniotic fluid,[161–163] of IL-6 in cord blood,[164] and of IL-1, IL-6, and interferon in neonatal blood of preterm infants in whom PVL or cerebral palsy develops.[154,165–167] Microglial expression of TNF-α and IL-6 immunoreactivity is found twice as commonly in the white matter of infants with PVL as in infants without injury to the region.[168,169]

In contrast to these potential deleterious effects, focal cerebral ischemia was found to be exacerbated in a mouse model of hypoxia-ischemia lacking TNF-α.[170] Injury-induced microglial activation was suppressed in the TNF-α knockout mice. These latter observations point to the complex interrelationships between cytokines and white matter injury.

Clinical Factors Associated With PVL

Perinatal events associated with postnatal cystic PVL and/or progressive white matter injury include a history of chorioamnionitis (see earlier discussion), prolonged rupture of membranes, peripartum hemorrhage, severe fetal acidemia, hypovolemia, sepsis, hypocarbia, hemodynamically significant PDA, postnatal infection/sepsis, and recurrent apnea and bradycardia.[122–130,159,171] A common feature of many of these conditions is a reduction in systemic blood pressure. Indeed, in one study, chorioamnionitis was associated with increased IL-6 and IL-1β concentrations in cord blood, elevated newborn heart rate, and decreased mean and diastolic blood pressures, and the cord blood IL-6 concentration correlated inversely with newborn systolic, mean, and diastolic blood pressures.[31] By contrast, in a study of 14 infants in whom PVL developed, only 4 (30%) had overt evidence of postnatal systemic hypotension, and asphyxia was an uncommon finding.[127] Other studies have also been unable to demonstrate a consistent association between hypotension and PVL.[172–174]

Prevention

From the preceding discussion, it is likely that prevention of PVL will be difficult. First, it is relatively uncommon; second, as noted previously, the pathogenesis of PVL is complex (Fig. 2.4); and third, the presentation is often subtle and detected only with neuroimaging. Although there is evidence pointing to an association between perinatal infection (chorioamnionitis) and PVL,[1,20,159] the precise mechanisms linking the two remain unclear; the positive predictive value of a history of chorioamnionitis and subsequent PVL is low, approximating 10%, and many cases of infection are asymptomatic with the diagnosis established only on histologic examination of the placenta.[3,78]

More specific potential strategies are as follows: (1) the appropriate treatment of infants with low blood pressure for a given gestational age with volume replacement therapy or inotropic support as clinically indicated, and (2) the careful ventilatory management of infants with respiratory distress so as to avoid hypocarbia. However, it is important to note that the mechanisms of white matter injury with hypocarbia also remain unclear. Thus ventilation-induced hypocarbia is often associated with higher mean airway pressures. Elevations in mean airway pressure are associated with impairment of venous return, a fall in cardiac output, as well as increases in sagittal sinus pressure.[30,175] The impairment of venous return, coupled with a

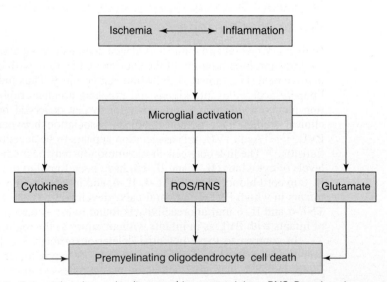

Fig. 2.4 Potential pathways leading to white matter injury. *RNS,* Reactive nitrogen species; *ROS,* reactive oxygen species.

concomitant decrease in CBF, as may occur with hypocarbia, would be expected to reduce cerebral perfusion pressure, including flow to white matter. The use of antioxidant therapy to counter free radical injury demonstrated in experimental models is another therapeutic possibility. However, antioxidant therapy has not been uniformly successful in the treatment of other neonatal conditions presumed to be related in part to free radical injury.[176]

Erythropoietin had previously been shown to be a promising candidate for neuroprotection in neonatal brain injury animal models. The mechanisms of neuroprotection have been suggested to be decreased apoptosis, inflammation, excitotoxicity, and glutamate toxicity on neurons and oligodendrocytes.[177] Erythropoietin also is known to stimulate neurogenesis, angiogenesis, and migration of regenerating neurons. Recent randomized controlled trials in very preterm infants have shown mixed outcomes of prophylactic early high-dose recombinant human erythropoietin. The Swiss EPO Neuroprotection Trial showed significantly reduced white and gray matter injury in a subset of infants with MRI, but the trial showed no improvement in neurodevelopmental outcomes at 2 years, including the primary outcome of the BSID Mental Developmental Index (MDI), and secondary motor, hearing, or visual outcomes.[178] Meanwhile, the Chinese EPO Neuroprotection trial show improved rates of moderate-severe neurologic disability (BSID-II MDI <70, cerebral palsy, deafness, or blindness) at 18 months corrected age.[179] The study in China continued treatment with EPO every 48 hours for 2 weeks, whereas the Swiss EPO Neuroprotection Trial completed 36 to 42 hours after birth. Additional investigations are ongoing in preterm infants.[180]

Outcome

Intraventricular Hemorrhage

The infant with severe IVH is at highest risk for adverse neurodevelopmental outcome (both motor and cognitive). This risk is related in part to the extent of the white matter involvement noted on cranial ultrasonography. Thus with a large IPE (>1 cm in diameter; see Fig. 2.1B) the outcome is invariably poor, with major motor and cognitive defects consistently noted at follow-up.[1,16,181] With smaller lesions (<1 cm in diameter), the outcome is less precise and a small percentage of patients (approximately 20%) may even have a normal outcome.[16]

However, as noted previously, the issue is much more complicated, and even infants with lesser grades of hemorrhage or with no hemorrhage seen on ultrasound are at risk for motor and cognitive deficits. One study showed that in those preterm infants with normal cranial sonogram findings, major neurologic disability was noted in 5% to 10% of infants, and a BSID MDI less than 70 was found in 25% of cases.[7] In another study of infants with lesser grades of hemorrhage (grades 1 and 2 IVH), major neurologic disabilities were noted in 13%, and MDI less than 70 was seen in 45% of cases.[8] Moreover, the comparable neurodevelopmental outcomes for infants with and without IVH in the indomethacin study clearly indicate that the genesis of brain injury in the sick premature infant is much more complex than can be deduced from the neonatal neurologic ultrasonographic appearance.

White Matter Injury

Although the ultrasonographic diagnosis of cystic PVL affects only a small fraction of VLBW infants (<5%), MRI performed at term shows that diffuse injury to white matter is much more common. This finding poses a significant burden in that the majority of affected infants have major long-term neurodevelopmental problems.[11,127,182–184] The most commonly described long-term motor sequela of PVL is spastic diplegia.[1] Later reports, however, describe a more severe deficit with involvement of all four extremities as well as visual and cognitive deficits.[185–189] This more severe outcome is consistent with the diffuse white matter injury noted on neuropathology in preterm infants who die with PVL as well as on MRI.[104,183] More severe white matter injury qualitatively or quantitatively measured by MRI predicts poor motor outcomes.[184–190] The genesis of the cognitive deficits in infants with PVL may be related to the associated developmental disturbances to cortical organization as a result of injury to subplate neurons or late migrating astrocytes.[1,109,191] Gray matter volumes are reduced in infants with substantial diffuse white matter injury identified on term-equivalent MRI in VLBW infants.[192] The latter findings may explain the substantial cognitive deficits noted at follow-up.[184]

Gaps in Knowledge

1. The mechanisms contributing to the motor deficits in up to 10% to 15% of infants and to the cognitive deficits in up to one-third of infants with normal sonogram findings and/or lower grades of IVH remain unclear but critical to delineate. Also, although prophylactic administration of indomethacin has been shown to result in a reduction in incidence of severe hemorrhage, it remains unclear why the incidence of cerebral palsy at 18 months in treated infants was comparable to that observed in control infants.[40] Furthermore, incidences of moderate to severe cognitive deficits were comparable in the two groups and were substantially higher than incidences of motor deficits.

2. Other than motor or cognitive disabilities, preterm survivors also have significant risks for language, behavioral, and neurosensory deficits; autism-spectrum disorders; and attention-deficit/hyperactivity disorder that are increasingly being recognized. The neuropathologic correlates are beginning to be identified, including the role of the cerebellar injury. For example, cerebellar hemorrhage may be more common than previously thought, especially as new MRI sequences are being added to routine imaging of preterm infants.[108,193] Severe IVH is much more common in infants without perinatal glucocorticoid exposure, identifying them as a target group for future interventions. Indomethacin remains the best intervention to use in this high-risk target population.

3. Although an association between placental inflammation and white matter injury has been demonstrated, it still remains unclear why the majority of infants born under such circumstances do not demonstrate overt white matter injury.

Conclusions

PV-IVH and adjacent white matter injury remain a significant problem in the premature infant, especially in the extremely preterm population. The potential mechanisms contributing to injury are complex and involve factors related to blood flow and its regulation as well as cellular mediators, including cytokines, free radical formation, and excitotoxic release. Although a reduction in the occurrence of severe IVH can be achieved with indomethacin, the reduction has not translated into long-term neurodevelopmental benefit. This fact reinforces the concept of a more diffuse insidious injury to brain in sick premature infants, a concept reinforced by MRI changes identified at follow-up.

REFERENCES

1. Volpe JJ. *Neurology of the Newborn.* 5th ed. Philadelphia: Saunders/Elsevier; 2008.
2. Shalak L, Perlman JM. Hemorrhagic-ischemic cerebral injury in the preterm infant: current concepts. *Clin Perinatol.* 2002;29(4):745–763.
3. Stoll BJ, Hansen NI, Bell EF, et al. Neonatal outcomes of extremely preterm infants from the NICHD Neonatal Research Network. *Pediatrics.* 2010;126(3):443–456.
4. Stoll BJ, Hansen NI, Bell EF, et al. Trends in care practices, morbidity, and mortality of extremely preterm neonates, 1993–2012. *JAMA.* 2015;314(10):1039–1051.
5. O'Shea TM, Allred EN, Kuban KC, et al. Intraventricular hemorrhage and developmental outcomes at 24 months of age in extremely preterm infants. *J Child Neurol.* 2012;27(1):22–29.
6. Bolisetty S, Dhawan A, Abdel-Latif M, et al. Intraventricular hemorrhage and neurodevelopmental outcomes in extreme preterm infants. *Pediatrics.* January 2014;133(1):55–62.
7. Laptook AR, O'Shea TM, Shankaran S, Bhaskar B. Adverse neurodevelopmental outcomes among extremely low birth weight infants with a normal head ultrasound: prevalence and antecedents. *Pediatrics.* 2005;115(3):673–680.

8. Patra K, Wilson-Costello D, Taylor HG, Mercuri-Minich N, Hack M. Grades I–II intraventricular hemorrhage in extremely low birth weight infants: effects on neurodevelopment. *J Pediatr.* 2006;149(2):169–173.
9. Ann Wy P, Rettiganti M, Li J, et al. Impact of intraventricular hemorrhage on cognitive and behavioral outcomes at 18 years of age in low birth weight preterm infants. *J Perinatol.* 2015;35(7): 511–515.
10. Melbourne L, Chang T, Murnick J, Zaniletti I, Glass P, Massaro AN. Clinical impact of term-equivalent magnetic resonance imaging in extremely low-birth-weight infants at a regional NICU. *J Perinatol.* 2016;36(11):985–989.
11. Inder TE, Anderson NJ, Spencer C, Wells S, Volpe JJ. White matter injury in the premature infant: a comparison between serial cranial sonographic and MR findings at term. *Am J Neuroradiol.* 2003;24(5):805–809.
12. Hambleton G, Wigglesworth JS. Origin of intraventricular haemorrhage in the preterm infant. *Arch Dis Child.* 1976;51(9):651–659.
13. Perlman JM, Rollins N. Surveillance protocol for the detection of intracranial abnormalities in premature neonates. *Arch Pediatr Adolesc Med.* 2000;154(8):822–826.
14. Papile LA, Burstein J, Burstein R, Koffler H. Incidence and evolution of subependymal and intraventricular hemorrhage: a study of infants with birth weights less than 1,500 gm. *J Pediatr.* 1978;92:529–534.
15. Gould SJ, Howard S, Hope PL, Reynolds EO. Periventricular intraparenchymal cerebral haemorrhage in preterm infants: the role of venous infarction. *J Pathol.* 1987;151(3):197–202.
16. Guzzetta F, Shackelford GD, Volpe S, Perlman JM, Volpe JJ. Periventricular intraparenchymal echodensities in the premature newborn: critical determinant of neurologic outcome. *Pediatrics.* 1986;78(6):995–1006.
17. Lou HC, Lassen NA, Friis-Hansen B. Impaired autoregulation of cerebral blood flow in the distressed newborn infant. *J Pediatr.* 1979;94(1):118–121.
18. Pryds O, Greisen G, Lou H, Friis-Hansen B. Heterogeneity of cerebral vasoreactivity in preterm infants supported by mechanical ventilation. *J Pediatr.* 1989;115(4):638–645.
19. Tsuji M, Saul JP, du Plessis A, et al. Cerebral intravascular oxygenation correlates with mean arterial pressure in critically ill premature infants. *Pediatrics.* 2000;106(4):625–632.
20. Soul JS, Hammer PE, Tsuji M, et al. Fluctuating pressure-passivity is common in the cerebral circulation of sick premature infants. *Pediatric Research.* 2007;61(4):467–473.
21. Goddard-Finegold J, Armstrong D, Zeller RS. Intraventricular hemorrhage, following volume expansion after hypovolemic hypotension in the newborn beagle. *J Pediatr.* 1982;100(5):796–799.
22. Ment LR, Stewart WB, Duncan CC, Lambrecht R. Beagle puppy model of intraventricular hemorrhage. *J Neurosurg.* 1982;57(2):219–223.
23. Goldberg RN, Chung D, Goldman SL, Bancalari E. The association of rapid volume expansion and intraventricular hemorrhage in the preterm infant. *J Pediatr.* 1980;96(6):1060–1063.
24. Hill A, Perlman JM, Volpe JJ. Relationship of pneumothorax to occurrence of intraventricular hemorrhage in the premature newborn. *Pediatrics.* 1982;69(2):144–149.
25. Perlman JM, McMenamin JB, Volpe JJ. Fluctuating cerebral blood-flow velocity in respiratory-distress syndrome. Relation to the development of intraventricular hemorrhage. *N Engl J Med.* 1983;309:204–209.
26. Mehrabani D, Gowen CW Jr, Kopelman AE. Association of pneumothorax and hypotension with intraventricular haemorrhage. *Arch Dis Child.* 1991;66(1 Spec No):48–51.
27. Bada HS, Korones SB, Perry EH, et al. Mean arterial blood pressure changes in premature infants and those at risk for intraventricular hemorrhage. *J Pediatr.* 1990;117(4):607–614.
28. Fabres J, Carlo WA, Phillips V, Howard G, Ambalavanan N. Both extremes of arterial carbon dioxide pressure and the magnitude of fluctuations in arterial carbon dioxide pressure are associated with severe intraventricular hemorrhage in preterm infants. *Pediatrics.* 2007;119:299–305.
29. Kaiser JR, Gauss CH, Pont MM, Williams DK. Hypercapnia during the first 3 days of life is associated with severe intraventricular hemorrhage in very low birth weight infants. *J Perinatol.* 2006;26(5):279–285.
30. Perlman JM, Volpe JJ. Are venous circulatory abnormalities important in the pathogenesis of hemorrhagic and/or ischemic cerebral injury? *Pediatrics.* 1987;80(5):705–711.
31. Yanowitz TD, Potter DM, Bowen A, Baker RW, Roberts JM. Variability in cerebral oxygen delivery is reduced in premature neonates exposed to chorioamnionitis. *Pediatric Res.* 2006;59(2):299–304.
32. Roberts D, Dalziel S. Antenatal corticosteroids for accelerating fetal lung maturation for women at risk of preterm birth. *Cochrane Database Syst Rev.* 2006;(3):CD004454.
33. Salhab WA, Wyckoff MH, Laptook AR, Perlman JM. Initial hypoglycemia and neonatal brain injury in term infants with severe fetal acidemia. *Pediatrics.* 2004;114(2):361–366.
34. Furukawa S, Sameshima H, Ikenoue T. Circulatory disturbances during the first postnatal 24 hours in extremely premature infants 25 weeks or less of gestation with histological fetal inflammation. *J Obstet Gynaecol Res.* 2008;34(1):27–33.
35. Takashima S, Tanaka K. Microangiography and fibrinolytic activity in subependymal matrix of the premature brain. *Brain Dev.* 1972;4:222.
36. Georgiadis P, Xu H, Chua C, et al. Characterization of acute brain injuries and neurobehavioral profiles in a rabbit model of germinal matrix hemorrhage. *Stroke.* 2008;39(12):3378–3388.
37. Russell GAB, Jeffers G, Cooke RWI. Plasma hypoxanthine: a marker for hypoxic-ischaemic induced periventricular leucomalacia? *Arch Dis Child.* 1992;67(4 Spec No):388–392.

38. Perlman JM, Risser R. Relationship of uric acid concentrations and severe intraventricular hemorrhage/leukomalacia in the premature infant. *J Pediatr*. 1998;132:436–439.
39. Allan WC, Vohr B, Makuch RW, Katz KH, Ment LR. Antecedents of cerebral palsy in a multicenter trial of indomethacin for intraventricular hemorrhage. *Arch Pediatr Adolesc Med*. 1997;151:580–585.
40. Schmidt B, Davis P, Moddemann D, et al. Long-term effects of indomethacin prophylaxis in extremely-low-birth-weight infants. *N Engl J Med*. 2001;344(26):1966–1972.
41. Perlman JM, Volpe JJ. Intraventricular hemorrhage in extremely small premature infants. *Am J Dis Child*. 1986;140(11):1122–1124.
42. Garite TJ, Rumney PJ, Briggs GG, et al. A randomized, placebo-controlled trial of betamethasone for the prevention of respiratory distress syndrome at 24 to 28 weeks' gestation. *Am J Obstet Gynecol*. 1992;166(2):646–651.
43. Jobe AH, Mitchell BR, Gunkel JH. Beneficial effects of the combined use or prenatal corticosteroids and postnatal surfactant on preterm infants. *Am J Obstet Gynecol*. 1993;168:508–513.
44. Kari MA, Hallman M, Eronen M, et al. Prenatal dexamethasone treatment in conjunction with rescue therapy of human surfactant: a randomized placebo-controlled multicenter study. *Pediatrics*. 1994;93:730–736.
45. Leviton A, Dammann O, Allred EN, et al. Antenatal corticosteroids and cranial ultrasonographic abnormalities. *Am J Obstet Gynecol*. 1999;181:1007–1017.
46. Maher JE, Cliver SP, Goldenberg RL, Davis RO, Copper RL. The effect of corticosteroid therapy in the very premature infant. *Am J Obstet Gynecol*. 1994;170(3):869–873.
47. Wright LL, Horbar JD, Gunkel H, et al. Evidence from multicenter networks on the current use and effectiveness of antenatal corticosteroids in low birth weight infants. *Am J Obstet Gynecol*. 1995;173(1):263–269.
48. Vinukonda G, Dummula K, Malik S, et al. Effect of prenatal glucocorticoids on cerebral vasculature of the developing brain. *Stroke*. August 2010;41(8):1766–1773.
49. Demarini S, Dollberg S, Hoath SB, Ho M, Donovan EF. Effects of antenatal corticosteroids on blood pressure in very low birth weight infants during the first 24 hours of life. *J Perinatol*. 1999;19(6 Pt 1):419–425.
50. Garland JS, Buck R, Leviton A. Effect of maternal glucocorticoid exposure on risk of severe intraventricular hemorrhage in surfactant-treated preterm infants. *J Pediatr*. 1995;126:272–279.
51. Crowther CA, McKinlay CJ, Middleton P, Harding JE. Repeat doses of prenatal corticosteroids for women at risk of preterm birth for improving neonatal health outcomes. *Cochrane Database Syst Rev*. 2015;(7):CD003935.
52. Wapner RJ, Sorokin Y, Mele L, et al. Long-term outcomes after repeat doses of antenatal corticosteroids. *N Engl J Med*. 2007;357(12):1190–1198.
53. Perlman JM, Riser RC, Gee JB. Pregnancy-induced hypertension and reduced intraventricular hemorrhage in preterm infants. *Pediatr Neurol*. 1997;17:29–33.
54. Leviton A, Pagano M, Kuban KC, Krishnamoorthy KS, Sullivan KF, Allred EN. The epidemiology of germinal matrix hemorrhage during the first half-day of life. *Dev Med Child Neurol*. 1991;33(2):138–145.
55. Kuban KC, Leviton A, Pagano M, Fenton T, Strassfeld R, Wolff M. Maternal toxemia is associated with reduced incidence of germinal matrix hemorrhage in premature babies. *J Child Neurol*. 1992;7(1):70–76.
56. Gagliardi L, Rusconi F, Da Fre M, et al. Pregnancy disorders leading to very preterm birth influence neonatal outcomes: results of the population-based ACTION cohort study. *Pediatr Res*. 2013;73(6):794–801.
57. Ancel PY, Marret S, Larroque B, et al. Are maternal hypertension and small-for-gestational age risk factors for severe intraventricular hemorrhage and cystic periventricular leukomalacia? Results of the EPIPAGE cohort study. *Am J Obstet Gynecol*. 2005;193(1):178–184.
58. Gould JB, Gluck L, Kulovich MV. The relationship between accelerated pulmonary maturity and accelerated neurological maturity in certain chronically stressed pregnancies. *Am J Obstet Gynecol*. 1977;127(2):181–186.
59. Hadi HA. Fetal cerebral maturation in hypertensive disorders of pregnancy. *Obstet Gynecol*. 1984;63(2):214–219.
60. van de Bor M, Verloove-Vanhorick SP, Brand R, Keirse MJ, Ruys JH. Incidence and prediction of periventricular-intraventricular hemorrhage in very preterm infants. *J Perinat Med*. 1987;15(4):333–339.
61. Leviton A, Paneth N, Susser M, et al. Maternal receipt of magnesium sulfate does not seem to reduce the risk of neonatal white matter damage. *Pediatrics*. 1997;99(4):E2.
62. Nelson KB, Grether JK. Can magnesium sulfate reduce the risk of cerebral palsy in very low birth-weight infants? *Pediatrics*. 1995;95(2):263–269.
63. Paneth N, Jetton J, Pinto-Martin J, Susser M. Magnesium sulfate in labor and risk of neonatal brain lesions and cerebral palsy in low birth weight infants. The Neonatal Brain Hemorrhage Study Analysis Group. *Pediatrics*. 1997;99(5):E1.
64. Canterino JC, Verma UL, Visintainer PF, Figueroa R, Klein SA, Tejani NA. Maternal magnesium sulfate and the development of neonatal periventricular leucomalacia and intraventricular hemorrhage. *Obstet Gynecol*. 1999;93(3):396–402.
65. Atkinson MW, Goldenberg RL, Gaudier FL, et al. Maternal corticosteroid and tocolytic treatment and morbidity and mortality in very low birth weight infants. *Am J Obstet Gynecol*. 1995;173(1):299–305.

66. Groome LJ, Goldenberg RL, Cliver SP, Davis RO, Copper RL. Neonatal periventricular-intra-ventricular hemorrhage after maternal beta-sympathomimetic tocolysis. *Am J Obstet Gynecol.* 1992;167:873–879.
67. Rouse DJ, Hirtz DG, Thom E, et al. A randomized, controlled trial of magnesium sulfate for the prevention of cerebral palsy. *N Engl J Med.* 2008;359(9):895–905.
68. Doyle LW, Crowther CA, Middleton P, Marret S, Rouse D. Magnesium sulphate for women at risk of preterm birth for neuroprotection of the fetus. *Cochrane Database Syst Rev.* 2009;(1): CD004661.
69. Doyle LW, Crowther CA, Middleton P, Marret S. Antenatal magnesium sulfate and neurologic outcome in preterm infants: a systematic review. *Obstet Gynecol.* 2009;113(6):1327–1333.
70. Committee Opinion No 652: Magnesium sulfate use in obstetrics. *Obstet Gynecol.* 2016;127(1): e52–e53.
71. Anderson GD, Bada HS, Shaver DC, et al. The effect of cesarean section on intraventricular hemor-rhage in the preterm infant. *Am J Obstet Gynecol.* 1992;166(4):1091–1101.
72. Low JA, Galbraith RS, Sauerbrei EE, et al. Maternal, fetal, and newborn complications associated with newborn intracranial hemorrhage. *Am J Obstet Gynecol.* 1986;154(2):345–351.
73. Strauss A, Kirz D, Modanlou HD, Freeman RK. Perinatal events and intraventricular/subependymal hemorrhage in the very low-birth weight infant. *Am J Obstet Gynecol.* 1985;151(8):1022–1027.
74. Ment LR, Oh W, Ehrenkranz RA, Philip AG, Duncan CC, Makuch RW. Antenatal steroids, delivery mode, and intraventricular hemorrhage in preterm infants. *Am J Obstet Gynecol.* 1995; 172(3):795–800.
75. Deulofeut R, Sola A, Lee B, Buchter S, Rahman M, Rogido M. The impact of vaginal delivery in premature infants weighing less than 1,251 grams. *Obstet Gynecol.* 2005;105(3):525–531.
76. Wadhawan R, Vohr BR, Fanaroff AA, et al. Does labor influence neonatal and neurodevelopmental outcomes of extremely-low-birth-weight infants who are born by cesarean delivery? *Am J Obstet Gynecol.* 2003;189(2):501–506.
77. Riskin A, Riskin-Mashiah S, Bader D, et al. Delivery mode and severe intraventricular hemorrhage in single, very low birth weight, vertex infants. *Obstet Gynecol.* 2008;112(1):21–28.
78. Hansen A, Leviton A. Labor and delivery characteristics and risks of cranial ultrasonographic abnormalities among very-low-birth-weight infants. *Am J Obstet Gynecol.* 1999;181:997–1006.
79. Brocato B, Holliday N, Whitehurst RM Jr, Lewis D, Varner S. Delayed cord clamping in preterm neonates: a review of benefits and risks. *Obstet Gynecol Surv.* 2016;71(1):39–42.
80. Backes CH, Rivera BK, Haque U, et al. Placental transfusion strategies in very preterm neonates: a systematic review and meta-analysis. *Obstet Gynecol.* 2014;124(1):47–56.
81. Rabe H, Diaz-Rossello JL, Duley L, Dowswell T. Effect of timing of umbilical cord clamping and other strategies to influence placental transfusion at preterm birth on maternal and infant outcomes. *Cochrane Database Syst Rev.* 2012;(8):CD003248.
82. Mercer JS, Erickson-Owens DA, Vohr BR, et al. Effects of placental transfusion on neonatal and 18 month outcomes in preterm infants: a randomized controlled trial. *J Pediatr.* 2016;168:50–55. e51.
83. Committee Opinion No. 684: Delayed umbilical cord clamping after birth. *Obstet Gynecol.* 2017; 129(1):e5–e10.
84. Elimian A, Goodman J, Escobedo M, Nightingale L, Knudtson E, Williams M. Immediate compared with delayed cord clamping in the preterm neonate: a randomized controlled trial. *Obstet Gynecol.* 2014;124(6):1075–1079.
85. Chiruvolu A, Tolia VN, Qin H, et al. Effect of delayed cord clamping on very preterm infants. *Am J Obstet Gynecol.* 2015;213(5):676.e671–e677.
86. Vohr B, Ment LR. Intraventricular hemorrhage in the preterm infant. *Early Hum Dev.* 1996;44:1–16.
87. Leviton A, VanMarter L, Kuban KC. Respiratory distress syndrome and intracranial hemorrhage: cause or association? Inferences from surfactant clinical trials. *Pediatrics.* 1989;84(5):915–922.
88. Perlman JM. Intraventricular hemorrhage. *Pediatrics.* 1989;84(5):913–915.
89. Ambalavanan N, Carlo WA, Wrage LA, et al. PaCO2 in surfactant, positive pressure, and oxygen-ation randomised trial (SUPPORT). *Arch Dis Child Fetal Neonatal Ed.* 2015;100(2):F145–F149.
90. Perlman J, Thach B. Respiratory origin of fluctuations in arterial blood pressure in premature infants with respiratory distress syndrome. *Pediatrics.* 1988;81(3):399–403.
91. Perlman JM, Goodman S, Kreusser KL, Volpe JJ. Reduction in intraventricular hemorrhage by elimination of fluctuating cerebral blood-flow velocity in preterm infants with respiratory distress syndrome. *N Engl J Med.* 1985;312(21):1353–1357.
92. Jobe AH. Pulmonary surfactant therapy. *N Engl J Med.* 1993;328(12):861–868.
93. Bedard MP, Shankaran S, Slovis TL, Pantoja A, Dayal B, Poland RL. Effect of prophylactic pheno-barbital on intraventricular hemorrhage in high-risk infants. *Pediatrics.* 1984;73(4):435–439.
94. Donn SM, Roloff DW, Goldstein GW. Prevention of intraventricular haemorrhage in preterm infants by phenobarbitone. A controlled trial. *Lancet.* 1981;2(8240):215–217.
95. Kuban KC, Leviton A, Krishnamoorthy KS, et al. Neonatal intracranial hemorrhage and phenobar-bital. *Pediatrics.* 1986;77:443–450.
96. Sinha S, Davies J, Toner N, Bogle S, Chiswick M. Vitamin E supplementation reduces frequency of periventricular haemorrhage in very preterm babies. *Lancet.* 1987;1(8531):466–471.
97. Morgan ME, Benson JW, Cooke RW. Ethamsylate reduces the incidence of periventricular haemor-rhage in very low birth-weight babies. *Lancet.* 1981;2(8251):830–831.
98. Bada HS, Green RS, Pourcyrous M, et al. Indomethacin reduces the risks of severe intraventricular hemorrhage. *J Pediatr.* 1989;115(4):631–637.

99. Ment LR, Oh W, Ehrenkranz RA, et al. Low-dose indomethacin and prevention of intraventricular hemorrhage: a multicenter randomized trial. *Pediatrics*. 1994;93(4):543–550.
100. Edwards AD, Wyatt JS, Richardson C, et al. Effects of indomethacin on cerebral haemodynamics in very preterm infants. *Lancet*. 1990;335(8704):1491–1495.
101. Pryds O, Greisen G, Johansen KH. Indomethacin and cerebral blood flow in premature infants treated for patent ductus arteriosus. *Eur J Pediatr*. 1988;147(3):315–316.
102. De Vries LS, Wigglesworth JS, Regev R, Dubowitz LM. Evolution of periventricular leukomalacia during the neonatal period and infancy: correlation of imaging and postmortem findings. *Early Hum Dev*. 1988;17(2-3):205–219.
103. Paneth N, Rudelli R, Monte W, et al. White matter necrosis in very low birth weight infants: neuropathologic and ultrasonographic findings in infants surviving six days or longer. *J Pediatr*. 1990;116(6):975–984.
104. de Vries LS, Regev R, Dubowitz LM. Late onset cystic leucomalacia. *Arch Dis Child*. 1986;61(3):298–299.
105. Perlman JM. White matter injury in the preterm infant: an important determination of abnormal neurodevelopment outcome. *Early Hum Dev*. 1998;53(2):99–120.
106. de Vries LS, Regev RR, Dubowitz LS, Whitelaw AA, Aber VR. Perinatal risk factors for the development of extensive cystic leukomalacia. *Am J Dis Child*. 1988;142(7):732–735.
107. Leviton A, Paneth N. White matter damage in preterm newborns—an epidemiologic perspective. *Early Hum Dev*. 1990;24(1):1–22.
108. Neubauer V, Djurdjevic T, Griesmaier E, Biermayr M, Gizewski ER, Kiechl-Kohlendorfer U. Routine magnetic resonance imaging at term-equivalent age detects brain injury in 25% of a contemporary cohort of very preterm infants. *PLoS one*. 2017;12(1):e0169442.
109. Volpe JJ. Brain injury in premature infants: a complex amalgam of destructive and developmental disturbances. *Lancet Neurol*. 2009;8(1):110–124.
110. Armstrong D, Norman MG. Periventricular leucomalacia in neonates. Complications and sequelae. *Arch Dis Child*. 1974;49(5):367–375.
111. Banker BQ, Larroche JC. Periventricular leukomalacia of infancy: a form of neonatal anoxic encephalopathy. *Arch Neurol*. 1962;7(5):386–410.
112. Dereuck J, Chattha AS, Richardson EP. Pathogenesis and evolution of periventricular leukomalacia in infancy. *Arch Neurol*. 1972;27(3):229–236.
113. Khwaja O, Volpe JJ. Pathogenesis of cerebral white matter injury of prematurity. *Arch Dis Child Fetal Neonatal Ed*. 2008;93(2):F153–F161.
114. Back SA. Brain injury in the preterm infant: new horizons for pathogenesis and prevention. *Pediatr Neurol*. 2015;53(3):185–192.
115. De Reuck J. The human periventricular arterial blood supply and the anatomy of cerebral infarctions. *European Neurology*. 1971;5(6):321–334.
116. Takashima S, Tanaka K. Development of cerebrovascular architecture and its relationship to periventricular leukomalacia. *Arch Neurol*. 1978;35(1):11–16.
117. De Reuck JL. Cerebral angioarchitecture and perinatal brain lesions in premature and full-term infants. *Acta Neurol Scand*. 1984;70:391–395.
118. Rorke LB. Anatomical features of the developing brain implicated in pathogenesis of hypoxic-ischemic injury. *Brain Pathol*. 1992;2(3):211–221.
119. Cavazzuti M, Duffy TE. Regulation of local cerebral blood flow in normal and hypoxic newborn dogs. *Ann Neurol*. 1982;11(3):247–257.
120. Szymonowicz W, Walker AM, Yu VY, Stewart ML, Cannata J, Cussen L. Regional cerebral blood flow after hemorrhagic hypotension in the preterm, near-term, and newborn lamb. *Pediatr Res*. 1990;28(4):361–366.
121. Young RS, Hernandez MJ, Yagel SK. Selective reduction of blood flow to white matter during hypotension in newborn dogs: a possible mechanism of periventricular leukomalacia. *Ann Neurol*. 1982;12(5):445–448.
122. Perlman JM, Volpe JJ. Episodes of apnea and bradycardia in the preterm newborn: impact on cerebral circulation. *Pediatrics*. 1985;76(3):333–338.
123. Low JA, Froese AF, Galbraith RS, Sauerbrei EE, McKinven JP, Karchmar EJ. The association of fetal and newborn metabolic acidosis with severe periventricular leukomalacia in the preterm newborn. *Am J Obstet Gynecol*. 1990;162(4):977–982.
124. Shankaran S, Langer JC, Kazzi SN, et al. Cumulative index of exposure to hypocarbia and hyperoxia as risk factors for periventricular leukomalacia in low birth weight infants. *Pediatrics*. 2006;118(4):1654–1659.
125. Greisen G, Munck H, Lou H. Severe hypocarbia in preterm infants and neurodevelopmental deficit. *Acta Paediatr Scand*. 1987;76(3):401–404.
126. Faix RG, Donn SM. Association of septic shock caused by early-onset group B streptococcal sepsis and periventricular leukomalacia in the preterm infant. *Pediatrics*. 1985;76(3):415–419.
127. Perlman JM, Risser R, Broyles RS. Bilateral cystic periventricular leukomalacia in the premature infant: associated risk factors. *Pediatrics*. 1996;97(6 I):822–827.
128. Fujimoto S, Togari H, Yamaguchi N, Mizutani F, Suzuki S, Sobajima H. Hypocarbia and cystic periventricular leukomalacia in premature infants. *Arch Dis Child*. 1994;(3 suppl):71.
129. Perlman JM, Hill A, Volpe JJ. The effect of patent ductus arteriosus on flow velocity in the anterior cerebral arteries: ductal steal in the premature newborn infant. *J Pediatr*. 1981;99(5):767–771.
130. Wiswell TE, Graziani LJ, Kornhauser MS, et al. Effects of hypocarbia on the development of cystic periventricular leukomalacia in premature infants treated with high-frequency jet ventilation. *Pediatrics*. 1996;98(5):918–924.

131. Back SA, Volpe JJ. Cellular and molecular pathogenesis of periventricular white matter injury. *Ment Retard Dev Disabil Res Rev.* 1997;3(1):96–107.

132. Yue X, Mehmet H, Penrice J, et al. Apoptosis and necrosis in the newborn piglet brain following transient cerebral hypoxia-ischaemia. *Neuropathol Appl Neurobiol.* 1997;23(1):16–25.

133. Yoon BH, Kim CJ, Romero R, et al. Experimentally induced intrauterine infection causes fetal brain white matter lesions in rabbits. *Am J Obstet Gynecol.* 1997;177(4):797–802.

134. Back SA, Han BH, Luo NL, et al. Selective vulnerability of late oligodendrocyte progenitors to hypoxia-ischemia. *J Neurosci.* 2002;22(2):455–463.

135. Segovia KN, McClure M, Moravec M, et al. Arrested oligodendrocyte lineage maturation in chronic perinatal white matter injury. *Ann Neurol.* 2008;63(4):520–530.

136. Buser JR, Maire J, Riddle A, et al. Arrested preoligodendrocyte maturation contributes to myelination failure in premature infants. *Ann Neurol.* 2012;71(1):93–109.

137. Billiards SS, Haynes RL, Folkerth RD, et al. Myelin abnormalities without oligodendrocyte loss in periventricular leukomalacia. *Brain Pathol.* 2008;18(2):153–163.

138. Chamnanvanakij S, Margraf LR, Burns D, Perlman JM. Apoptosis and white matter injury in preterm infants. *Pediatr Dev Pathol.* 2002;5(2):184–189.

139. Haynes RL, Folkerth RD, Keefe RJ, et al. Nitrosative and oxidative injury to premyelinating oligodendrocytes in periventricular leukomalacia. *J Neuropathol Exp Neurol.* 2003;62(5):441–450.

140. Oka A, Belliveau MJ, Rosenberg PA, Volpe JJ. Vulnerability of oligodendroglia to glutamate: pharmacology, mechanisms, and prevention. *J Neurosci.* 1993;13(4):1441–1453.

141. Yonezawa M, Back SA, Gan X, Rosenberg PA, Volpe JJ. Cystine deprivation induces oligodendroglial death: rescue by free radical scavengers and by a diffusible glial factor. *J Neurochem.* 1996;67(2):566–573.

142. Ozawa H, Nishida A, Mito T, Takashima S. Development of ferritin-positive cells in cerebrum of human brain. *Pediatr Neurol.* 1994;10(1):44–48.

143. Folkerth RD, Haynes RL, Borenstein NS, et al. Developmental lag in superoxide dismutases relative to other antioxidant enzymes in premyelinated human telencephalic white matter. *J Neuropathol Exp Neurol.* 2004;63(9):990–999.

144. Gerstner B, DeSilva TM, Genz K, et al. Hyperoxia causes maturation-dependent cell death in the developing white matter. *J Neurosci.* 2008;28(5):1236–1245.

145. Gerstner B, Sifringer M, Dzietko M, et al. Estradiol attenuates hyperoxia-induced cell death in the developing white matter. *Ann Neurol.* 2007;61(6):562–573.

146. Rosenberg PA, Dai W, Gan XD, et al. Mature myelin basic protein-expressing oligodendrocytes are insensitive to kainate toxicity. *J Neurosci Res.* January 15 2003;71(2):237–245.

147. Yoshioka A, Bacskai B, Pleasure D. Pathophysiology of oligodendroglial excitotoxicity. *J Neurosci Res.* 1996;46(4):427–437.

148. Follett PL, Rosenberg PA, Volpe JJ, Jensen FE. NBQX attenuates excitotoxic injury in developing white matter. *J Neurosci.* 2000;20(24):9235–9241.

149. Salter MG, Fern R. NMDA receptors are expressed in developing oligodendrocyte processes and mediate injury. *Nature.* 2005;438(7071):1167–1171.

150. Bona E, Andersson AL, Blomgren K, et al. Chemokine and inflammatory cell response to hypoxia-ischemia in immature rats. *Pediatr Res.* 1999;45(4 Pt 1):500–509.

151. Selmaj K, Raine CS, Farooq M, Norton WT, Brosnan CF. Cytokine cytotoxicity against oligodendrocytes: apoptosis induced by lymphotoxin. *J Immunol.* 1991;147(5):1522–1529.

152. Andrews T, Zhang P, Bhat NR. TNFα potentiates IFNγ-induced cell death in oligodendrocyte progenitors. *J Neurosci Res.* 1998;54(5):574–583.

153. Dommergues MA, Patkai J, Renauld JC, Evrard P, Gressens P. Proinflammatory cytokines and interleukin-9 exacerbate excitotoxic lesions of the newborn murine neopallium. *Ann Neurol.* 2000;47(1):54–63.

154. Hansen-Pupp I, Harling S, Berg AC, Cilio C, Hellstrom-Westas L, Ley D. Circulating interferon-gamma and white matter brain damage in preterm infants. *Pediatr Res.* 2005;58:946–952.

155. Saija A, Princi P, Lanza M, Scalese M, Aramnejad E, Sarro AD. Systemic cytokine administration can affect blood-brain barrier permeability in the rat. *Life Sciences.* 1995;56(10):775–784.

156. Westlin WF, Gimbrone MA Jr. Neutrophil-mediated damage to human vascular endothelium. Role of cytokine activation. *Am J Pathol.* 1993;142(1):117–128.

157. Ando M, Takashima S, Mito T. Endotoxin, cerebral blood flow, amino acids and brain damage in young rabbits. *Brain Dev.* 1988;10(6):365–370.

158. Gilles FH, Leviton A, Kerr CS. Endotoxin leucoencephalopathy in the telencephalon of the newborn kitten. *J Neurol Sci.* 1976;27(2):183–191.

159. Zupan V, Gonzalez P, Lacaze-Masmonteil T, et al. Periventricular leukomalacia: risk factors revisited. *Dev Med Child Neurol.* 1996;38(12):1061–1067.

160. Leviton A, Paneth N, Reuss ML, et al. Maternal infection, fetal inflammatory response, and brain damage in very low birth weight infants. *Pediatr Res.* 1999;46(5):566–575.

161. Hillier SL, Witkin SS, Krohn MA, Watts DH, Kiviat NB, Eschenbach DA. The relationship of amniotic fluid cytokines and preterm delivery, amniotic fluid infection, histologic chorioamnionitis, and chorioamnion infection. *Obstet Gynecol.* 1993;81(6):941–948.

162. Baud O, Emilie D, Pelletier E, et al. Amniotic fluid concentrations of interleukin-1β, interlenkin-6 and TNF-α in chorioamnionitis before 32 weeks of gestation: histological associations and neonatal outcome. *BJOG.* 1999;106(1):72–77.

163. Saito S, Kasahara T, Kato Y, Ishihara Y, Ichijo M. Elevation of amniotic fluid interleukin 6 (IL-6), IL-8 and granulocyte colony stimulating factor (G-CSF) in term and preterm parturition. *Cytokine.* 1993;5(1):81–88.

164. Yoon BH, Romero R, Yang SH, et al. Interleukin-6 concentrations in umbilical cord plasma are elevated in neonates with white matter lesions associated with periventricular leukomalacia. *Am J Obstet Gynecol.* 1996;174(5):1433–1440.
165. Grether JK, Nelson KB. Maternal infection and cerebral palsy in infants of normal birth weight. *JAMA.* 1997;278(3):207–211.
166. Grether JK, Nelson KB, Dambrosia JM, Phillips TM. Interferons and cerebral palsy. *J Pediatr.* 1999;134(3):324–332.
167. Wu YW, Colford JM. Chorioamnionitis as a risk factor for cerebral palsy: a meta-analysis. *JAMA.* 2000;284(11):1417–1424.
168. Yoon BH, Romero R, Kim CJ, et al. High expression of tumor necrosis factor-alpha and interleukin-6 in periventricular leukomalacia. *Am J Obstet Gynecol.* 1997;177(2):406–411.
169. Deguchi K, Mizuguchi M, Takashima S. Immunohistochemical expression of tumor necrosis factor alpha in neonatal leukomalacia. *Pediatr Neurol.* 1996;14(1):13–16.
170. Bruce AJ, Boling W, Kindy MS, et al. Altered neuronal and microglial responses to excitotoxic and ischemic brain injury in mice lacking TNF receptors. *Nat Med.* 1996;2(7):788–794.
171. Glass HC, Bonifacio SL, Chau V, et al. Recurrent postnatal infections are associated with progressive white matter injury in premature infants. *Pediatrics.* 2008;122(2):299–305.
172. Graziani LJ, Spitzer AR, Mitchell DG, et al. Mechanical ventilation in preterm infants: neurosonographic and developmental studies. *Pediatrics.* 1992;90(4):515–522.
173. Trounce JQ, Shaw DE, Levene MI, Rutter N. Clinical risk factors and periventricular leucomalacia. *Arch Dis Child.* 1988;63(1):17–22.
174. Weindling AM, Wilkinson AR, Cook J, Calvert SA, Fok TF, Rochefort MJ. Perinatal events which precede periventricular haemorrhage and leukomalacia in the newborn. *BJOG.* 1985;92(12):1218–1223.
175. Mirro R, Busija D, Green R, Leffler C. Relationship between mean airway pressure, cardiac output, and organ blood flow with normal and decreased respiratory compliance. *J Pediatr.* 1987;111(1):101–106.
176. Phelps DL, Rosenbaum AL, Isenberg SJ, Leake RD, Dorey FJ. Tocopherol efficacy and safety for preventing retinopathy of prematurity: a randomized, controlled, double-masked trial. *Pediatrics.* 1987;79(4):489–500.
177. Juul SE, Ferriero DM. Pharmacologic neuroprotective strategies in neonatal brain injury. *Clin Perinatol.* 2014;41(1):119–131.
178. Natalucci G, Latal B, Koller B, et al. Effect of early prophylactic high-dose recombinant human erythropoietin in very preterm infants on neurodevelopmental outcome at 2 years: a randomized clinical trial. *JAMA.* 2016;315(19):2079–2085.
179. Song J, Sun H, Xu F, et al. Recombinant human erythropoietin improves neurological outcomes in very preterm infants. *Ann Neurol.* July 2016;80(1):24–34.
180. Juul SE, Mayock DE, Comstock BA, Heagerty PJ. Neuroprotective potential of erythropoietin in neonates; design of a randomized trial. *Matern Health Neonatol Perinatol.* 2015;1:27.
181. Stewart AL, Reynolds EOR, Hope PL, et al. Probability of neurodevelopmental disorders estimated from ultrasound appearance of brains of very preterm infants. *Dev Med Child Neurol.* 1987;29(1):3–11.
182. Fazzi E, Lanzi G, Gerardo A, Ometto A, Orcesi S, Rondini G. Neurodevelopmental outcome in very-low-birth-weight infants with or without periventricular haemorrhage and/or leucomalacia. *Acta Paediatr.* 1992;81(10):808–811.
183. Rogers B, Msall M, Owens T, et al. Cystic periventricular leukomalacia and type of cerebral palsy in preterm infants. *J Pediatr.* 1994;125(1):S1–S8.
184. Woodward LJ, Anderson PJ, Austin NC, Howard K, Inder TE. Neonatal MRI to predict neurodevelopmental outcomes in preterm infants. *NEJM.* 2006;355(7):685–694.
185. Melhem ER, Hoon AH Jr, Ferrucci JT Jr, et al. Periventricular leukomalacia: relationship between lateral ventricular volume on brain MR images and severity of cognitive and motor impairment. *Radiology.* 2000;214(1):199–204.
186. De Vries LS, Eken P, Groenendaal F, Van Haastert IC, Meiners LC. Correlation between the degree of periventricular leukomalacia diagnosed using cranial ultrasound and MRI later in infancy in children with cerebral palsy. *Neuropediatrics.* 1993;24(5):263–268.
187. De Vries LS, Connell JA, Dubowitz LMS, Oozeer RC, Dubowitz V, Pennock JM. Neurological, electrophysiological and MRI abnormalities in infants with extensive cystic leukomalacia. *Neuropediatrics.* 1987;18(2):61–66.
188. Jacobson LK, Button GN. Periventricular leukomalacia: an important cause of visual and ocular motility dysfunction in children. *Surv Ophthalmol.* 2000;45(1):1–13.
189. Scher MS, Dobson V, Carpenter NA, Guthrie RD. Visual and neurological outcome of infants with periventricular leukomalacia. *Dev Med Child Neurol.* 1989;31(3):353–365.
190. Guo T, Duerden EG, Adams E, et al. Quantitative assessment of white matter injury in preterm neonates: association with outcomes. *Neurology.* 2017.
191. Volpe JJ. Encephalopathy of prematurity includes neuronal abnormalities. *Pediatrics.* 2005;116:221–225.
192. Inder TE, Huppi PS, Warfield S, et al. Periventricular white matter injury in the premature infant is followed by reduced cerebral cortical gray matter volume at term. *Ann Neurol.* 1999;46(5):755–760.
193. Gano D, Ho ML, Partridge JC, et al. Antenatal exposure to magnesium sulfate is associated with reduced cerebellar hemorrhage in preterm newborns. *J Pediatr.* 2016;178:68–74.

CHAPTER 3

Posthemorrhagic Hydrocephalus Management Strategies

Andrew Whitelaw

- **Posthemorrhagic hydrocephalus is characterized by deposition of extracellular matrix proteins weeks following intraventricular hemorrhage.**
- **Periventricular white matter may be progressively injured by raised intracranial pressure, inflammation and free radical injury.**
- **There is not one standard approach to treating post hemorrhagic hydrocephalus.**
- **Ventricular lavage remains an experimental therapy.**

Hemorrhage into the ventricles of the brain is one of the most serious complications of premature birth despite improvements in the survival of premature infants. Large intraventricular hemorrhage (IVH) has a high risk of neurologic disability, and more than 50% of children with IVH go on to have progressive ventricular dilation.[1] Increasing survival of extremely premature infants is associated with posthemorrhagic ventricular dilation (PHVD) with high morbidity and considerable mortality.[2] Overall, approximately two-thirds of these children have cerebral palsy and about one-third have multiple impairments.[3,4] The term posthemorrhagic hydrocephalus is generally reserved for cases in which PHVD is persistent and associated with excessive head enlargement. This condition still does not have a safe and effective "cure," but advances in our understanding of the pathophysiology and experience from clinical trials allow us to suggest some guidelines on assessment and management and to identify gaps in knowledge where further advances are needed.

CASE HISTORY: INFANT A

A mother in her third pregnancy suffered a placental abruption at 28 weeks and delivered a male infant weighing 877 g at delivery. He was intubated at birth and received surfactant prophylactically. He was ventilated at low pressures and had a low oxygen requirement until, on day 2, he suffered a pulmonary hemorrhage with a period of hypotension (mean arterial pressure below 25 mm Hg for 2 hours), which was corrected with the use of dopamine and blood transfusion. His respiratory status stabilized within hours. On day 3 a cranial ultrasound scan showed bilateral IVH (Fig. 3.1A). He progressed from minimal ventilation settings to nasal continuous positive airway pressure. He then had scans twice a week. Ventricular dimensions progressively enlarged until day 18 (see Fig. 3.1B). Head circumference had increased by 1.5 cm over 7 days. A lumbar puncture (LP) produced 12 mL (10 mL/kg) of port wine–colored cerebrospinal fluid (CSF). This procedure reduced head circumference by 0.3 cm. Two days later, head circumference had increased by 0.5 cm from the postpuncture

Continued

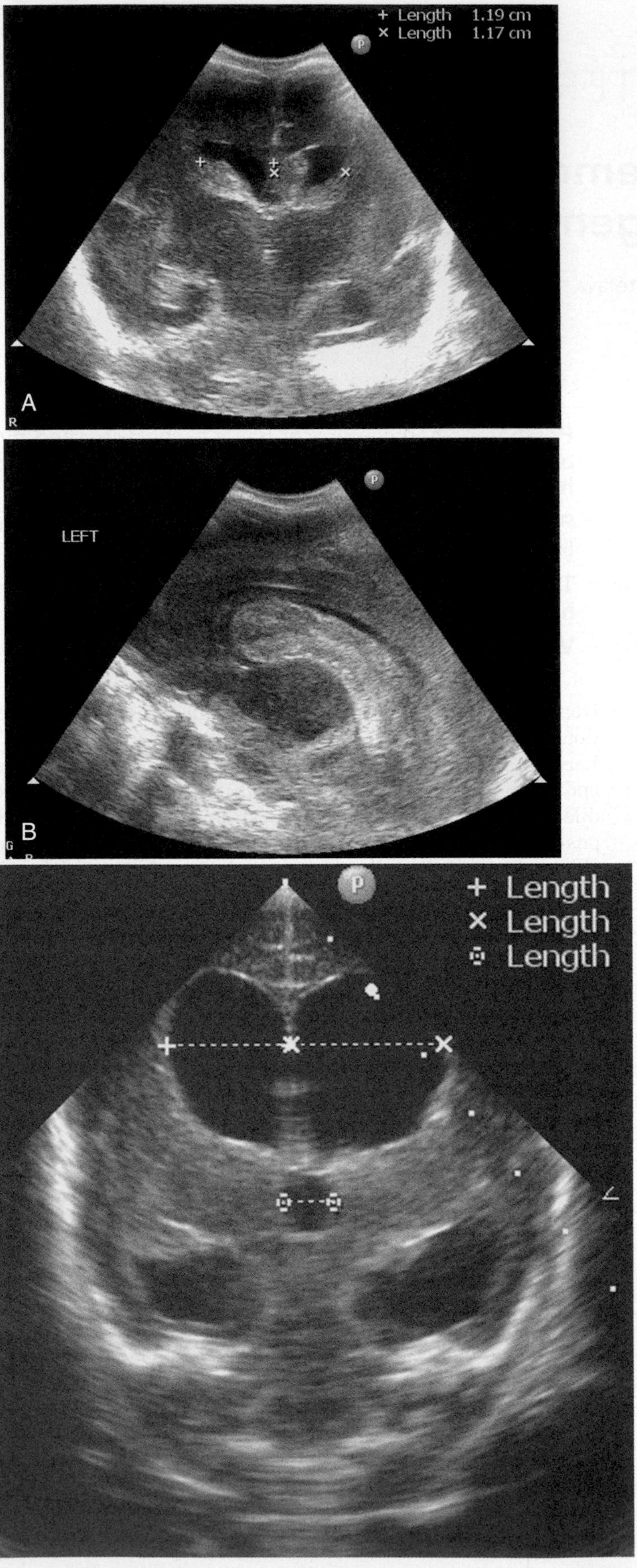

Fig. 3.1 **Cranial ultrasound scans from Infant A (Case History).** A, Midcoronal view obtained on day 3, showing hemorrhage in both lateral ventricles. B, Left parasagittal view, obtained on day 3, showing extensive blood clot within the left lateral ventricle. C, Midcoronal view, obtained on day 18, showing enlargement of both lateral ventricles and the third ventricle.

CASE HISTORY: INFANT A—cont'd

measurement. A second LP was carried out, which again produced 12 mL (10 mL/kg) of CSF. Head circumference decreased by 0.3 cm but then increased by 0.5 cm from the postpuncture measurement 2 days later. A third LP produced only 6 mL of CSF before flow stopped. Head circumference did not decrease, the fontanelle remained full, and ultrasonography confirmed that the ventricles were still "ballooned."

As there was a need for repeated tapping of CSF and repeated LP was becoming impractical, an Ommaya reservoir (ventricular access device) was inserted frontally in the right ventricle with the patient under general anesthesia. At the time of its insertion, 13 mL (10 mL/kg) of CSF was removed. To avoid raised pressure and resultant CSF leak with a risk of infection, the reservoir was tapped daily, at 10 mL/kg per day for 5 days. Thereafter the reservoir was tapped as required to control excessive expansion or suspected pressure symptoms. Head circumference enlargement necessitated tapping 10 mL/kg every 1 to 2 days. Pressure measurement at the start of tapping typically showed a pressure of 6 to 7 mm Hg. After 10 mL/kg had been removed, pressure had fallen to 3 mm Hg. Clinically, apnea increased at the time of head expansion and decreased after tapping.

This regimen of tapping as required was reviewed every 7 days to confirm that head enlargement in 1 week had not been excessive. CSF protein was initially 4.1 g/L. Tapping the reservoir continued to be necessary for 6 weeks, and on a few days, it was obvious that 10 mL/kg had been insufficient to control head enlargement and the subsequent tap had been increased to 15 mL/kg. CSF protein continued to remain high (1.8–2.0 g/L), and tapping was continued for a further 2 weeks, by which time CSF protein had decreased to 1.45 g/L and the infant's weight had risen to nearly 2500 g. Nasal catheter oxygen was no longer required. A ventriculoperitoneal low-pressure shunt was inserted when Infant A reached full-term gestational age. Postoperatively there was no pulmonary problem, CSF leak, or infection but Infant A initially needed to be placed on a considerable head-up tilt to facilitate adequate shunt function and control head circumference. Although control of head circumference and suspected pressure had been maintained, magnetic resonance imaging (MRI) at term showed considerable ventricular dilation with some loss of periventricular white matter.

Question 1: What Measurements of Ventricular Size Are Used in Diagnosis of PHVD?

The chances of progressive ventricular dilation increase with the amount of blood visible in the ventricles. With a small IVH (grade II on Papile scale[5] or IIa on De Vries grading[6]), measurement of ventricular size once a week for 4 weeks and then at discharge is appropriate; with a large IVH (grade III on Papile scale[5] or IIb on De Vries grading[6]), twice-weekly ultrasonography is needed because dilation is likely and may be rapid. Although large, balloon-shaped ventricles are obvious without formal measurements, quantitative documentation is essential if serial scans are being done by different ultrasonographers as well as in epidemiologic studies and clinical trials. Reference ranges for measurement of the width (midline to lateral border) of the lateral ventricles at the midcoronal level were first published in 1981.[7] Since 1984, an "action line," defined as width 4 mm higher than the 97th centile width for age, has been used as a definition of serious PHVD in therapeutic trials[3,4] and as a secondary outcome in randomized trials of neonatal intensive care interventions (Fig. 3.2A). This measurement has the advantage of being highly reproducible among observers because it is relatively unaffected by anterior or posterior angulation of the scan head as the lateral wall of the ventricle in this orientation runs fairly parallel to the midline. The frequency of PHVD using this definition is 1 in 3000 births among residents of Bristol, United Kingdom. However, ventricular enlargement is

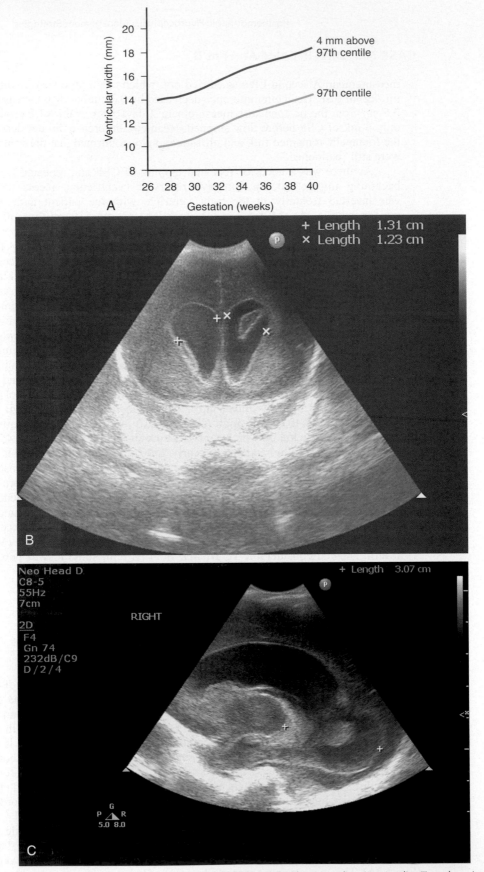

Fig. 3.2   A, 97th centile for ventricular width with the 97th centile plus 4-mm line ("action line") as the criterion for diagnosis of posthemorrhagic ventricular dilation. B and C, Cranial ultrasound scans from Infant A (Case History) obtained on day 18. Frontal coronal view (B) showing the anterior horn width marked with calipers (×). Right parasagittal view (C) showing the thalamo-occipital dimension with calipers (×). (A, Modified from Levene M. Measurement of the growth of the lateral ventricles in preterm infants with real-time ultrasound. *Arch Dis Child.* 1981;56(12):900–904.)

not always sideways, and sometimes the most marked change is posterior enlargement or a change from thin slit to round balloon. With this in mind, Davies and colleagues[8] published reference ranges for anterior horn width (to capture the change in shape to balloon) (95th centile approximately 3 mm), thalamo-occipital width (to capture posterior enlargement) (95th centile approximately 25 mm) (Fig. 3.2B), and third ventricle width (95th centile approximately 2 mm). My colleagues and I have found the anterior horn, thalamo-occipital, and third ventricle widths to be practical and useful but with greater interobserver variation. We have used all three measurements since 2003, requiring all three measurements (bilaterally) to be 1 mm over the 95th centile as a criterion for PHVD.

Question 2: How Can Ventricular Dilation Driven By Cerebrospinal Fluid Under Pressure Be Distinguished From Ventricular Dilation Caused By Loss of Periventricular White Matter?

The distinction of CSF under pressure and the loss of periventricular white matter as the cause of ventricular dilation are important because removing fluid that has accumulated as a replacement for dead brain is unlikely to improve outcome.

CSF-driven ventricular enlargement can be slow or rapid, it is characterized by balloon-shaped lateral ventricles, and if CSF pressure is measured, it is found to be raised or near the upper limit of normal (mean 3 mm Hg, upper limit 6 mm Hg[9]). Furthermore, head circumference growth over time is accelerated, although it may lag ventricular enlargement by 1 to 2 weeks. In contrast, ventricular enlargement from atrophy is always slow, it is more irregular in outline rather than balloon shaped, and if CSF pressure is measured, it is found not to be raised. Head circumference velocity is either normal or slow but is not accelerated. Nonprogressive mild ventricular dilation at term is a marker of periventricular leukomalacia.

Question 3: How Is Excessive Head Enlargement Defined?

Head circumference normally enlarges by approximately 1 mm/day between 26 weeks of gestation and 32 weeks, and about 0.7 mm/day between 32 and 40 weeks.[10] We regard a persistent increase of 2 mm/day as excessive. Measuring head circumference accurately, although "low-tech," is not as easy as it sounds. The relevant measurement is the maximum fronto-occipital circumference. Detecting a difference of 1 mm from day to day is difficult, and we do not react to a difference of 2 mm from 1 day to the next unless there is other evidence of raised intracranial pressure. However, an increase of 4 mm over 2 days is more likely to be real, and an increase of 14 mm over 7 days is definitely excessive.

Question 4: How Is Raised Intracranial Pressure Recognized?

It is possible to detect a change in palpation of the fontanelle from concave to bulging and to document excessive head enlargement. The preterm skull is very compliant and can easily accommodate an increase in CSF by expanding with separation of the sutures. When CSF pressure was measured with an electronic transducer in infants in whom ventricles were expanding after IVH, the mean CSF pressure was approximately 9 mm Hg, 3 times the mean in normal infants.[10] There was a considerable range, with ventricle and head expansion in some infants at a pressure of 5 to 6 mm Hg, and in a small number with CSF pressure around 15 mm Hg. A CSF pressure of 9 mm Hg does not necessarily produce clinical signs but may be associated with an increase in apnea or vomiting, hypotonia, hypertonia, or decreased alertness.

Obtaining serial calculations of the Doppler flow-velocity resistance index (RI) on the anterior cerebral artery is a useful and practical way of detecting impairment of cerebral perfusion by raised intracranial pressure and can easily be done during ultrasound imaging. The resistance index is calculated as follows: (systolic velocity – diastolic velocity)/systolic velocity. This measurement is independent of the angle of insonation. If intracranial pressure rises to a level exceeding the infant's compensation, end-diastolic velocity tends to decrease, eventually becoming zero (the RI is then 1.0) (Fig. 3.3). Serial increases in RI above 0.85 while the ventricles are rapidly expanding would be evidence that pressure is rising.[11] This statement assumes that the infant does not have a significant left-to-right shunt at the ductal level and that the partial pressure of carbon dioxide (Pco_2) has not decreased recently, because both of these physiologic changes could increase RI. Severe intracranial hypertension may cause reversed end-diastolic velocities. The sensitivity of the RI can be increased by applying pressure to the fontanelle during the examination. An infant who is close to the limit of cranial compliance responds with a large decrease in end-diastolic velocities—that is, an increase in RI.[12] Amplitude-integrated electroencephalography (EEG) may show a deterioration, with electroencephalographic activity becoming less frequent as dilation increases and improving with effective CSF drainage.[13]

Question 5: What Is Infant A's Prognosis?

The prognosis at diagnosis of PHVD using the preceding criteria is influenced by the presence of identifiable parenchymal lesions. The Ventriculomegaly Trial and the PHVD Drug Trial used the 4 mm plus 97th centile definition of PHVD and had standardized follow-up. Of children in whom ultrasonographic examination shows no persistent echodensities or echolucencies (cysts), approximately 40% will have cerebral palsy and about 25% will have multiple impairments.[3,4] Cerebral MRI at term is increasingly used to assess infants with PHVD because this technique can reveal parenchymal injury that cannot be easily demonstrated with ultrasonography.[14] Lesions detected by MRI include abnormal signal in the white matter without cyst formation, gray matter abnormality, and cerebellar secondary atrophy. In Infant

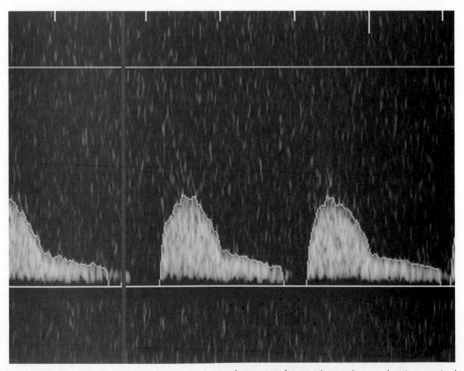

Fig. 3.3 Cerebral blood flow velocity Doppler spectra from an infant with posthemorrhagic ventricular dilation and an intracranial pressure of 15 mm Hg. There is loss of end-diastolic velocities. When the pressure was reduced to 6 mm Hg, end-diastolic velocities returned.

A's case, there were no ultrasonographic abnormalities in the parenchyma, and thus the risk of some level of cerebral palsy would be no higher than 40%.

Question 6: What Is the Mechanism of PHVD?

After a large IVH, multiple blood clots can obstruct the ventricular system or channels of reabsorption, initially leading to a phase of CSF accumulation.[15] Although tissue plasminogen activator (TPA) can be demonstrated in posthemorrhagic CSF, fibrinolysis is very inefficient in the CSF, which has low levels of plasminogen and high levels of plasminogen activator inhibitor.[16,17] This potentially reversible obstruction by thrombi may lead to a chronic obliterative, fibrosing arachnoiditis, and subependymal gliosis[18] involving deposition of extracellular matrix proteins in the foramina of the fourth ventricle and the subarachnoid space. Fig. 3.4A shows the brainstem and cerebellum of an infant with PHVD who died at age 2 months. A layer of collagenous connective tissue surrounds the brainstem. Fig. 3.4B shows perivascular deposition of the extracellular matrix protein, laminin, in the subependymal region in another infant with PHVD who also died at age 2 months.

Transforming growth factor β (TGF-β) is likely to be a key mediator of this process because TGF-β is involved in the initiation of wound healing and fibrosis.[19] TGF-β elevates the expression of genes encoding fibronectin, various types of collagen,[20,21] and other extracellular matrix components,[22] and is involved in a number of serious diseases in which there is excessive deposition of collagen, including diabetic nephropathy and cirrhosis.[23] TGF-β has three isoforms, β1, β2, and β3. TGF-β1 is stored in platelets. Thus IVH, by definition, provides a store of TGF-β1 for many weeks in the CSF. TGF-β is elevated in the CSF of adults with hydrocephalus after subarachnoid hemorrhage, and intrathecal administration of TGF-β to mice resulted in hydrocephalus.[24,25] My colleagues and I have demonstrated that TGF-β1 and TGF-β2 concentrations in CSF from infants with posthemorrhagic ventricular dilation are 10 to 20 times those in nonhemorrhagic CSF and that the concentration of TGF-β in CSF is higher in those shunted later.[26] Heep and colleagues[27] have confirmed elevations of TGF-β1 in posthemorrhagic hydrocephalus CSF as well as a product of TGF-β, amino-terminal propeptide of type I collagen.[27] Chow and associates[28] have demonstrated elevation of TGF-β2 and nitrated chondroitin sulfate proteoglycans (an extracellular matrix protein) in CSF from preterm infants with posthemorrhagic hydrocephalus.[28]

A rat pup model of PHVD has also provided evidence of the involvement of TGF-β and its downstream products, fibronectin, laminin, and vitronectin.[29,30] Transgenic mice that overexpress TGF-β1 in the central nervous system are born with hydrocephalus.[31] Thus there is a strong possibility of a role for the TGF-βs in the development and/or maintenance of hydrocephalus after ventricular hemorrhage. However, two drugs that inhibit TGF-β, pirfenidone and losartan, did not reduce ventricular size or improve neuromotor performance in a rat pup model of PHVD.[32]

Question 7: How Can PHVD Injure White Matter?

Damage to periventricular white matter is probably exacerbated by ischemia owing to raised intracranial pressure and parenchymal compression, by oxidative stress caused by the generation of free radicals, and by the actions of inflammatory cytokines.

Raised Intracranial Pressure, Parenchymal Compression, and Ischemia

PHVD raises CSF pressure to, on average, three times normal.[9] Fig. 3.3 shows that in an infant with PHVD, an intracranial pressure of 15 mm Hg was high enough to prevent cerebral blood flow during diastole; cerebral perfusion was restored when the pressure was reduced to 6 mm Hg. A reduction of perfusion of this magnitude raises the risk of ischemic injury. There is also evidence that distortion of periventricular axons as the result of ventricular dilation may cause injury independently of ischemia.[33]

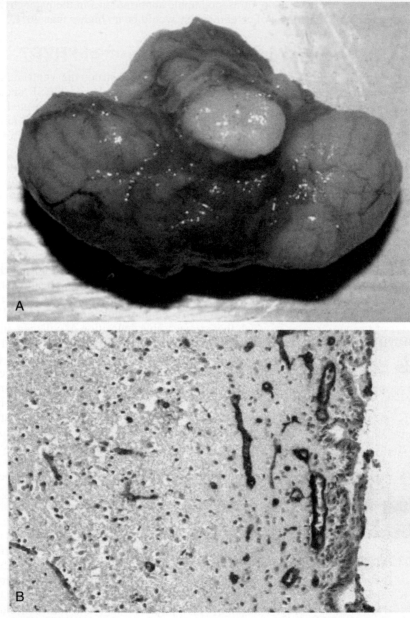

Fig. 3.4 A, Brainstem and cerebellum of an infant with posthemorrhagic ventricular dilation (PHVD) who died at age 2 months. In addition to the staining from old blood, there are gray strands of connective tissue wrapped around the brainstem. B, Histologic section from the subependymal region of the brain of another infant with PHVD who also died at age 2 months. Immunostaining shows increased perivascular deposition of the extracellular matrix protein laminin.

Free Radical–Mediated Injury

Nonprotein-bound iron is readily detectable in the CSF of neonates with PHVD.[34] Hemoglobin that enters the CSF releases large amounts of iron, which is likely to exceed the protein-binding capacity of the CSF and lead to the generation of hydroxyl free radicals from hydrogen peroxide via the Fenton reaction. Inder and coworkers[35] demonstrated products of lipid peroxidation in the CSF of infants with periventricular leukomalacia. Further evidence of potential oxidative stress comes from the finding of raised concentrations of hypoxanthine in the CSF of infants with PHVD.[36] Under conditions of ischemia, xanthine dehydrogenase is modified to form xanthine oxidase, which uses oxygen as the electron acceptor.[37] On restoration of cerebral perfusion, xanthine oxidase–mediated oxidation of xanthine and hypoxanthine generates superoxide and hydrogen peroxide, which cause oxidative damage. Oligodendrocyte progenitors, abundant in the periventricular white matter of premature infants, are highly susceptible to oxidative damage.[38]

Proinflammatory Cytokines

Clinical evidence suggests that inflammation causes damage to immature white matter.[39] The concentration of tumor necrosis factor α, interleukin (IL) 1β, IL-6, IL-8, and interferon-γ are significantly elevated in the CSF of infants with PHVD.[40] Tumor necrosis factor α and IL-1β have both been implicated in the development of periventricular leukomalacia,[41] and it seems likely that these proinflammatory cytokines also contribute to white matter damage in PHVD.

Loss of White Matter and Gray Matter

In the rat model of PHVD, there is a significant negative correlation between the extent of ventricular dilation and the thickness of both the corpus callosum and the frontal cortex.[42] The development of hydrocephalus is associated with a mean reduction in the thickness of the corpus callosum of 48% and of the frontal cortex of 31%. Loss of white matter is also marked in the lateral periventricular region; loss of myelin and axons is associated with a reduced density of oligodendrocytes.[42]

Question 8: What Interventions Have Been Used in PHVD, and Is There Any Evidence That They Improve Outcome?

Box 3.1 lists therapeutic interventions that have been used in infants with PHVD.

Ventriculoperitoneal Shunt Surgery

Ventriculoperitoneal shunt (VPS) surgery is the conventional approach to other types of established hydrocephalus. Treatment of PHVD is more difficult than that of other types of hydrocephalus because the large amount of blood in the ventricles, combined with the small size and instability of the patient, make an early Ventriculoperitoneal (VP) shunt operation impossible. In one series of 19 infants with PHVD requiring shunt surgery, there were 29 shunt blockages and 12 infections.[43] The risk of shunt blockage was increased if the CSF protein concentration was more than 1.5 g/L at the time of shunt insertion. In a series of 36 infants who underwent shunt placement for PHVD, shunt blockage and infection occurred only in those who had shunt placement before 35 days of age.[44] There is a considerable complication rate throughout a child's life from VPS surgery, and the child is permanently dependent on the shunt system. A VPS is a treatment but not a cure, and the child is vulnerable to shunt dysfunction. Shunt blockage after the cranial sutures have fused can rapidly raise intracranial pressure, resulting in permanent cerebral damage. Sudden blindness and death have been recorded in such circumstances. Repeated shunt revisions are associated with a worsening of neurologic outcome.[45] Shunt infection is another complication that can further injure the developing brain.

Objectives in Treating PHVD

The objectives of treatment for PHVD are as follows:
1. To reduce secondary injury to the brain from pressure, distortion, free radicals, and inflammation.
2. To minimize iatrogenic injury from interventions, especially in those infants in whom PHVD resolves after a period of weeks.
3. To minimize the need for a VP shunt.

3

> **Box 3.1** THERAPEUTIC INTERVENTIONS USED IN INFANTS WITH POSTHEMORRHAGIC HYDROCEPHALUS
>
> - Repeated early lumbar punctures/ventricular taps
> - Diuretic drugs to reduce cerebrospinal fluid (CSF) production
> - Intraventricular fibrinolytic therapy
> - External ventricular drain
> - Ventricular reservoir and repeated taps
> - Ventriculosubgaleal shunt
> - Third ventriculostomy
> - Choroid plexus coagulation
> - Ventriculoperitoneal shunt after CSF clears and CSF protein level <1.5 g/L
>
> NONE IS BOTH SAFE AND EFFECTIVE

Repeated Lumbar Punctures or Ventricular Taps

Repeated LPs were suggested as a way of controlling pressure, preventing progressive ventricular enlargement, and removing some of the red blood cells and protein from the CSF. Kressuer and associates[46] showed that a minimum of 10 mL/kg needed to be removed for the removal to have a significant effect on ventricular size. In our experience, only a minority of infants with PHVD have consistently communicating PHVD with a sufficient yield of CSF. Tapping of ventricular CSF must therefore be considered. A policy of repeated early tapping of lumbar or ventricular CSF for PHVD has been tested in four controlled clinical trials.[47] Overall, there was no evidence that this approach reduced the rate of VPS surgery or disability, and there was a 7% infection rate among the infants who underwent repeated tapping in the Ventriculomegaly Trial.[4]

Drug Treatment to Reduce CSF Production

Faced with this lack of effect and risk of infection from invasive procedures, pharmacologic treatment to reduce CSF production seemed an excellent approach. Acetazolamide had been in clinical use for benign intracranial hypertension and appeared to have acceptable adverse effects as long as electrolyte and acid-base balances were monitored. Results from uncontrolled studies were positive about the effect of acetazolamide in PHVD. Experimentally, acetazolamide produced an initial increase in cerebral blood flow mediated by an increase in tissue carbon dioxide (CO_2) and inhibition of respiratory elimination of CO_2.[48] Clinical investigation of infants with chronic lung disease of prematurity showed that acetazolamide produced an increase in P_{CO_2}.[49] Eventually a large multicenter randomized trial of acetazolamide combined with furosemide (which also reduces CSF production) was carried out. Not only was there no clinical benefit, but the group receiving the combined drug treatment had significantly worse outcome in terms of shunt surgery and death or disability.[50]

Intraventricular Fibrinolytic Therapy

The idea of injecting a fibrinolytic agent intraventricularly grew out of Pang's experimental PHVD model, in which blood was injected intraventricularly into dogs. In this model, hydrocephalus developed in 80% of subjects, but if urokinase was injected intraventricularly, only 10% demonstrated hydrocephalus.[51] The idea was supported by laboratory work showing weak endogenous fibrinolytic activity in posthemorrhagic CSF[16,17] and by the relative safety of low-dose fibrinolytic therapy administered locally. A number of small nonrandomized trials of intraventricular streptokinase, urokinase, and TPA, as well as two small randomized trials, have collectively shown that there is no reduction in VPS surgery and there is a risk of secondary intraventricular bleeding in infants receiving these agents.[52]

External Ventricular Drain

The insertion of an external ventricular drain is a logical way of providing continuous relief from raised pressure, preventing distortion from ventricular enlargement,

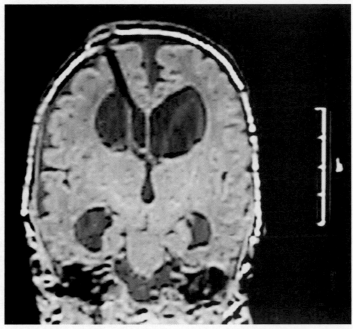

Fig. 3.5 T1-weighted coronal magnetic resonance image showing ventricular dilation with a subcutaneous Ommaya reservoir and catheter to the right lateral ventricle.

and removing protein and red blood cells. This approach has certainly been used in a small number of centers, but to our knowledge it has not been tested in a randomized trial.[53] The concern among neurosurgeons has been the risk of infection from prolonged presence of a ventricular drain.

Tapping Via an Ommaya Reservoir

The most widely used approach we have encountered in neonatal units that treat a considerable number of infants with PHVD is the insertion of ventricular access device—for example, an Ommaya reservoir (Fig. 3.5)—in those cases in which repeated tapping is necessary to control excessive head enlargement and suspected raised pressure. This approach approximates that used in the conservative arm of the Ventriculomegaly Trial and the PHVD Drug Trial and, in our view, should be regarded as standard treatment now. Not all infants with PHVD demonstrate excessive head enlargement or signs of raised pressure, so this is a selective approach. Once it becomes obvious that repeated CSF tapping is necessary, the surgically inserted reservoir enables it to be done whenever the need arises even in a small peripheral neonatal unit without neurosurgical or tertiary care neonatologists. This approach has been published but not yet tested in a randomized trial.[54] It is clear that in a unit with a sufficient volume of patients, a ventricular access device can be inserted into any extremely small infant (e.g., 700 g) with a very low complication rate. In Bristol a total of 100 such procedures have been carried out in preterm infants over 10 years with no cases of perioperative mortality and only one infection. There is currently a trial (ISRCTN43171322) of this approach comparing low-threshold intervention (ventricular width >97th centile and frontal horn 6 mm) with high-threshold intervention (ventricular width 4 mm over the 97th centile and frontal horn 10 mm).

Ventriculosubgaleal Shunt

This procedure involves insertion of a ventricular catheter with a subcutaneous reservoir connected to a distal catheter ending in the subgaleal space. There is usually a valve in a subgaleal shunt. Ventricular fluid can then accumulate outside the skull but under the skin. Absorption of CSF is slow from this site and a marked swelling becomes obvious on one side of the skull. This procedure is seen as an alternative to an Ommaya ventricular reservoir. The advantage is that ventricular drainage and control of intracranial pressure can occur continuously, whereas drainage and control of pressure are intermittent with tapping a ventricular reservoir. One advantage of using a reservoir is that the frequency and volume of taps can be increased or decreased according to need. This cannot be done with a subgaleal shunt. The subcutaneous swelling can sometimes interfere with measuring changes in head circumference, so interpretation has to allow for this and frequent scans are needed.

Limbrick et al.[55] reviewed 95 infants with PHVD treated either with a ventricular reservoir or a subgaleal shunt. One of 30 subgaleal shunts became infected compared with 4 of 65 ventricular reservoirs. There was no difference in the proportion requiring a permanent ventriculoperitoneal shunt.

Third Ventriculostomy

Third ventriculostomy is carried out endoscopically and can be a good treatment for other types of hydrocephalus, especially aqueduct stenosis. The endoscope is inserted into the ventricular system and then into the third ventricle. A hole is made in the midline of the floor of the third ventricle, with care to avoid the arteries on either side. This communication between the third ventricle and the subarachnoid space allows CSF to bypass obstruction in the aqueduct and foramina of the fourth ventricle. However, in PHVD, the problem is reabsorption of CSF and is not usually restricted to the aqueduct and fourth ventricle. Experience with third ventriculostomy in PHVD has been limited and the results disappointing.[56]

Choroid Plexus Coagulation

Choroid plexus coagulation is carried out endoscopically and is based on most CSF production arising from the choroid plexus within the lateral ventricles and third ventricle. Because the problem with PHVD is primarily failed reabsorption and not overproduction of CSF, it would seem unlikely that this approach would be successful in PHVD. Choroid plexus coagulation has never been subjected to a controlled trial in PHVD.[57]

Drainage, Irrigation, and Fibrinolytic Therapy

Drainage, irrigation, and fibrinolytic therapy (DRIFT), also known as ventricular lavage, is an approach that grew out of the unsatisfactory results of the preceding treatments and the emerging evidence that free radical injury and inflammation result from intraventricular blood and injure the brain over many weeks (Fig. 3.6). The objectives are to remove as much as possible of the intraventricular blood and to gently decompress the ventricles earlier.

The procedure involves insertion of right frontal and left occipital ventricular catheters. TPA is injected intraventricularly at a dose 0.5 mg/kg that is insufficient to produce a systemic effect, and it is left for approximately 8 hours. The occipital ventricular catheter is connected to a sterile closed ventricular drainage system, and the height of the drainage reservoir is adjusted to keep intracranial pressure below 7 mm Hg. Artificial Cerebrospinal Fluid (Torbay Pharmaceutical, Torbay, UK) is then pumped into the frontal ventricular catheter at 20 mL/hr with continuous intracranial pressure monitoring. The drainage fluid initially looks like cola but gradually clears to look like white wine, at which point irrigation is stopped and the catheters are removed. This process commonly takes 72 hours but can require up to 7 days.

Ventricular lavage has been tested in a randomized trial that recruited 77 preterm infants with PHVD; 39 received DRIFT and 38 received standard treatment (LP followed by ventricular reservoir to be tapped to control expansion and pressure). There was no reduction in the proportion of either group who underwent surgical shunt placement or died.[58] All survivors were followed up at 2 years corrected age. Of the 39 patients in the DRIFT group, 21 (54%) were severely disabled or dead compared with 27 of the 38 (71%) in the standard treatment group. Eleven of 35 survivors assessed with the Bayley scale (31%) in the DRIFT group had severe cognitive disability compared with 19 of 32 (59%)

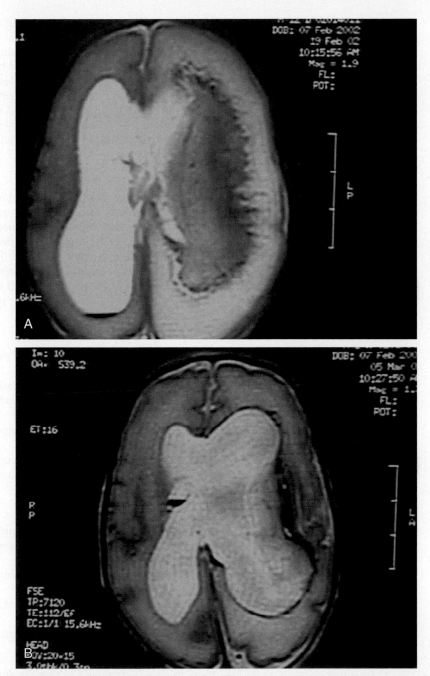

Fig. 3.6   T2-weighted magnetic resonance images of an infant with posthemorrhagic ventricular dilation. A, This image shows extensive intraventricular debris, parenchymal injury and edema of the left ventricle, and gravitation of blood to the occipital pole of the right ventricle. B, Image in the same infant after DRIFT (drainage, irrigation, and fibrinolytic therapy) showing that the intraventricular debris has been removed and the hemispheric edema reduced.

in the standard group.[59] There was significantly more secondary intraventricular bleeding in the DRIFT group, but the bleeding was not associated with increased disability.

At 10 years of age, mean cognitive quotient was 69 in the DRIFT group compared with 54 in the standard group. Twenty-one of 32 patients (66%) who received DRIFT were alive with no severe cognitive disability compared with only 11 of 30 (37%) in the standard group.[60] This difference in cognitive development corresponds to well over a year, educationally important. Ventricular lavage is the only intervention for PHVD that has been objectively shown to improve any outcome, but it is a demanding and invasive procedure requiring close collaboration among neonatologist, neuroimaging service, and neurosurgeon.

Schulz et al.[61] described a simpler method of ventricular lavage, using an endoscope in the operating room, in 19 neonates with PHVD. They lavaged both lateral and the third ventricles with 2 to 3 L of Ringer solution in a single session. This approach may be more suitable for dissemination but needs more objective evaluation. Although there are good grounds for wanting to remove harmful substances in CSF by ventricular lavage, the possibility of also removing necessary substances such as growth factors exists. Injection of stem cells at the end of ventricular lavage offers a possible solution.

Stem Cell Therapy

Using a rat model of IVH, Ang et al. have shown that intraventricular injection of umbilical cord–derived mesenchymal stem cells reduces PHVD and inflammatory markers while improving myelination and neuromotor function when administered 2 days, but not 7 days, after IVH.[62] This impressive effect may be due to upregulation of brain-derived neurotrophic factor (BDNF).[63] This group is now conducting a trial of intraventricular human umbilical cord–derived mesenchymal stem cells in infants within 7 days of diagnosis of grade III or IV IVH (NCT02274428).[64]

Conclusions

1. Posthemorrhagic hydrocephalus is characterized by deposition of extracellular matrix proteins weeks after intraventricular hemorrhage.
2. Raised intracranial pressure, distortion, inflammation, and free radical injury from iron are mechanisms by which periventricular white matter can be progressively injured.
3. Eight different therapeutic approaches have been used without objective evidence of efficacy and safety.
4. Although ventricular lavage, in a small randomized trial, reduced cognitive disability, this is still an experimental treatment requiring more evidence.

Gaps in Knowledge

Gaps in knowledge about PHVD can be summarized in the following questions:
1. How important is injury from free radicals, and can chelation improve neurologic outcome or reduce shunt dependence?
2. Does very early drainage of CSF to prevent distortion and pressure improve neurologic outcome or reduce shunt dependence?
3. Can ventricular lavage be made more efficient, easier, and safer so that it can be tested in more centers?
4. Can stem cell therapy early after IVH reduce PHVD and its consequences?

REFERENCES

1. Volpe JJ. *Neurology of the Newborn*. 5th ed. Philadelphia: WB Saunders; 2008:428–493.
2. Murphy BP, Inder TE, Rooks V, et al. Posthemorrhagic ventricular dilatation in the premature infant: natural history and predictors of outcome. *Arch Dis Child*. 2002;87:F37–F41.
3. Ventriculomegaly Trial Group. Randomised trial of early tapping in neonatal posthaemorrhagic ventricular dilatation. *Arch Dis Child*. 1990;65:3–10.
4. International PHVD. Drug Trial Group. International randomised trial of acetazolamide and furosemide in posthaemorrhagic ventricular dilatation. *Lancet*. 1998;352:433–440.
5. Papile LA, Burstein J, Burstein R, Koffler H. Incidence and evolution of subependymal and intraventricular hemorrhage: a study of infants with birth weights less than 1,500 gm. *J Pediatr*. 1978;92:529–534.
6. De Vries LS, Dubowitz LM, Dubowitz V, et al. Predictive value of cranial ultrasound in the newborn baby: a reappraisal. *Lancet*. 1985;20;2(8447):137–140.
7. Levene M. Measurement of the growth of the lateral ventricle in preterm infants with real-time ultrasound. *Arch Dis Child*. 1981;56:900–904.
8. Davies MW, Swaminathan M, Chuang SL, et al. Reference ranges for linear dimensions of intracranial ventricles in preterm neonates. *Arch Dis Child*. 2000;82:F218–F223.

9. Kaiser A, Whitelaw A. Cerebrospinal fluid pressure during posthemorrhagic ventricular dilatation in newborn infants. *Arch Dis Child*. 1985;60:920–923.

10. Fenton TR. A new growth chart for preterm babies: Babson and Benda's chart updated with recent data and a new format. *BMC Pediatrics*. 2003;3:13.

11. Quinn MW, Ando Y, Levene MI. Cerebral arterial and venous flow-velocity measurements in posthaemorrhagic ventricular dilatation. *Dev Med Child Neurol*. 1992;34:863–869.

12. Taylor GA, Madsen JR. Neonatal hydrocephalus: hemodynamic response to fontanelle compression: correlation with intracranial pressure and need for shunt placement. *Radiology*. 1996;201:685–689.

13. Olischar M, Klebermass K, Hengl B, et al. Cerebrospinal fluid drainage in posthaemorrhagic ventricular dilatation leads to improvement in amplitude-integrated electroencephalographic activity. *Acta Paediatr*. 2009;98:1002–1009.

14. Inder TE, Wells SJ, Mogridge NB, et al. Defining the nature of the cerebral abnormalities in the premature infant: a qualitative magnetic resonance imaging study. *J Pediatr*. 2003;143:171–179.

15. Hill A, Shackelford GD, Volpe JJ. A potential mechanism of pathogenesis for early post-hemorrhagic hydrocephalus in the premature newborn. *Pediatrics*. 1984;73:19–21.

16. Whitelaw A, Mowinckel MC, Abildgaard U. Low levels of plasminogen in cerebrospinal fluid after intraventricular haemorrhage: a limiting factor for clot lysis? *Acta Paediatr*. 1995;84:933–936.

17. Hansen A, Whitelaw A, Lapp C, Brugnara C. Cerebrospinal fluid plasminogen activator inhibitor-1: a prognostic factor in posthaemorrhagic hydrocephalus. *Acta Paediatr*. 1997;86:995–998.

18. Larroche JC. Posthemorrhagic hydrocephalus in infancy. *BioNeonate*. 1972;20:287–299.

19. Beck LS, Chen TL, Amman AJ, et al. Accelerated healing of ulcer wounds in the rabbit ear by recombinant human transforming growth factor beta-1. *Growth Factors*. 1990;2:273–282.

20. Ignotz RA, Massague J. Transforming growth factor beta stimulates the expression of fibronectin and collagen and their incorporation into the extracellular matrix. *J Biol Chem*. 1986;261:4337–4345.

21. Roberts AB, Sporn MB, Assoian RK, et al. Transforming growth factor type β: rapid induction of fibrosis and angiogenesis in vivo and stimulation of collagen formation in vitro. *Proc Natl Acad Sci USA*. 1986;83:4167–4171.

22. Border WA, Ruoslahti E. Transforming growth factor-beta 1 induces extracellular matrix formation in glomerulonephritis. *Cell Differ Dev*. 1990;32:425–431.

23. Castilla A, Prieto J, Fausto N. Transforming growth factors beta 1 and alpha in chronic liver disease. Effects of interferon alfa therapy. *N Engl J Med*. 1991;324:933–940.

24. Kitazawa K, Tada T. Elevation of transforming growth factor beta-1 level in cerebrospinal fluid of patients with communicating hydrocephalus after subarachnoid hemorrhage. *Stroke*. 1994;25:1400–1404.

25. Tada T, Kanaji M, Kobayashi S. Induction of communicating hydrocephalus in mice by intrathecal injection of human recombinant transforming growth factor beta-1. *J Neuroimmunol*. 1994;50:153–158.

26. Whitelaw A, Christie S, Pople I. Transforming growth factor β-1: a possible signal molecule for posthemorrhagic hydrocephalus? *Pediatr Res*. 1999;46:576–580.

27. Heep A, Bartmann P, Stoffel-Wagner B, et al. Cerebrospinal fluid obstruction and malabsorption in human neonatal hydrocephaly. *Childs Nerv Syst*. 2006;22:1249–1255.

28. Chow LC, Soliman A, Zandian M, et al. Accumulation of transforming growth factor-beta2 and nitrated chondroitin sulfate proteoglycans in cerebrospinal fluid correlates with poor neurologic outcome in preterm hydrocephalus. *Biol Neonate*. 2005;88:1–11.

29. Cherian SS, Love S, Silver IA, et al. Posthemorrhagic ventricular dilation in the neonate: development and characterization of a rat model. *J Neuropathol Exp Neurol*. 2003;62:292–303.

30. Cherian S, Thoresen M, Silver IA, et al. Transforming growth factor-betas in a rat model of neonatal posthaemorrhagic hydrocephalus. *Neuropathol Appl Neurobiol*. 2004;30:585–600.

31. Wyss-Coray T, Feng L, Masliah E, et al. Increased central nervous system production of extracellular matrix components and development of hydrocephalus in transgenic mice overexpressing transforming growth factor-beta 1. *Am J Pathol*. 1995;147:53–67.

32. Aquilina K, Hobbs C, Tucker A, et al. Do drugs that block transforming growth factor beta reduce posthaemorrhagic ventricular dilatation in a neonatal rat model? *Acta Paediatr*. 2008;97:1181–1186.

33. Del Bigio MR. Neuropathological changes caused by hydrocephalus. *Acta Neuropathol*. 1993;85:573–585.

34. Savman K, Nilsson UA, Blennow M, et al. Non-protein-bound iron is elevated in cerebrospinal fluid from preterm infants with posthemorrhagic ventricular dilatation. *Pediatr Res*. 2001;49:208–212.

35. Inder T, Mocatta T, Darlow B, et al. Elevated free radical products in the cerebrospinal fluid of VLBW infants with cerebral white matter injury. *Pediatr Res*. 2002;52:213–218.

36. Bejar R, Saugstad OD, James H, Gluck L. Increased hypoxanthine concentrations in cerebrospinal fluid of infants with hydrocephalus. *J Pediatr*. 1983;103:44–48.

37. Nishino T, Tamura I. The mechanism of conversion of xanthine dehydrogenase to oxidase and the role of the enzyme in reperfusion injury. *Adv Exp Med Biol*. 1991;309A:327–333.

38. Back SA, Luo NL, Borenstein NS, et al. Late oligodendrocyte progenitors coincide with the developmental window of vulnerability for human perinatal white matter injury. *J Neurosci*. 2001;21:1302–1312.

39. Leviton A, Paneth N, Reuss ML, et al. Maternal infection, fetal inflammatory response, and brain damage in very low birth weight infants. *Pediatr Res*. 1999;46:566–575.

40. Savman K, Blennow M, Hagberg H, et al. Cytokine responses in cerebrospinal fluid from preterm infants with posthaemorrhagic ventricular dilatation. *Acta Paediatr*. 2002;91:1357–1363.

41. Kadhim H, Tabarki B, Verellen G, et al. Inflammatory cytokines in the pathogenesis of periventricular leukomalacia. *Neurology*. 2001;56:1278–1284.

42. Cherian S, Whitelaw A, Thoresen M, Love S. The pathogenesis of neonatal post-hemorrhagic hydrocephalus. *Brain Pathol*. 2004;14:305–311.

43. Hislop JE, Dubowitz LM, Kaiser AM, et al. Outcome of infants shunted for post-haemorrhagic ventricular dilatation. *Dev Med Child Neurol*. 1988;30:451–456.

44. Taylor AG, Peter JC. Advantages of delayed VP shunting in post-haemorrhagic hydrocephalus seen in low-birth-weight infants. *Childs Nerv Syst*. 2001;17:328–333.

45. Tuli S. Risk factors for repeated cerebrospinal shunt failures in pediatric patients with hydrocephalus. *J Neurosurg*. 2000;92:31–38.

46. Kreusser KL, Tarby TJ, Kovnar E, et al. Serial lumbar punctures for at least temporary amelioration of neonatal posthemorrhagic hydrocephalus. *Pediatrics*. 1985;75:719–724.

47. Whitelaw A. Repeated lumbar or ventricular punctures in newborns with intraventricular hemorrhage. *Cochrane Database Syst Rev*. 2001;(1):CD000216.

48. Thoresen M, Whitelaw A. Effect of acetazolamide on cerebral blood flow velocity and CO_2 elimination in normotensive and hypotensive newborn piglets. *Biol Neonate*. 1990;58:200–207.

49. Cowan F, Whitelaw A. Acute effects of acetazolamide on cerebral blood flow velocity and pCO_2 in the newborn infant. *Acta Paediatr Scand*. 1991;80:22–27.

50. Whitelaw A, Kennedy CR, Brion LP. Diuretic therapy for newborn infants with posthemorrhagic ventricular dilatation. *Cochrane Database Syst Rev*. 2001;(2):CD002270.

51. Pang D, Sclabassi RJ, Horton JA. Lysis of intraventricular blood clot with urokinase in a canine model: Part 3. Effects of intraventricular urokinase on clot lysis and posthemorrhagic hydrocephalus. *Neurosurgery*. 1986;19:553–572.

52. Whitelaw A, Odd DE. Intraventricular streptokinase after intraventricular hemorrhage in newborn infants. *Cochrane Database Syst Rev*. 2007;(4):CD000498.

53. Berger A, Weninger M, Reinprecht A, et al. Long-term experience with subcutaneously tunneled external ventricular drainage in preterm infants. *Childs Nerv Syst*. 2000;16:103–109.

54. de Vries LS, Liem KD, van Dijk K, Dutch Working Group of Neonatal Neurology, et al. Early versus late treatment of posthaemorrhagic ventricular dilatation: results of a retrospective study from five neonatal intensive care units in The Netherlands. *Acta Paediatr*. 2002;91:212–217.

55. Limbrick DD Jr, Mathur A, Johnston JM, et al. Neurosurgical treatment of progressive posthemorrhagic ventricular dilation in preterm infants: a 10-year single-institution study. *J Neurosurg Pediatr*. 2010;6(3):224–230.

56. Buxton N, Macarthur D, Mallucci C, et al. Neuroendoscopic third ventriculostomy in patients less than 1 year old. *Pediatr Neurosurg*. 1998;29:73–76.

57. Pople IK, Edwards RJ, Aquilina K. Endoscopic methods of hydrocephalus treatment. *Neurosurg Clin N Am*. 2001;12:719–735.

58. Whitelaw A, Evans D, Carter M, et al. Randomized clinical trial of prevention of hydrocephalus after intraventricular hemorrhage in preterm infants: brain-washing versus tapping fluid. *Pediatrics*. 2007;119:e1071–e1078.

59. Whitelaw A, Jary S, Kmita G, et al. Randomized trial of drainage, irrigation and fibrinolytic therapy for premature infants with posthemorrhagic ventricular dilatation: developmental outcome at 2 years. *Pediatrics*. 2010;125:e852–e858.

60. Odd D, Jary S, Lea C, et al. Drainage, irrigation and fibrinolytic therapy (DRIFT) for premature infants with posthaemorrhagic ventricular dilatation; neurodisability at school-age. Presented at the Neonatal Society; 23rd June 2016; Cambridge. www.neonatalsociety.ac.uk.

61. Schulz M, Bührer C, Pohl-Schickinger A, et al. Neuroendoscopic lavage for the treatment of intraventricular hemorrhage and hydrocephalus in neonates. *J Neurosurg Pediatr*. June 2014;13(6):626–635.

62. Park WS, Sung SI, Ahn SY, et al. Optimal timing of mesenchymal stem cell therapy for neonatal intraventricular hemorrhage. *Cell Transplant*. 2016;25(6):1131–1144.

63. Ahn SY, Chang YS, Sung DK, et al. Pivotal role of brain derived neurotrophic factor secreted by mesenchymal stem cells in severe intraventricular hemorrhage in the newborn rats. *Cell Transplant*. 2017;26(1):145–156.

64. Ahn SY, Chang YS, Park WS. Stem cells for neonatal brain disorders. *Neonatology*. 2016;109(4):377–383.

CHAPTER 4

Hypothermia for Neonatal Hypoxic-Ischemic Encephalopathy: Different Cooling Regimens and Infants Not Included in Prior Trials

Adrienne Bingham and Abbot R. Laptook

4

- There is strong rationale for further investigation of therapeutic hypothermia.
- A longer duration of cooling or a lower temperature for cooling when treating hypoxic-ischemic encephalopathy can be associated with harm.
- There is biologic and clinical rationale for initiating therapeutic hypothermia after 6 hours of age and this deserves clinical testing.
- Cooling on transport is effective when performed with a device that can control core temperature.
- There is little data to indicate benefit from hypothermia for hypoxic-ischemic encephalopathy among with infants with a mild encephalopathy, preterm infants or infants in low or middle-income countries.

Therapeutic hypothermia is an effective therapy for neonatal encephalopathy when the likelihood of a hypoxic-ischemic origin is high. Multiple randomized trials demonstrated that relatively small reductions in core temperature either alone, or in combination with reduced head temperature, reduced death or disability at 18 months.[1–6] The Cochrane meta-analysis indicates that therapeutic hypothermia reduced the composite outcome of death or major neurodevelopmental disability in survivors from 61% in noncooled infants compared with 46% in infants treated with hypothermia, yielding a risk ratio of 0.75 (95% confidence interval [CI] 0.68–0.83).[7] Components of the primary outcome were also reduced by hypothermia; death was decreased from 34% to 25% (risk ratio 0.75, 95% CI 0.64–0.88), and disability was reduced from 24.9% to 19.2% (risk ratio 0.77, 95% CI 0.63–0.94). Disability was typically severe and could be any of cognitive, motor, or sensory deficits. Neuroprotective effects of therapeutic hypothermia persisted even at 6 to 7 years.[8,9] The importance of this therapy extends beyond the benefits provided to infants and their families; it signifies that hypoxic-ischemic brain injury is modifiable and has accelerated testing other potential neuroprotective interventions either with or without therapeutic hypothermia.[10] Given the beneficial effects of hypothermia, the Committee on the Fetus and Newborn of the American Academy of Pediatrics has provided an overview of the available data and expectations for centers that provide this therapy.[11]

Hypothermia regimens have multiple components (Box 4.1) that contribute to three phases of the therapy: induction, maintenance, and rewarming. Induction represents the time from initiation of cooling to reaching target temperature; maintenance represents the duration of keeping the infant at the target temperature; and rewarming represents the reestablishment of a normothermic temperature. The initial trials of hypothermia[1–6] used remarkably similar cooling regimens. Specifically, the age of initiation was always less than 6 hours after birth, the extent of temperature reduction was 33.5°C for whole-body cooling

> **Box 4.1** COMPONENTS OF A THERAPEUTIC HYPOTHERMIA REGIMEN
>
> - Age of initiation of cooling
> - Target temperature
> - Duration of cooling
> - Rate of rewarming
> - Mode of cooling

and 34.5°C for head combined with body cooling, the duration of cooling was 72 hours, and the rate of rewarming was 0.5°C/hr. The similarity in hypothermia regimens facilitated meta-analyses of multiple trials to provide more accurate estimates of patient outcomes.[7] The only major component of cooling regimens that differed among the initial trials was the mode of cooling: whole-body versus head with body cooling. Meta-analysis indicated that outcomes are similar irrespective of the mode of cooling.[7]

Rationale for Further Investigations of Therapeutic Hypothermia

There are several justifications to perform further study of hypothermia even when the results of multiple trials demonstrated reductions in death or disability.[1–6] First, the Cochrane meta-analysis indicates that 46% of infants treated with hypothermia either die or are diagnosed with moderate or severe impairment.[7] There is obviously a need for improvement in outcome. Additional trials of hypothermia could be viewed as diverting valuable research resources from investigation of other potential neuroprotective agents, such as erythropoietin, xenon, and melatonin.[10] This raises the second justification that refinement of the cooling regimen holds promise that outcomes could be further improved since hypothermia was studied as a package with little variability in the components of the regimen. Furthermore, many of the hypothermia components used in the first series of trials[1–6] represented "a best estimate" based on animal investigation and pilot human studies. Third, the application of therapeutic hypothermia was limited to a specific group of newborns—that is, those with a diagnosis of hypoxia-ischemia presenting at less than 6 hours of age and with a gestational age of at least 36 weeks. These trials did not address other cohorts of newborns (preterm, mild encephalopathy, or cooling in low-resource countries).

This chapter addresses two major domains concerning therapeutic hypothermia. First, will there be clinical trials designed to improve the hypothermia regimen? Second, will there be clinical trials and observational studies that address extending hypothermia to infants not enrolled in the first series of hypothermia trials?[1–6] These domains are consistent with the priorities for investigation of neuroprotective therapies for newborn infants published by the National Institute of Child Health Consensus Workshop on therapeutic hypothermia.[12]

What Is the Optimal Temperature and Duration for Therapeutic Hypothermia?

The depth of temperature reduction used in the first series of hypothermia trials[1–6] was extrapolated from preclinical investigation and pilot studies in newborns. Recognition that small changes in brain temperature modified the extent of hypoxic-ischemic brain injury in adult animals[13] prompted perinatal animal investigations to examine the effects of depth and duration of "modest hypothermia" at varying times after brain hypoxia-ischemia. Modest hypothermia encompassed a range of temperature reductions from as little as 2°C to as much as 5°C using newborn swine, rat pups, and fetal sheep.[14–18] This range reflected concerns regarding a possible trade-off between the potential benefit of lower temperature and adverse effects of hypothermia, which increase with greater reductions in core temperature.[19] An interesting caveat in using animal investigation to plan clinical trials is that the basal temperature of newborn animals differs; for example, the resting temperature of newborn

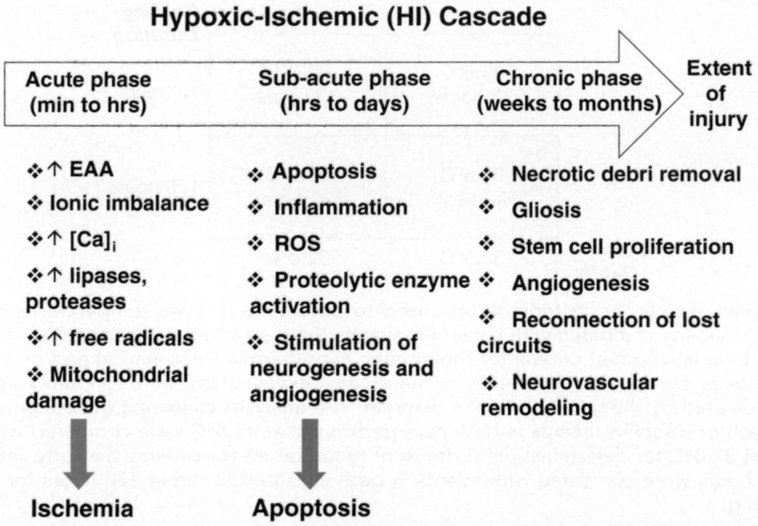

Hypoxic-Ischemic (HI) Cascade

Acute phase (min to hrs)	Sub-acute phase (hrs to days)	Chronic phase (weeks to months)	Extent of injury
❖ ↑ EAA	❖ Apoptosis	❖ Necrotic debri removal	
❖ Ionic imbalance	❖ Inflammation	❖ Gliosis	
❖ ↑ [Ca]$_i$	❖ ROS	❖ Stem cell proliferation	
❖ ↑ lipases, proteases	❖ Proteolytic enzyme activation	❖ Angiogenesis	
❖ ↑ free radicals	❖ Stimulation of neurogenesis and angiogenesis	❖ Reconnection of lost circuits	
❖ Mitochondrial damage		❖ Neurovascular remodeling	

Ischemia   Apoptosis

Fig. 4.1   There are multiple mechanisms that mediate brain injury among term infants; the temporal profile of these mechanisms overlaps but extends for periods of hours to days. (Data from Ferriero DM. Neonatal brain injury. N Engl J Med. 2004;351[19]:1985–1995.)

swine is 38.5°C to 39.0°C, whereas the nesting temperature of newborn rat pups is 36.0°C to 36.5°C. Comparison of the extent of neuroprotection associated with hypothermia using animals needs an awareness of the relative temperature reduction and the absolute temperature achieved. The optimal temperature to use for hypothermic intervention in clinical trials was not known but was guided by existing animal data and the assessment of incremental reductions in core temperature in pilot human studies of head cooling combined with body cooling[20,21] and whole-body cooling.[22] Based on this body of work, clinical trials of head cooling combined with body cooling and whole-body cooling alone were conducted at a rectal temperature of 34.5°C and an esophageal temperature of 33.5°C, respectively.[1,2]

The optimal duration of hypothermia was also uncertain when the first series of clinical trials of hypothermia were undertaken in newborn infants.[1–6] Available data were derived primarily from adult animals and indicated that increasing the duration of hypothermia reduced brain injury compared with shorter cooling intervals.[23–25] Although not studied as extensively in newborn animals, 21-day-old rat pups subjected to hypoxia-ischemia had reduced brain injury when cooling was extended to 72 hours compared with 6 hours.[26] Pilot studies in preparation to study hypothermia after brain ischemia in fetal sheep by Gunn et al. indicated rebound epileptiform activity when cooling was stopped after 48 hours but not observed if cooling was continued for 72 hours.[17] Based on these series of studies, clinical trials of head cooling with mild body cooling and whole-body cooling used a 72-hour cooling intervention.

The absence of strong evidence for the depth and duration of cooling and the approximate 46% of infants with an outcome of death or disability despite hypothermia therapy provided unequivocal rationale for further investigation. The rationale became even stronger with a growing appreciation that the temporal profile of the pathways to injury is not confined to the early hours following hypoxia-ischemia but extends to days following the insult (Fig. 4.1).[27,28]

In response to these knowledge gaps, the National Institute of Child Health and Human Development (NICHD) Neonatal Research Network (NRN) conducted a randomized clinical trial of cooling to a lower temperature and for a longer duration (Optimizing Cooling Trial, NCT 01192776).[29] The Optimizing Cooling Trial was a randomized 2 × 2 factorial design performed at 18 centers to determine if longer cooling (120 hours), deeper cooling (32.0°C), or both initiated before 6 hours of age are superior to cooling at 33.5°C for 72 hours among infants of at least 36 weeks' gestation with moderate or severe hypoxic-ischemic encephalopathy (HIE) (Fig. 4.2). The primary outcome was death or disability at 18 to 22 months adjusted for

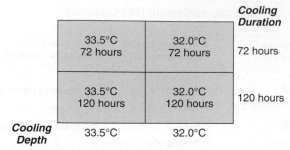

Fig. 4.2 The figure depicts the factorial design used to determine if lower temperatures or longer cooling reduces death or disability compared with cooling regimens that use a target temperature of 33.5°C and duration of 72 hours. Infants who met criteria for therapeutic hypothermia (biochemical and/or clinical criteria followed by moderate or severe encephalopathy on neurologic examination) were randomly assigned to one of four groups as indicated by the four cells of the diagram. The analyses examined the margins of the figure for differences in death or disability. Infants in both cells performed at 33.5°C were compared with infants in both cells performed at 32.0°C for determination of depth of temperature for cooling. Similarly, infants in both cells performed at 72 hours were compared with infants in both cells performed at 120 hours for determination of duration for cooling.

center and level of encephalopathy. The trial was closed to patient enrollment after 364 of a planned 726 infants were enrolled based on recommendations of an independent Data Safety Monitoring Committee. In-hospital mortality rates for cooling of 72 compared with 120 hours' duration were 11% and 16%, respectively (adjusted risk ratio [aRR] 1.37, 95% CI 0.92–2.04). In-hospital mortality rates for cooling at 33.5°C compared with 32.0°C were 12% and 16%, respectively (aRR 1.24, 95% CI 0.69–2.25). Although not statistically different, the risk ratio and boundary of the 95% CI suggest that longer cooling maybe associated with an increase in mortality. Cooling for 120 hours was associated with more arrhythmias, anuria, and a longer length of hospital stay compared with 72 hours of cooling, whereas cooling to 32.0°C was associated with a higher use of inhaled nitric oxide, extracorporeal membrane oxygenation, longer use of supplemental oxygen, and a higher incidence of bradycardia compared with cooling to 33.5°C. A preliminary report of the 18-month follow-up indicated that death or disability occurred in 32% of infants cooled for 72 hours and 32% for infants cooled for 120 hours (aRR 0.92, 95% CI 0.68–1.25), 32% of infants cooled to 33.5°C, and 31% for infants cooled to 32.0°C (aRR 0.92, 95% CI 0.68–1.26).[30]

The results of this trial indicate that among infants of at least 36 weeks' gestation with HIE, longer cooling was not superior to 72 hours of cooling and deeper cooling was not superior to cooling to 33.5°C. Despite the paucity of data to support the depth and duration of hypothermia in the first series of cooling trials,[1-6] the Optimizing Cooling Trial supports the continued practice of whole-body hypothermia at 33.5°C for 72 hours and drift from this practice could be associated with increased mortality and morbidity.

How Late Can Hypothermia be Initiated?

The time of initiation of hypothermia represents the component of a hypothermia regimen studied in the most systematic fashion in preclinical investigations. Gunn et al. performed a series of fetal sheep studies where 30 minutes of brain ischemia was followed by 72 hours of hypothermia (cooling cap positioned on the fetal head in utero) initiated at 1.5, 5.5 and 8.5 hours following ischemia.[17,31,32] A neuronal loss score in different brain regions was assessed at 48 hours after completion of hypothermia and demonstrated that the extent of neuroprotection was time sensitive. Earlier cooling was neuroprotective (initiation at 1.5 more so than 5.5 hours) but later cooling (initiation at 8.5 hours) was not. These experiments provided the rationale for initiation of cooling within 6 hours of birth in the first series of human cooling trials.[1-6] These trials, however, could not determine if initiation of

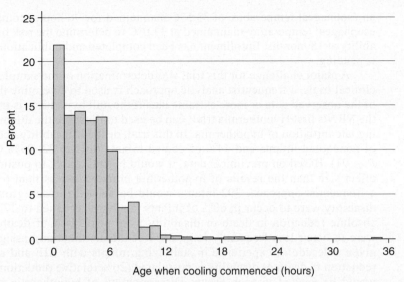

Fig. 4.3 The age of initiation of cooling among 1331 infants provided therapeutic hypothermia in the TOBY registry. (Reprinted with permission from Azzopardi, Strohm B, Linsell L, et al. Implementation and conduct of therapeutic hypothermia for perinatal asphyxial encephalopathy in the UK—analysis of national data. *PLoS One.* 2012;7[6]:e38504.)

cooling earlier in the 6-hour window is more effective since the vast majority of enrolled infants had hypothermia initiated between 4 and 5 hours. A single-center retrospective cohort analysis of hypothermia reported that initiation of cooling at 3 hours or earlier is associated with higher psychomotor developmental scores using the Bayley II Scales of Infant Development compared with cooling initiated after 3 hours.[33]

Although these data suggest that studying initiation of hypothermia after 6 hours of age would not be of benefit, there is strong biologic and clinical rationale for further investigation. As noted for the preclinical studies of the depth of temperature reduction, data from animal models may not be readily extrapolated to newborns. A therapeutic window of 6 hours in fetal sheep seems reasonably established, but there is no information of the duration of the therapeutic window in newborns with HIE because all cooling trials initiated hypothermia by 6 hours.[7] Whether in utero preconditioning events prolong the therapeutic window is unknown.[34,35] Enrollment in clinical trials of hypothermia at less than 6 hours of age assumes that hypoxic-ischemic events occur proximate to delivery. However, precise timing of hypoxic-ischemia in utero among newborns with HIE may be inaccurate in the absence of a sentinel event, and prior trials likely enrolled infants beyond 6 hours from hypoxia-ischemia. Other important considerations are births in rural communities remote from centers that provide hypothermia, evolution of encephalopathy after 6 hours of age, and late recognition of encephalopathy. All these variables may limit application of hypothermia within a putative narrow therapeutic window. However, initiation of hypothermia after 6 hours has been reported despite the absence of evidence. A comprehensive registry established in the United Kingdom reported on the implementation of hypothermia among 1331 infants born between December 2006 and July 2011; initiation of hypothermia between 6 and 12 hours of age occurred in approximately 9% to 10% of infants and beyond 12 hours of age in 2.2% of infants (Fig. 4.3).[36]

Given the knowledge gap concerning initiation of hypothermia beyond 6 hours, the NRN has conducted a randomized trial to obtain an unbiased estimate of the probability of benefit or harm from "late" initiation of hypothermia (NCT 00614744). Infants at least 36 weeks of gestational age with moderate or severe HIE assessed at or after 6 hours up to 24 hours of age were randomly assigned to an esophageal temperature of 33.5°C maintained for 96 hours, compared with an esophageal temperature maintained at 37.0°C to determine the risk of death or disability at 18 months. Enrollment has been completed and publication of the results is pending.

A major challenge for this trial was determination of the sample size. In most clinical trials, a frequentist analytic approach is used to determine the probability of the observed data or more extreme data if the null hypothesis is true. Results of the NRN's first Hypothermia trial[2] can be used to illustrate the dilemma for studying late initiation of hypothermia. In this trial, death or disability occurred in 62% of noncooled infants and 44% of cooled infants (aRR 0.72, 95% CI 0.54–0.95, $P = .01$). Based on preclinical data, it would be reasonable to postulate a smaller effect size than the results of hypothermia initiated at less than 6 hours. Using a frequentist approach, 392 infants would be needed in each group if death or disability were to occur in 60% of infants randomly assigned to 37°C and a 10% absolute reduction in death or disability were postulated. If death or disability were to occur less frequently (e.g., 30% of infants randomly assigned to 37°C) given a decade of experience in stabilizing infants with HIE and a 6% absolute reduction in death or disability is postulated (20% relative reduction), 859 infants would be needed in each group. Dissemination of hypothermia at less than 6 hours of age across the neonatology community made it prohibitive to plan such a large trial.

An alternative approach is to use a Bayesian analysis, which provides different information for hypothesis testing than a frequentist analysis and was prespecified in the NRN trial of late initiation of hypothermia. A Bayesian analysis provides the probability that the hypothesis is true based on the observed data. It is a formal statistical method to assess the range of treatment effects compatible with the best available evidence and is recommended for trials with limited sample size.[37] In contrast to a traditional frequentist analysis, a Bayesian analysis uses preexisting data (pilot studies, clinical trials, observational reports, and animal work) to establish a prior distribution representing the probability of a hypothesized treatment effect (Fig. 4.4A). The position of the prior distribution along an axis of risk ratio values depends on the available data at the start of the trial; if there are few data available concerning the intervention, the prior distribution can be centered at 1.0, indicating an equal number of infants may benefit or be harmed (neutral prior). If existing data support benefit, or alternatively, harm of the intervention before the trial, the prior distribution can be shifted to a risk ratio that best represents the available data (enthusiastic or skeptical prior distribution). The prior distribution is then combined with the observed data from the trial to yield a posterior probability of treatment effect (Fig. 4.4B). The latter can be characterized by the area under the curve less than aRR of 1.0 and represents the posterior probability of a treatment benefit (e.g., reduction in death or disability). The level of probability that clinicians feel justified to use a specific therapy in practice will reflect the severity of the outcome targeted by the intervention and possible hazard associated with the treatment. A Bayesian analysis can thereby provide clinicians with the best estimate of treatment effect when definitive results using a frequentist approach are not feasible.

Should Infants With Mild HIE Receive Hypothermia Therapy?

Infants with mild encephalopathy were not part of the inclusion criteria of the initial randomized trials of therapeutic hypothermia[1-6] based on reported favorable outcome of infants with mild encephalopathy. An excellent example of the latter is an observational, prospective cohort of 226 infants of at least 37 weeks' gestation with evidence of HIE born between 1974 and 1979 from western Canada.[38] The relationship between stage of encephalopathy (mild n = 79, moderate n = 119, severe n = 28) and subsequent neurodevelopmental and school-age follow-up was based on the most *severe stage* during the first week of life. Among infants with mild HIE, there were no deaths or handicap (cerebral palsy, sensory impairment, cognitive delay, or

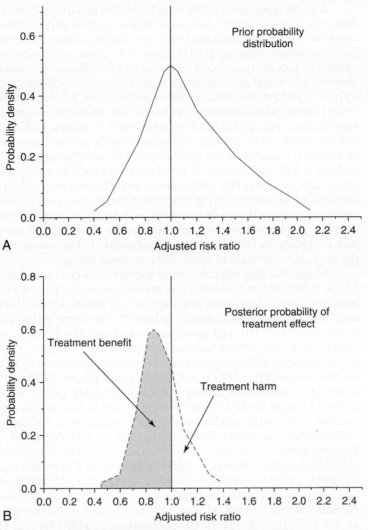

Fig. 4.4   A, A theoretical prior distribution representing the probability of a hypothesized treatment effect. This example is a neutral prior distribution centered at a risk ratio of 1.0 and indicates an equal number of infants would be expected to be benefited by the treatment or its comparison group. Such a prior distribution could be used in testing late initiation of hypothermia given the paucity of data available when the trial was planned. B, Plot of the posterior probability of treatment effect derived by combining the prior distribution with the trial results. In this example, the distribution is shifted to the left of a risk ratio of 1.0 and can be characterized by a point estimate. The area under the curve that is less than a risk ratio on 1.0 *(stripped area)* represents the posterior probability of a reduction in a specified outcome (e.g., death or disability). The area under the curve that is greater than a risk ratio on 1.0 represents the posterior probability of an increase in an outcome.

severe seizures) at 3.5 years. A delay of more than 6 months in gross motor skills occurred in 5% of mild HIE survivors, indicating the potential for subtle injury. At 8 years, psychoeducational assessments were compared among 56 of the 79 children who had mild HIE and 155 children representing a peer group.[39] There were no differences between children who had mild HIE and the peer group for intelligence quotients (IQs), visual motor integration, receptive vocabulary, and the percent of children with delays in reading, spelling, and math. Subsequent reports indicate that children with mild encephalopathy who did not have cerebral palsy may have subtle differences from infants who did not experience mild HIE; infants with mild HIE had lower mean IQ scores (Wechsler Intelligence Scale) than controls (99 ± 17 vs. 109 ± 12, respectively).[40] Children with mild encephalopathy assessed at 9 to 10 years were reported to have more problematic behavior compared with controls, including social problems, anxiety and depression, attention regulation, and thought problems.[41]

With the completion of the initial hypothermia trials,[1-6] observations emerged from retrospective reports that some infants not provided hypothermia had adverse short-term outcomes, including seizures, feeding difficulties, and abnormal magnetic resonance imaging (MRI) scans.[42-44] These observations prompted some centers to provide therapeutic hypothermia for infants with mild HIE despite the absence of clinical trials to provide evidence of benefit or harm from this therapy.[43,45] Furthermore, none of these publications provided early childhood neurodevelopmental assessments. Although not intended, two of the first series of hypothermia trials enrolled a limited number of infants with mild HIE[5,6] and follow-up results for the primary outcome of death or disability were reported. Death or disability occurred in one trial[5] but not the other[6] among infants with mild HIE, making it difficult to reconcile these observations. The recognition of morbidities associated with mild HIE in the era of hypothermia may reflect establishment of the level of encephalopathy at less than 6 hours compared with the worst stage of encephalopathy in the first week (prehypothermia) because progression of encephalopathy is known to occur. Alternatively, the limitations of retrospective reports, lack of definitions for mild HIE, and variability in the assessment of encephalopathy may also contribute to some of these observations.

Prospective data regarding mild hypothermia determined at less than 6 hours of age is limited but provocative. A preliminary report from a multicenter research initiative described the short-term outcomes of infants with mild HIE following perinatal acidosis and/or resuscitation at birth.[46] This investigation used a standardized definition of mild HIE and examiners were trained to promote consistency among centers. Fifty-four infants had complete data and 28 infants (52%) had abnormalities of any of the following predefined short-term outcomes: an amplitude integrated electroencephalogram (EEG) before 9 hours of age, an MRI scan, and a discharge neurologic examination. Brain MRI abnormalities (17%) were mostly limited to focal changes in the cerebral cortex, except in two infants who showed abnormalities in the basal ganglia/thalamus. The majority of the discharge examination abnormalities represented persistent features of encephalopathy (22 of 54, 41%). Eighteen-month follow-up of this cohort is in progress. A prospective observational cohort from Ireland evaluated cognitive function at 5 years among infants of at least 37 weeks' gestation with HIE.[47] Children with a history of mild neonatal HIE (n = 22) had lower cognitive outcome than control infants (n = 30) for full-scale IQ (median, interquartile range, 99 [94–112] vs. 117 [110–124], $P = .001$), verbal IQ (105 [99–111] vs. 116 [112–125], $P = .001$), and performance IQ (103 [98–112] vs. 115 [107–124], $P = .004$). Although lower, the scores among children with mild HIE were close to the standardized mean and standard deviation for the test (100 ± 15). These findings support a randomized trial of hypothermia for mild HIE to determine if cognitive function can be improved.

Should Hypothermia Be Used in Preterm Infants With HIE?

Most clinical trials of hypothermia studied newborns with HIE who were at least 36 weeks' gestation.[1-4,6] One trial[5] and one pilot trial[48] enrolled a total of seven infants at 35^0 to 35^6 weeks. The Committee on the Fetus and Newborn of the American Academy of Pediatrics concluded that the efficacy of therapeutic hypothermia for infants <35 weeks gestation is lacking.[11] However, the risks and benefits of therapeutic hypothermia for infants 35 0/7 to 35 6/7 weeks' gestation cannot be determined with limited enrollment in randomized trials and further study is justified.

A major knowledge gap is the absence of definitive data on the neuropathology of hypoxic-ischemic brain injury in moderate and late preterm infants. Do the data resemble those of a term infant, for whom the pathology is dominated by selective neuronal necrosis, followed by parasagittal cerebral injury, and least commonly focal ischemic necrosis?[49] Alternatively, do the data resemble those of white matter injury and arrest of the oligodendrocyte lineage, which is the major hypoxic-ischemic lesion in extremely preterm infants?[50,51] Despite this knowledge gap, there is biologic rationale for considering therapeutic hypothermia as a treatment option for preterm infants. Brain ischemia followed by hypothermia in fetal sheep at preterm gestations indicated that cooling protects oligodendrocytes, the critical target for brain injury in preterm infants. However, protection was also noted for the brain injury pattern observed in term infants.[52] These results have provided justification to extend the use of therapeutic hypothermia to preterm infants in the presence of hypoxia-ischemic events at birth.[53]

Cooling preterm infants has been reported from single-center experiences. One publication reported on 6 newborns at a gestational age of 34 0/7 to 35 5/7 weeks with HIE who were provided hypothermia treatment.[54] All six infants survived and 25% had a severe disability at 2 years using the Bayley Scales of Infant Development (second edition). In contrast, a pilot study of head cooling in 4 infants with a gestational age of 32 to 35 weeks with HIE had a very different outcome.[55] One infant died, two survivors had severe cognitive deficits and cerebral palsy, and one survivor had moderate cerebral palsy with a Bayley Scale of Infant Development cognitive score of 90. The authors concluded that hypothermia should not be provided to preterm infants outside a clinical trial. In a larger single-center retrospective report, 31 preterm (gestational age 34–35 weeks) and 32 term infants with HIE were provided therapeutic hypothermia and compared for safety and short-term outcomes.[56] Preterm infants had more adverse events (hyperglycemia, leukopenia), more extensive injury on MRI scans, and more deaths. Intracranial hemorrhage occurred only in preterm infants (intraparenchymal, n = 2; intraventricular, n = 1). None of the infants underwent neurodevelopmental follow-up. This report demonstrates that the safety profile of hypothermia therapy in preterm infants may differ from term infants, in whom it is well tolerated; this underscores the need for a randomized controlled trial. The NRN has initiated a randomized trial of hypothermia for infants with a gestational age of 33 0/7 to 35 6/7 weeks (NCT 01793129). Major challenges for this trial will be sufficient sample size (similar to the Late Initiation of Hypothermia study) in addition to establishing a diagnosis of HIE among preterm infants in whom neurologic features may overlap with those of encephalopathy.

How Should Cooling on Transport Be Conducted?

HIE will affect births in Level I facilities owing to obstetric events that cannot be anticipated (e.g., placental abruption, ruptured uterus, maternal trauma). Therapeutic hypothermia should not be performed in every hospital because HIE is characterized by multisystem organ dysfunction and requires neonatal intensive care units with the necessary expertise, consultants, and diagnostic services to manage the full spectrum of morbidities associated with encephalopathy. The therapeutic window during which hypothermia is thought to be effective is time sensitive and necessitates close working relationships between tertiary centers and referral institutions for proper stabilization and recognition of encephalopathy. However, geographic constraints and postnatal age of recognition may limit application of hypothermia and has led to initiation of hypothermia during transport.

Initial attempts at cooling on transport involved either passive cooling (removal of exogenous heat sources) or active cooling (application of gel packs or ice to the body). Although this approach allows a higher percent of infants to have therapy initiated before 6 hours of age, only 44% of infants had core temperatures within the targeted range for therapeutic hypothermia on admission to tertiary centers using a statewide database.[57] Some admission temperatures were exceedingly low, and risk hazard and other temperatures were negligibly reduced with presumably little neuroprotective benefit. This reflects a lack of standardization of the cooling process on transport. Other methods of passive cooling have been used (mattresses with phase-changing material, cooling fans) with similar results.[58] In contrast, investigators in the United Kingdom developed consensus guidelines for passive cooling at referring hospitals and on transport that were evaluated in a prospective study.[59] These investigators were able to demonstrate that 67% of infants were in the target range of 33°C to 34°C on arrival at the tertiary center. Although guidelines for passive cooling represent a step forward to initiate hypothermia earlier and more effectively, they will still be challenging for many referral hospitals and transport teams. This reflects the fact that moderate or severe HIE in infants represents a rare event that occurs in 1.5 per 1000 live births in population-based studies.[60]

Continuous monitoring of core temperature and a device that can regulate core temperature are critical to initiating effective and safe hypothermia on transport to a desired target. A randomized, nonmasked clinical trial of cooling on transport for infants with HIE has been performed among nine neonatal intensive care units in California (NCT 01683383).[61] Infants were randomly assigned to receive cooling according to usual center practices compared with servo control of temperature using the Tecotherm Neo (Inspiration Healthcare, Leicester, United Kingdom). Usual center practices included passive cooling (removing exogenous heat sources) and/or active cooling (ice or gel packs), and rectal or esophageal temperatures were recorded at 15-minute intervals using indwelling temperature probes. The Tecotherm device was used to continuously adjust either rectal or esophageal temperature via indwelling probes. The percent of all core temperatures recorded within the target range of 33°C to 34°C indicated large group differences: the median and interquartile range for the device arm was 73% (17%–88%) compared with 0% (0%–52%) for the usual center practices (Fig. 4.5). Servo control of temperature is markedly more effective than nondevice methods of initiating hypothermia on transport.

An issue not addressed in reports of cooling on transport is whether infants are appropriate candidates for the treatment. All clinical trials enrolled infants who manifested moderate or severe encephalopathy attributable to hypoxia-ischemia.[1–6] Training transport teams to recognize HIE is critical, but geographic constraints may limit the opportunity of transport teams to assess infants before 6 hours. Outreach education for referring providers is used by many centers. However, distinguishing subtle aspects of encephalopathy may be challenging for examiners who encounter such infants every 1 to 3 years even with intermittent education refreshers. Harnessing technology by the use of video conferencing and smart phones can enable real-time communication between referring providers and personnel at tertiary centers to improve decisions regarding initiation of cooling on transport.

Is Therapeutic Hypothermia Neuroprotective When Used in Low- and Middle-Income Countries?

The primary causes of neonatal mortality worldwide are prematurity (28%), infections (26%), and hypoxia-ischemia (23%, commonly termed asphyxia). It is estimated that approximately 1 million newborns die each year from neonatal encephalopathy in low- and middle-income countries.[62,63] Unfortunately, direct extrapolation from clinical trials of therapeutic hypothermia performed in high-income countries[1–6] to low- and middle-income countries cannot be done. This reflects performance of hypothermia trials in tertiary centers of high-income countries with the infrastructure to care for the multisystem organ dysfunction characteristic of HIE. In addition, patient populations at risk for HIE may be substantially different between high- compared with low- and middle-income countries. In the latter, antenatal care is poor, intrauterine growth restriction is common, and the incidence of perinatal infections and meconium aspiration syndrome is much higher.

A number of randomized controlled trials have been reported from low- and middle-income countries and have been pooled for meta-analysis.[64] Seven trials including 567 infants were included in the meta-analysis. Many of these trials were small and of poor quality. Most infants did not receive mechanical ventilation and cooling devices varied (cooling caps, gel packs, ice water bottles, and mattresses with phase-changing material). Cooling therapy was not associated with a reduction in neonatal mortality. Only three trials reported neurodevelopmental outcome; follow-up rates were poor and the confidence intervals of reported outcomes were

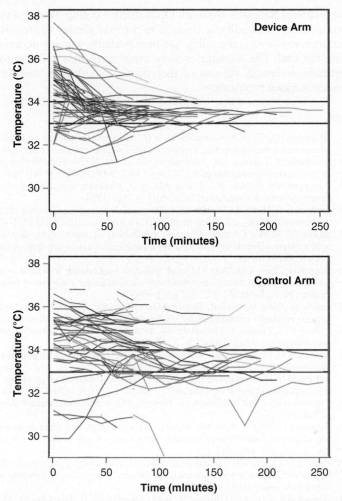

Fig. 4.5 Core temperature (rectal or esophageal) patterns during transport of infants whose temperature was adjusted with a servo-controlled device (Device arm, *upper panel*) or via usual care practices using either passive or active cooling without a device (Control arm, *lower panel*). The target temperature range was 33.0°C to 34.0°C; each infant is represented by an individual line. (Reprinted with permission from Akula VP, Joe P, Thusu K, et al. A randomized clinical trial of therapeutic hypothermia mode during transport for neonatal encephalopathy. *J Pediatr.* 2015;166(4):856–861.)

wide such that important clinical differences could not be excluded. Although hypothermia treatment achieved group differences in temperature among these trials, the benefit of cooling remains unclear. Larger, better-designed randomized clinical trials of therapeutic hypothermia are underway in low- and middle-income countries (Hypothermia for Encephalopathy in Low- and Middle-Income Countries trial [HELIX trial], NCT 02387385).

Conclusions

It is tempting to extrapolate from clinical trials that established efficacy and safety of hypothermia for HIE[1–6] to other clinical scenarios related to HIE. There have been multiple editorials suggesting the extension of the use of therapeutic hypothermia for indications outside clinical trials.[53,65] This is understandable given the associated mortality and lifelong, serious morbidity associated with HIE. However, well-designed, carefully performed clinical trials of hypothermia to determine if (1) there are better hypothermia regimens or (2) cooling works in other groups of infants with similar efficacy and safety profiles are needed to prevent drifts in practice without evidence and unintended adverse effects. The lesson learned from the Neonatal Research Network Optimizing Cooling Trial is a strong reminder that extrapolation to conditions thought to provide greater neuroprotection, lower temperature, and/or longer cooling had unexpectedly worse outcomes, resulting in stopping the trial. The message is very clear: until new information is available and critically reviewed, the use of therapeutic hypothermia should follow published, evidence-based protocols.

REFERENCES

1. Gluckman PD, Wyatt JS, Azzopardi D, et al. Selective head cooling with mild systemic hypothermia after neonatal encephalopathy: multicentre randomised trial. *Lancet*. 2005;365(9460):663–670.
2. Shankaran S, Laptook AR, Ehrenkranz RA, et al. Whole-body hypothermia for neonates with hypoxic-ischemic encephalopathy. *N Engl J Med*. 2005;353(15):1574–1584.
3. Azzopardi DV, Strohm B, Edwards AD, et al. Moderate hypothermia to treat perinatal asphyxial encephalopathy. *N Engl J Med*. 2009;361(14):1349–1358.
4. Simbruner G, Mittal RA, Rohlmann F, Muche R. Systemic hypothermia after neonatal encephalopathy: outcomes of neo.nEURO.network RCT. *Pediatrics*. 2010;126(4):e771–e778.
5. Jacobs SE, Morley CJ, Inder TE, et al. Whole-body hypothermia for term and near-term newborns with hypoxic-ischemic encephalopathy: a randomized controlled trial. *Arch Pediatr Adolesc Med*. 2011;165(8):692–700.
6. Zhou WH, Cheng GQ, Shao XM, et al. Selective head cooling with mild systemic hypothermia after neonatal hypoxic-ischemic encephalopathy: a multicenter randomized controlled trial in China. *J Pediatr*. 2010;157(3):367–372, 372.e361–e363.
7. Jacobs SE, Berg M, Hunt R, Tarnow-Mordi WO, Inder TE, Davis PG. Cooling for newborns with hypoxic ischaemic encephalopathy. *Cochrane Database Syst Rev (Online)*. 2013;1:CD003311.
8. Shankaran S, Pappas A, McDonald SA, et al. Childhood outcomes after hypothermia for neonatal encephalopathy. *N Engl J Med*. 2012;366(22):2085–2092.
9. Azzopardi D, Strohm B, Marlow N, et al. Effects of hypothermia for perinatal asphyxia on childhood outcomes. *N Engl J Med*. 2014;371(2):140–149.
10. Robertson NJ, Tan S, Groenendaal F, et al. Which neuroprotective agents are ready for bench to bedside translation in the newborn infant? *J Pediatr*. 2012;160(4):544–552.e544.
11. Committee on Fetus and Newborn. Hypothermia and neonatal encephalopathy. *Pediatrics*. 2014;133(6):1146–1150.
12. Higgins RD, Raju T, Edwards AD, et al. Hypothermia and other treatment options for neonatal encephalopathy: an executive summary of the Eunice Kennedy Shriver NICHD workshop. *J Pediatr*. 2011;159(5):851–858.e851.
13. Busto R, Dietrich WD, Globus MY, Valdes I, Scheinberg P, Ginsberg MD. Small differences in intraischemic brain temperature critically determine the extent of ischemic neuronal injury. *J Cereb Blood Flow Metab*. 1987;7(6):729–738.
14. Laptook AR, Corbett RJ, Sterett R, Burns DK, Garcia D, Tollefsbol G. Modest hypothermia provides partial neuroprotection when used for immediate resuscitation after brain ischemia. *Pediatr Res*. 1997;42(1):17–23.
15. Thoresen M, Bagenholm R, Loberg EM, Apricena F, Kjellmer I. Posthypoxic cooling of neonatal rats provides protection against brain injury. *Arch Dis Child Fetal Neonatal Ed*. 1996;74(1):F3–F9.
16. Trescher WH, Ishiwa S, Johnston MV. Brief post-hypoxic-ischemic hypothermia markedly delays neonatal brain injury. *Brain Dev*. 1997;19(5):326–338.
17. Gunn AJ, Gunn TR, de Haan HH, Williams CE, Gluckman PD. Dramatic neuronal rescue with prolonged selective head cooling after ischemia in fetal lambs. *J Clin Invest*. 1997;99(2):248–256.
18. Bona E, Hagberg H, Loberg EM, Bagenholm R, Thoresen M. Protective effects of moderate hypothermia after neonatal hypoxia-ischemia: short- and long-term outcome. *Pediatr Res*. 1998;43(6):738–745.
19. Schubert A. Side effects of mild hypothermia. *J Neurosurg Anesthesiol*. 1995;7(2):139–147.
20. Gunn AJ, Gluckman PD, Gunn TR. Selective head cooling in newborn infants after perinatal asphyxia: a safety study. *Pediatrics*. 1998;102(4 Pt 1):885–892.
21. Battin MR, Penrice J, Gunn TR, Gunn AJ. Treatment of term infants with head cooling and mild systemic hypothermia (35.0 degrees C and 34.5 degrees C) after perinatal asphyxia. *Pediatrics*. 2003;111(2):244–251.
22. Shankaran S, Laptook A, Wright LL, et al. Whole-body hypothermia for neonatal encephalopathy: animal observations as a basis for a randomized, controlled pilot study in term infants. *Pediatrics*. 2002;110(2 Pt 1):377–385.
23. Carroll M, Beek O. Protection against hippocampal CA1 cell loss by post-ischemic hypothermia is dependent on delay of initiation and duration. *Metab Brain Dis*. 1992;7(1):45–50.
24. Colbourne F, Corbett D. Delayed and prolonged post-ischemic hypothermia is neuroprotective in the gerbil. *Brain Res*. 1994;654(2):265–272.
25. Coimbra C, Wieloch T. Moderate hypothermia mitigates neuronal damage in the rat brain when initiated several hours following transient cerebral ischemia. *Acta Neuropathol*. 1994;87(4):325–331.
26. Sirimanne ES, Blumberg RM, Bossano D, et al. The effect of prolonged modification of cerebral temperature on outcome after hypoxic-ischemic brain injury in the infant rat. *Pediatr Res*. 1996;39(4 Pt 1):591–597.

4

27. Ferriero DM. Neonatal brain injury. *N Engl J Med*. 2004;351(19):1985–1995.
28. Yenari MA, Han HS. Neuroprotective mechanisms of hypothermia in brain ischaemia. *Nat Rev Neurosci*. 2012;13(4):267–278.
29. Shankaran S, Laptook AR, Pappas A, et al. Effect of depth and duration of cooling on deaths in the NICU among neonates with hypoxic ischemic encephalopathy: a randomized clinical trial. *JAMA*. 2014;312(24):2629–2639.
30. Shankaran S, Laptook A, Pappas A, et al. Randomized Controlled Trial (RCT) of optimizing cooling strategies for neonatal hypoxic-ischemic encephalopathy. *Pediatric*. 2016. Academic Societies' meeting abstracts, Abstract#4470.1.
31. Gunn AJ, Gunn TR, Gunning MI, Williams CE, Gluckman PD. Neuroprotection with prolonged head cooling started before postischemic seizures in fetal sheep. *Pediatrics*. 1998;102(5):1098–1106.
32. Gunn AJ, Bennet L, Gunning MI, Gluckman PD, Gunn TR. Cerebral hypothermia is not neuroprotective when started after postischemic seizures in fetal sheep. *Pediatr Res*. 1999;46(3):274–280.
33. Thoresen M, Tooley J, Liu X, et al. Time is brain: starting therapeutic hypothermia within three hours after birth improves motor outcome in asphyxiated newborns. *Neonatology*. 2013;104(3):228–233.
34. Galle AA, Jones NM. The neuroprotective actions of hypoxic preconditioning and postconditioning in a neonatal rat model of hypoxic-ischemic brain injury. *Brain Res*. 2013;1498:1–8.
35. Hassell KJ, Ezzati M, Alonso-Alconada D, Hausenloy DJ, Robertson NJ. New horizons for newborn brain protection: enhancing endogenous neuroprotection. *Arch Dis Child Fetal Neonatal Ed*. 2015;100(6):F541–F552.
36. Azzopardi D, Strohm B, Linsell L, et al. Implementation and conduct of therapeutic hypothermia for perinatal asphyxial encephalopathy in the UK–analysis of national data. *PLoS One*. 2012;7(6): e38504.
37. Lilford RJ, Thornton JG, Braunholtz D. Clinical trials and rare diseases: a way out of a conundrum. *BMJ*. 1995;311(7020):1621–1625.
38. Robertson C, Finer N. Term infants with hypoxic-ischemic encephalopathy: outcome at 3.5 years. *Dev Med Child Neurol*. 1985;27(4):473–484.
39. Robertson CM, Finer NN, Grace MG. School performance of survivors of neonatal encephalopathy associated with birth asphyxia at term. *J Pediatr*. 1989;114(5):753–760.
40. van Kooij BJ, van Handel M, Nievelstein RA, Groenendaal F, Jongmans MJ, de Vries LS. Serial MRI and neurodevelopmental outcome in 9- to 10-year-old children with neonatal encephalopathy. *J Pediatr*. 2010;157(2):221–227.e222.
41. van Handel M, Swaab H, de Vries LS, Jongmans MJ. Behavioral outcome in children with a history of neonatal encephalopathy following perinatal asphyxia. *J Pediatr Psychol*. 2010;35(3):286–295.
42. DuPont TL, Chalak LF, Morriss MC, Burchfield PJ, Christie L, Sanchez PJ. Short-term outcomes of newborns with perinatal acidemia who are not eligible for systemic hypothermia therapy. *J Pediatr*. 2013;162(1):35–41.
43. Massaro AN, Murthy K, Zaniletti I, et al. Short-term outcomes after perinatal hypoxic ischemic encephalopathy: a report from the Children's Hospitals Neonatal Consortium HIE focus group. *J Perinatol*. 2015;35(4):290–296.
44. Gagne-Loranger M, Sheppard M, Ali N, Saint-Martin C, Wintermark P. Newborns referred for therapeutic hypothermia: association between initial degree of encephalopathy and severity of brain injury (what about the newborns with mild encephalopathy on admission?). *Am J Perinatol*. 2016;33(2):195–202.
45. Kracer B, Hintz SR, Van Meurs KP, Lee HC. Hypothermia therapy for neonatal hypoxic ischemic encephalopathy in the state of California. *J Pediatr*. 2014;165(2):267–273.
46. Garfinkle J, Chalak LF, Prempunpong C, et al. Prospective research in infants with mild encephalopathy—the PRIME study. *Pediatric*. 2016;153. Academic Societies' meeting abstracts, Abstract#4116.
47. Murray DM, O'Connor CM, Ryan CA, Korotchikova I, Boylan GB. Early EEG grade and outcome at 5 years after mild neonatal hypoxic ischemic encephalopathy. *Pediatrics*. 2016;138(4):e20160659.
48. Eicher DJ, Wagner CL, Katikaneni LP, et al. Moderate hypothermia in neonatal encephalopathy: efficacy outcomes. *Pediatr Neurol*. 2005;32(1):11–17.
49. Volpe JJ. *Neurology of the Newborn*. 5th ed. Philadelphia, PA: Saunders Elsevier; 2008.
50. Back SA, Riddle A, McClure MM. Maturation-dependent vulnerability of perinatal white matter in premature birth. *Stroke*. 2007;38(2 suppl):724–730.
51. Volpe JJ, Kinney HC, Jensen FE, Rosenberg PA. The developing oligodendrocyte: key cellular target in brain injury in the premature infant. *Int J Dev Neurosci*. 2011;29(4):423–440.
52. Bennet L, Roelfsema V, George S, Dean JM, Emerald BS, Gunn AJ. The effect of cerebral hypothermia on white and grey matter injury induced by severe hypoxia in preterm fetal sheep. *J Physiol*. 2007;578(Pt 2):491–506.
53. Austin T, Shanmugalingam S, Clarke P. To cool or not to cool? Hypothermia treatment outside trial criteria. *Arch Dis Child Fetal Neonatal Ed*. 2013;98(5):F451–F453.
54. Smit E, Liu X, Jary S, Cowan F, Thoresen M. Cooling neonates who do not fulfil the standard cooling criteria—short- and long-term outcomes. *Acta Paediatr*. 2015;104(2):138–145.
55. Walsh WF, Butler D, Schmidt JW. Report of a pilot study of cooling four preterm infants 32–35 weeks gestation with HIE. *J Neonatal Perinatal Med*. 2015;8:47–51.
56. Rao R, Trivedi S, Vesoulis Z, Liao SM, Smyser CD, Mathur AM. Safety and short-term outcomes of therapeutic hypothermia in preterm neonates 34–35 weeks gestational age with hypoxic-ischemic encephalopathy. *J Pediatr*. 2016.
57. Akula VP, Gould JB, Davis AS, Hackel A, Oehlert J, Van Meurs KP. Therapeutic hypothermia during neonatal transport: data from the California Perinatal Quality Care Collaborative (CPQCC) and California Perinatal Transport System (CPeTS) for 2010. *J Perinatol*. 2013;33(3):194–197.

4

58. Robertson NJ, Kendall GS, Thayyil S. Techniques for therapeutic hypothermia during transport and in hospital for perinatal asphyxial encephalopathy. *Semin Fetal Neonatal Med.* 2010;15(5):276–286.

59. Kendall GS, Kapetanakis A, Ratnavel N, Azzopardi D, Robertson NJ. Passive cooling for initiation of therapeutic hypothermia in neonatal encephalopathy. *Arch Dis Child Fetal Neonatal Ed.* 2010;95(6):F408–F412.

60. Kurinczuk JJ, White-Koning M, Badawi N. Epidemiology of neonatal encephalopathy and hypoxic-ischaemic encephalopathy. *Early Hum Dev.* 2010;86(6):329–338.

61. Akula VP, Joe P, Thusu K, et al. A randomized clinical trial of therapeutic hypothermia mode during transport for neonatal encephalopathy. *J Pediatr.* 2015;166(4):856–861.e851–852.

62. Lawn JE, Cousens S, Zupan J. Lancet Neonatal Survival Steering Team. 4 million neonatal deaths: when? Where? Why? *Lancet.* 2005;365(9462):891–900.

63. Liu L, Oza S, Hogan D, et al. Global, regional, and national causes of child mortality in 2000–13, with projections to inform post-2015 priorities: an updated systematic analysis. *Lancet.* 2015;385(9966):430–440.

64. Pauliah SS, Shankaran S, Wade A, Cady EB, Thayyil S. Therapeutic hypothermia for neonatal encephalopathy in low- and middle-income countries: a systematic review and meta-analysis. *PLoS One.* 2013;8(3):e58834.

65. Saliba E. Should we extend the indications for therapeutic hypothermia? *Acta Paediatr.* 2015; 104(2):114–115.

4

CHAPTER 5

General Supportive Management of the Term Infant With Neonatal Encephalopathy Following Intrapartum Hypoxia-Ischemia

Ericalyn Kasdorf and Jeffrey M. Perlman

- Early identification of the infant at risk for evolving hypoxic-ischemic encephalopathy and initiation of therapeutic hypothermia is critical in overall management.
- Glucose should be checked shortly after birth and corrected promptly as needed.
- Carbon dioxide should be maintained within a normal range to avoid exacerbation of brain injury.
- Judicious fluid management is necessary in this population at risk for renal injury and oliguria.
- Hyperthermia should be avoided, and passive or active cooling may be considered for infants traveling long distances to a cooling center.
- Adjunctive therapies to therapeutic hypothermia, such as xenon or erythropoietin administration, are promising but larger clinical studies are needed.

CASE HISTORY

HI was a 3200-g, 38-week male infant born to a 28-year-old G2P1 (gravida 2, para 1) mother following an uncomplicated pregnancy. Labor was complicated by a maternal temperature of 38.5°C for which the mother received antibiotics, a prolonged second stage of labor associated with variable decelerations, and a bradycardic episode that resulted in an emergency cesarean section. Meconium staining of the amniotic fluid was noted. The infant was hypotonic at delivery and without respiratory effort. Resuscitation included intubation and positive-pressure ventilation (PPV). The initial heart rate was 50 beats/min but increased rapidly to >100 beats/min within 30 seconds of the start of PPV. The infant's color improved, and he took a first gasp at 4 minutes and made a first respiratory effort at 8 minutes. A rectal temperature in the delivery room was 38.2°C. The Apgar scores were 1, 4, and 7 at 1, 5, and 10 minutes, respectively. The infant was transferred to the neonatal intensive care unit (NICU) for further management. The cord arterial blood gas analysis revealed a partial pressure of carbon dioxide (P_{CO_2}) of 101 mm Hg, pH of 6.78, and base deficit of −23 mEq/L. The initial arterial blood gas analysis at 30 minutes revealed a P_{aO_2} of 146 mm Hg (on 50% oxygen), P_{CO_2} of 30 mm Hg, and pH of 7.12. The initial blood glucose level was 32 mg/dL. The hypoglycemia was treated with a 2-mL/kg bolus of dextrose 10% in water ($D_{10}W$), and subsequent glucose concentration was 84 mg/dL. The initial clinical assessment revealed a lethargic infant with a low-level sensory response. The anterior fontanel was soft. The capillary refill time

Continued

CASE HISTORY—cont'd

was approximately 2 seconds. Pertinent cardiovascular findings were a heart rate of 134 beats/min and blood pressure of 44/24 mm Hg with a mean of 34 mm Hg. The infant was intubated and placed on modest ventilator support with equal but coarse breath sounds. The abdomen was soft and without masses. The central nervous examination revealed pupils that were 3 mm and reactive. There were weak gag and suck reflexes, along with central hypotonia with proximal weakness. The reflexes were present and symmetric. The encephalopathy at this stage was categorized as Sarnat stage 2. Because of the history and clinical findings, the infant underwent an amplitude-integrated electroencephalography (aEEG) examination that revealed a moderately suppressed pattern without seizure activity. The infant met criteria for cooling, which was initiated at approximately 4 hours of age. At 12 hours of age the infant began to exhibit subtle seizure activity with blinking of the eyes, mouth smacking, and horizontal eye deviation associated with desaturation episodes. A clinical diagnosis of seizures was made, and the infant received a loading dose of phenobarbital (40 mg/kg). The seizures persisted over the next 12 hours and the infant was given phosphenytoin and additional phenobarbital and a midazolam drip was started before control of the clinical as well as the electrographic seizures was achieved. The encephalopathy peaked on day of life (DOL) 2, and the infant remained in Sarnat stage 2 encephalopathy. The supportive management included fluid restriction; the initial urine output was less than 1 mL/kg per hour for the first 24 hours but increased thereafter, and by DOL 3 the infant was in a diuretic phase. Sodium was initially 136 mEq/L, reached a nadir of 128 mEq/L on DOL 3, but corrected over the next 36 hours. The initial serum bicarbonate level was 18 mEq/L with an anion gap of 16. Both resolved spontaneously by DOL 3. The infant received assisted ventilation until DOL 3, and the P_{CO_2} values ranged between 40 and 50 mm Hg. Additional abnormalities included low calcium and magnesium levels (DOL 2) and mildly elevated liver enzymes. Low-dose dopamine treatment was started for approximately 24 hours for a low mean blood pressure. The infant was treated with antibiotics for 7 days for presumed sepsis, although the blood culture results remained negative. Parenteral nutrition was initiated on DOL 3, tube feedings were started on DOL 4, and the infant was able to achieve full nipple feedings on DOL 14. The neurologic findings improved, although they were still abnormal with central hypotonia and increased deep tendon reflexes at the time of discharge. Magnetic resonance imaging (MRI) on DOL 7 revealed marked hyperintensity on the diffusion-weighted images within the putamen and thalamus bilaterally. Findings of repeat electroencephalography (EEG) were pertinent for mild background slowing. Finally, the placental pathology was consistent with acute chorioamnionitis. The infant was discharged on DOL 16.

This case illustrates typical evolving neonatal encephalopathy following intrapartum hypoxia-ischemia against the background of placental infection/inflammation. The brain injury that develops is an evolving process that is initiated during the insult and extends into a recovery period, the latter referred to as the "reperfusion phase" of injury.[1-3] Management of such an infant should be initiated in the delivery room with effective resuscitation and continued through the evolving process. Management consists of identification of the infant as at high risk for developing evolving brain injury, supportive therapy to facilitate adequate perfusion and nutrients to the brain, and neuroprotective strategies, including therapeutic hypothermia as well as therapy targeted at the cellular level to ameliorate the processes of ongoing brain injury (see Chapter 4). These management components are briefly discussed in this chapter.

Introduction

Hypoxic-ischemic encephalopathy (HIE) is an infrequent event with a range of reported incidences but likely occurring in less than 1 of 1000 live term deliveries in the developed world. HIE secondary to intrapartum asphyxia is a widely recognized cause of long-term neurologic sequelae, including cerebral palsy.[4] Severe and prolonged interruption of placental blood flow will ultimately lead to asphyxia, the biochemical process characterized by worsening hypoxia, hypercarbia, and acidosis (in the more severe cases defined as an umbilical arterial cord pH ≤7.00).[5] During the acute phase of asphyxia, the ability to autoregulate cerebral blood flow (CBF) to maintain cerebral perfusion is lost. When this state occurs, CBF becomes entirely dependent on blood pressure to maintain perfusion pressure, a term known as a *pressure-passive cerebral circulation.*[1] With interruption of placental blood flow the fetus will attempt to maintain CBF by redistributing cardiac output not only to the brain but also to the adrenal glands and myocardium. This redistribution occurs at the expense of blood flow to kidneys, intestine, and skin.[5] Even a moderate decrease in blood pressure at this stage could lead to severely compromised CBF. With ongoing hypoxia-ischemia, CBF declines, leading to deleterious cellular effects. With oxygen depletion a number of cellular alterations occur, including replacement of oxidative phosphorylation with anaerobic metabolism, diminution of adenosine triphosphate (ATP), intracellular acidosis, and accumulation particularly of calcium. The ultimate deleterious effects include the release of excitatory neurotransmitters, such as glutamate, free radical production from fatty acid peroxidation, and nitric oxide (NO)–mediated neurotoxicity, all resulting in cell death.[4,5] Following resuscitation and the reestablishment of CBF and oxygenation, a phase of secondary energy failure occurs. In the experimental paradigm this phase transpires from 6 to 48 hours after the initial insult and is thought to be related to extension of the preceding mechanisms, leading to mitochondrial dysfunction.[2] It is clear that during asphyxia, not only the brain but also many other vital organs are at risk for injury. For this reason, postresuscitation management of the infant who has suffered intrapartum hypoxia-ischemia must also focus on supporting those systemic organs that may have been injured. Future therapies must also target the cellular injury that occurs following asphyxia.

Delivery Room Management

The use of room air or supplemental oxygen in the delivery room has been previously identified as a gap in knowledge that is crucial to resolve. Resuscitation of the depressed neonate is aimed at restoring blood flow and oxygen delivery to the tissues. The most current international guidelines continue to recommend initiation of resuscitation with room air or blended oxygen in term infants, with the goal of achieving oxygen saturations in the interquartile range of preductal saturations measured in healthy term babies born vaginally at sea level (Table 5.1).[6] This concept is based in part on meta-analyses of five studies.[7,8] The 2005 Cochrane meta-analysis showed a significant reduction in the rate of death in infants resuscitated with room

Table 5.1 TARGETED PREDUCTUAL SPo$_2$ AFTER BIRTH

Time After Birth (min)	SPo$_2$ Level (%)
1	60–65
2	65–70
3	70–75
4	75–80
5	80–85
10	85–95

Adapted from Wyckoff MH, Aziz K, Escobedo MB, et al. Part 13: Neonatal Resuscitation: 2015 American Heart Association Guidelines Update for Cardiopulmonary Resuscitation and Emergency Cardiovascular Care. Reprinted with permission *Circulation.* 2015;132:S543-S560 ©2015 American Heart Association, Inc.

air in comparison with 100% oxygen (relative risk [RR] 0.71, 95% confidence interval [CI] 0.54–0.94). Of note, there was no significant difference in incidence of grade II or III HIE (based on Sarnat staging) between groups.[8] A subsequent meta-analysis, performed by Rabi and colleagues, included two additional studies and also demonstrated lower mortality in the room air group than in the 100% oxygen resuscitation group in the first week of life (odds ratio [OR] 0.7, 95% CI 0.5–0.98), and at 1 month (OR 0.63, 95% CI 0.42–0.94). Again, there was no difference between groups in incidence of grade II or III HIE.[9] It remains unclear why this discordance exists as more severe encephalopathy may have been anticipated in the oxygen-treated group if brain injury and mortality are linked. Clearly the mechanisms contributing to death in the oxygen group are unclear and important to determine. Interestingly, use of 100% oxygen has been associated with increased biochemical markers of oxidative stress and delay to first cry and sustained respiration.[10]

In relation to long-term follow-up, Saugstad et al. had previously shown no difference in neurologic handicap at 18 to 24 months of life (albeit with a high dropout rate) between term and preterm infants resuscitated with room air versus those resuscitated with 100% oxygen.[11] Importantly, most of the patients were from a low-resource limited setting, which combined with the high dropout rate, limits the generalizability of these data. A more recent meta-analysis by Saugstad et al. that included the aforementioned study with an additional two follow-up studies again showed no significant difference in neurodevelopmental outcome at follow-up ranging from 11 to 24 months.[12]

There have been few studies comparing room air with 100% oxygen specifically during resuscitation of infants with HIE. One study performed in the era before cooling demonstrated increased risk of adverse outcome, defined as death or severe neurodevelopmental disability, by 24 months of age in infants diagnosed with asphyxia and exposed to severe hyperoxemia in the first 2 hours of life (defined as arterial partial pressure of oxygen [Pao_2] >200 mm Hg).[13] Another more recent study of infants with perinatal acidemia or an acute perinatal event in addition to a 10-minute Apgar score of 5 or less or ongoing need for assisted ventilation at 10 minutes and hyperoxemia on admission (defined as a Pao_2 >100 mm Hg) demonstrated an association with moderate-severe HIE and abnormal brain MRI scans. This population included both infants treated with whole-body hypothermia as well as controls.[14]

Some experimental studies do suggest benefit associated with oxygen use over room air as it relates to the brain and systemic circulation. Thus resuscitation with 100% oxygen is associated with more rapid restoration of hypoxia-depressed CBF, improved cerebral perfusion, and significantly lower levels of excitatory amino acid levels in striatum, as well as more favorable short- and long-term outcomes in surviving adult mice.[15,16] Additionally, in mice exposed to hypoxia-ischemia associated with circulatory arrest, resuscitation with 100% oxygen resulted in significantly greater rates of return of spontaneous circulation than that with room air.[17] These observations may be important to consider in resuscitation of the neonate with sustained bradycardia in the delivery room that is reflective of circulatory hypoperfusion.

There is a critical need for ongoing studies with long-term follow-up assessing the use of room air versus supplemental oxygen, especially in the setting of HIE. Three of the largest studies that have driven the international guidelines and recommendations were conducted in developing countries where antenatal and peripartum care and neonatal mortality rates differ from those in the developed world.[8]

Early Identification of Infants at Highest Risk for Development of Hypoxic-Ischemic Brain Injury

The initial step in management is early identification of those infants at greatest risk for progression to HIE. This is a highly relevant issue because the therapeutic window—that is, the interval following hypoxia-ischemia during which interventions might be efficacious in reducing the severity of ultimate brain injury—is likely to be short. It is estimated on the basis of experimental studies to vary from soon following the insult to approximately 6 hours.[18–20] Given this presumed short window of opportunity, infants must be identified as soon as possible after delivery to facilitate the implementation of early interventions as described in the case history. What put this infant at high risk for neurologic injury? There was clinical evidence to suggest chorioamnionitis, there was fetal bradycardia before delivery, the infant was severely depressed, there was the need for resuscitation in the delivery room (i.e., intubation and positive-pressure ventilation), and there was evidence of severe fetal acidemia, followed by evidence of early abnormal neurologic findings and abnormal cerebral function as demonstrated by amplitude-integrated EEG.[21–23] Indeed the infant progressed to stage 2 encephalopathy with seizures.

Supportive Care

A summary of supportive management is given in Fig. 5.1.

Ventilation

Assessment of adequate respiratory function is critical in the infant with HIE. Inadequate ventilation and frequent apneic episodes are not uncommon in severely affected infants, necessitating assisted ventilation. Changes in $Paco_2$ are important to monitor carefully as hypercarbia increases and hypocarbia decreases CBF.[24] Some experimental animal studies had previously suggested that a modest elevation in $Paco_2$ (50–55 mm Hg) at the time of hypoxia-ischemia was associated with better outcome than when the $Paco_2$ is within the normal (mid-30s) range.[25] However, this is a complex issue because progressive hypercarbia in ventilated premature infants is associated with loss of autoregulation.[26] Moreover, in the management of preterm infants with respiratory distress syndrome (RDS), the presence of hypocarbia has been associated with periventricular leukomalacia (PVL) (see Chapter 2). In term infants, there is increasing evidence that hypocarbia is associated with adverse outcome, especially in the setting of HIE. In a study of term infants diagnosed with intrapartum asphyxia, severe hypocapnia (defined as $Paco_2$ <20 mm Hg) led to increased risk of adverse outcome defined as death or severe neurodevelopmental disability at 12 months of age.[13] A secondary study of the National Institute of Child

Delivery Room

- Resuscitation beginning with room air ± supplemental oxygen if needed

Temperature

- Avoid hyperthermia

Ventilation

- Maintain $Paco_2$ in normal range

Perfusion

- Promptly treat hypotension
- Avoid hypertension

Fluid and Metabolic Status

- Initial fluid restriction
- Follow serum sodium concentration and fluid balance
- Follow serial glucoses and correct promptly when abnormal

Fig. 5.1 Summary of supportive management for neonatal encephalopathy after hypoxia-ischemia.

Health and Human Development (NICHD) whole-body hypothermia trial demonstrated an association of minimum $Paco_2$ and cumulative exposure to $Paco_2$ less than 35 mm Hg with adverse neurodevelopmental outcome at 18 to 22 months of age.[27] A post hoc analysis of the Cool Cap Study showed similar results, with hypocapnia in the first 72 hours after randomization (defined as $Paco_2$ <30 mm Hg) associated with an increased risk of death or severe neurodevelopmental disability at 18 months of age.[28] The authors of this study appropriately speculated that the etiology for frequent hypocapnia is unclear, it may be related to less carbon dioxide (CO_2) production in the setting of severe brain injury versus excessive support with mechanical ventilation and/or resuscitation. With these data in mind, it is recommended that the $Paco_2$ be maintained in the normal range in mechanically ventilated infants at risk for HIE. This goal may be difficult to achieve in clinical practice as infants with HIE often demonstrate hypocapnia. In a study of term infants with HIE, with only 11.5% of infants were normocapnic through the first 3 days of life; 29% were moderately hypocapnic and 5.8% were severely hypocapnic.[29]

Maintenance of Adequate Perfusion

Given the presence of a pressure-passive cerebral circulation as discussed earlier, management strategy should aim to maintain the arterial blood pressure within a normal range for age and gestation. It is not uncommon for infants with hypoxia-ischemia to exhibit hypotension. The hypotension may be related to myocardial dysfunction, to endothelial cell damage, or rarely to volume loss. The treatment should be directed toward the cause—that is, inotropic support should be given for myocardial dysfunction, and volume replacement for intravascular depletion.[30] On rare occasions infants may be hypertensive, though this may be observed in association with seizures.

Fluid Status

Hypoxic-ischemic infants often progress to a fluid overload state. Delivery room management may contribute to this problem as many infants receive fluid volume as part of the resuscitation process. Animal studies have suggested that fluid volume infusion at time of resuscitation may be detrimental in some cases. Thus in the asphyxiated neonatal piglet model, animals that received volume infusion during resuscitation demonstrated increased pulmonary edema and decreased lung compliance 2 hours after resuscitation.[31] The fluid overload seen after delivery may be related to renal failure secondary to acute tubular necrosis or to the syndrome of inappropriate antidiuretic hormone release (SIADH). Clinically such infants present with an increase in weight, low urine output, and hyponatremia. Indeed, in our case example, all these findings were present and treatment consisted of fluid restriction until diuresis was achieved and the gradual introduction of sodium supplementation on DOL 2. Others have treated the oliguria with theophylline on the theory that adenosine acts as a vasoconstrictive metabolite following hypoxia-ischemia, which contributes to a decreased glomerular filtration rate. In two randomized controlled studies, asphyxiated infants received a single dose of theophylline (8 mg/kg) within the first hour of life in an attempt to block this vasoconstriction. Theophylline was associated with a decrease in serum creatinine and urinary β_2-microglobulin concentrations as well as enhancement of creatinine clearance.[32,33] A meta-analysis of four studies, including these two, assessing the use of prophylactic theophylline for the prevention of renal dysfunction in term infants with asphyxia showed a reduced incidence of severe renal dysfunction.[34] These studies, however, were conducted before the era of therapeutic hypothermia. Additionally, theophylline levels were not measured in two of the four studies. Cleary more data are needed to better assess potential side effects, as well as to understand the drugs' effects in conjunction with therapeutic hypothermia.

Control of Blood Glucose Concentration

In the context of cerebral hypoxia-ischemia, experimental studies suggest that both hyperglycemia and hypoglycemia may exacerbate brain damage. In adult experimental models as well as in humans, hyperglycemia accentuates brain damage, whereas in immature animals subjected to cerebral hypoxia-ischemia, significant hyperglycemia to a blood glucose concentration of 600 mg/dL entirely prevented brain damage.[35] Conversely, the effects of hypoglycemia in experimental neonatal models vary, as do the mechanisms of the hypoglycemia. Thus insulin-induced hypoglycemia is detrimental to immature rat brain subjected to hypoxia-ischemia. However, if fasting induces hypoglycemia, a high degree of protection is noted.[36] This protective effect is thought to be secondary to the increased concentrations of ketone bodies, which presumably serve as alternative substrates to the immature brain.

In the clinical setting, hypoglycemia when associated with hypoxia-ischemia is detrimental to the brain. Thus term infants delivered in the presence of severe fetal acidemia (umbilical arterial pH <7.0) who presented with an initial blood glucose concentration lower than 40 mg/dL were 18 times more likely to progress to moderate or severe encephalopathy compared with infants with a glucose greater than 40 mg/dL.[37] In another post hoc analysis of the Cool Cap Study, unfavorable outcome at 18 months was seen more commonly in infants with hypoglycemia (≤40 mg/dL) and hyperglycemia (≥150 mg/dL) within the first 12 hours following randomization.[38] Interestingly, multiorgan dysfunction, as measured by liver and renal function, and hematologic studies, was more severely abnormal in the hypoglycemic population.[39] Hypoglycemia was another risk factor for adverse outcome in our case as the infant presented with an initial blood glucose concentration of 32 mg/dL. In the ongoing management of hypoxia-ischemia, a glucose level should be screened shortly after birth, corrected promptly as needed, and monitored closely.

Temperature

In both animal and human studies, ischemic brain injury has been shown to be influenced by temperature; elevation either during or following the insult exacerbates brain injury, whereas a modest reduction in temperature reduces the extent of injury (see Chapter 4).[40] The potential risks associated with an elevated temperature were highlighted in an observational secondary study of the NICHD whole-body cooling trial.[41] This study found that an increased temperature in the control group following hypoxia-ischemia was associated with a higher risk of adverse outcome. The odds ratio of death or disability at 18 to 22 months of age was increased 3.6- to 4-fold for each 1°C increase in the highest quartile of skin or esophageal temperatures (see also Chapter 4).[41] In this same cohort, this effect persisted into childhood, with an increased odds of death or IQ less than 70 at age 6 to 7 years for infants with an average esophageal or skin temperature in the upper quartile in the first 3 days of life.[42] Therefore it is important to pay close attention to temperature in the infant with a hypoxic-ischemic event. At the time of delivery, the infant's temperature may be in the normal range or may be elevated in the context of clinical chorioamnionitis with maternal fever, making temperature a highly relevant issue. This raises the important question of how to manage temperature immediately following resuscitation of a near-term or term infant. Should the goal be to maintain the temperature in a normal range until it is evident that the neonate is a potential candidate for therapeutic hypothermia? On the other hand, the clinician could consider initiating passive cooling even at the time of delivery, with discontinuation of use of the radiant warmer in the delivery room. In a study of passive cooling initiated before and during transport to a referral center for evaluation for therapeutic hypothermia, passive cooling resulted in initiation of therapy 4.6 hours earlier than if therapy had been started at the cooling center.[43] This concept is especially relevant because many infants who may be treated with therapeutic hypothermia are born at referring centers. Thus in a study of 45 term infants with moderate or severe HIE treated at a single center with selective head cooling, 96% were outborn, and the time to initiate cooling was 4.69 ± 0.79 hours.[44] Another study comparing active cooling with a servo-controlled mattress to passive cooling during transport demonstrated a later age at cooling and greater temperature instability in the passively cooled group; 27% of infants in the passive group did not achieve the target temperature and 34% of infants were overcooled. Given these results, transport teams travelling long distances with infants to a cooling center should develop protocols for the transfer of such infants, so as to avoid a delay in cooling and to improve temperature stability.[45]

Seizures

Hypoxic-ischemic cerebral injury is one of the most common causes of early-onset neonatal seizures. Although seizures are a consequence of the underlying brain injury, seizure activity in itself may also contribute to ongoing injury. Experimental evidence strongly suggests that repetitive seizures disturb brain growth and development as well as increase the risk for subsequent epilepsy.[46,47] Human studies, however, show conflicting evidence. Glass et al. demonstrated that clinical seizures in the setting of HIE in the era before therapeutic hypothermia were associated with worse cognitive and motor outcome at age 4 years.[48] The Cool Cap Study also demonstrated that the presence of aEEG seizures at time of enrollment was independently associated with an unfavorable outcome, defined as death or severe disability at 18 months.[49] It remains unclear if seizures may be truly damaging to the newborn brain or if they are simply reflective of the degree of brain injury. In contrast, a secondary analysis of the NICHD whole-body cooling trial demonstrated that the presence of clinical seizures at any time during the hospitalization was not associated with death or moderate or severe disability at 18 months of life.[50] This conflicting evidence, along with the observation that not all clinical seizures have an electrographic correlate, highlights that the optimal management of seizures in the neonatal period in the setting of HIE remains unclear (see also Chapter 7).[51–53] In many centers clinical and/or electrographic seizures are treated with an anticonvulsant, usually phenobarbital, and treatment is continued if seizures persist until the anticonvulsant therapy (e.g., phenobarbital, phosphenytoin, or midazolam) has been optimized. Large randomized controlled trials are warranted to guide evidence-based management for monitoring and management of seizures associated with HIE.

Prophylactic Barbiturates

Experimental studies lend support to the potential role of prophylactic phenobarbital in combination with hypothermia. In the neonatal rat model of HIE, rats treated with both 40 mg/kg phenobarbital and hypothermia had better early and late outcomes than hypothermia-only treatment. Early outcomes included better sensorimotor performance and less cortical damage in the phenobarbital-treated group. Late beneficial outcomes included better sensorimotor performance and lower neuropathology scores.[54] The prophylactic administration of high-dose barbiturates to infants at highest risk for developing HIE was evaluated in small studies before the era of therapeutic hypothermia and the results were conflicting. In one randomized study, the administration of thiopental initiated within 2 hours of birth and infused for 24 hours did not alter the frequency of seizures, intracranial pressure, or short-term neurodevelopmental outcome at 12 months.[55] Of importance was the observation that systemic hypotension occurred significantly more often in the treated group. In another randomized study, 40 mg/kg body weight of phenobarbital administered intravenously to asphyxiated infants between 1 and 6 hours of life was associated with subsequent neuroprotection. In this study there was no difference in the frequency of seizures between the two groups in the neonatal period; however 73% of the pretreated infants compared with 18% of the control group ($P < .05$) demonstrated normal neurodevelopmental outcome at 3-year follow-up. No adverse effect of phenobarbital administration was observed.[56] There have been additional studies demonstrating a decrease in the incidence of seizures in infants treated with prophylactic phenobarbital. In one small study of term and near-term asphyxiated infants, phenobarbital administered within 6 hours of life resulted in a seizure frequency of 8% in the treatment group versus 40% in the control group ($P = .01$). Mortality and neurologic outcome at discharge were not statistically different between the two groups.[57]

Similarly, in a second study, infants who were given 40 mg/kg of prophylactic phenobarbital during whole-body cooling had fewer clinical seizures than a control group of infants (15% vs. 82%, $P < .0001$). There was, however, no reduction in neurodevelopmental impairment at latest follow-up (range 18–49 months).[58] The most recent Cochrane review of prophylactic barbiturate administration following perinatal asphyxia demonstrated an overall reduction in seizures with treatment but no significant change in mortality.[59] This review also highlights the paucity of data regarding long-term outcome. It is clear more studies are needed with long-term follow-up to assess the potential protective effect of prophylactic phenobarbital when used in combination with hypothermia.

Potential Neuroprotective Strategies Aimed at Ameliorating Secondary Brain Injury

In addition to hypothermia (see Chapter 4), the following potential neuroprotective strategies have been considered (Fig. 5.2).

Oxygen Free Radical Inhibitors and Scavengers

Another proposed therapeutic approach for the elimination of oxygen free radicals generated during and after hypoxia-ischemia is to administer specific enzymes known to degrade highly reactive radicals to a nonreactive component.[1] In newborn animals, neuroprotection has been demonstrated when superoxide dismutase mimetics have been administered several hours before the hypoxic-ischemic insult.[60] A second group of free radical inhibitors shown to be effective in experimental animals are agents that inhibit the production of xanthines, such as allopurinol and oxypurinol.[1] In a clinical study, asphyxiated infants who received allopurinol demonstrated lower blood concentrations of oxygen free radicals than control infants.[61,62] However, a 2012 Cochrane review of three trials, involving 114 infants with encephalopathy treated with allopurinol, concluded there was no significant difference between treated and control groups in the risk of death during infancy or of neonatal seizures.[63] With such a small number of patients included in these studies, larger studies may be needed to determine whether there is truly lack of benefit. Follow-up from two of these randomized studies showed no difference in long-term outcomes at 4 to 8 years of age between treated infants and controls.[64] A third proposed treatment has used targeted blockade of free radical formation, specifically hydroxyl radical, from free iron during reperfusion.[1] Thus deferoxamine, a chelating agent, prevents the formation of free radicals from iron, reduces the severity of brain injury, and improves cerebral metabolism in animal models of hypoxia-ischemia when given during reperfusion.[62] Other animal studies have shown less benefit from deferoxamine treatment, including a study investigating the combination of the antioxidant effect of deferoxamine with the antiapoptotic effect of erythropoietin.[65] In summary, none of these interventions targeting free radicals have revealed clinical promise. Melatonin has recently been suggested as a potential adjunctive therapy because of its antioxidant properties. Aly et al. recently described a small study of 30 term infants with HIE and 15 controls. Half of the infants with HIE were randomly assigned to the

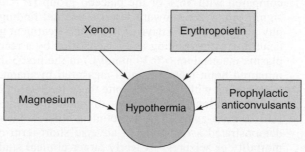

Fig. 5.2 Potential strategies to evaluate in high-risk infants treated with therapeutic hypothermia.

10 mg/kg enteral melatonin plus hypothermia group and the other half to hypothermia alone. The melatonin/hypothermia group had fewer seizures on follow-up EEG at 2 weeks and fewer white matter abnormalities on MRI obtained after 2 weeks of life compared with the hypothermia group alone.[66] Larger studies with later follow-up are needed, but these initial results show promise.

Excitatory Amino Acid Antagonists

Given the important role of excessive stimulation of neuronal surface receptors by glutamate in promoting a cascade of events leading to cellular death, it has been logical to identify pharmacologic agents that would either inhibit glutamate release or block its postsynaptic action.[1] Glutamate receptor antagonists (i.e., N-methyl-D-aspartate [NMDA] subtypes) have been extensively investigated in experimental animals. Noncompetitive antagonists provided a reduction in brain damage in adult animals even when administered up to 24 hours after the insult. The available NMDA antagonists include dizocilpine (MK-801), magnesium, xenon, phencyclidine (PCP), dextromethorphan, and ketamine.[1] Most of the previously mentioned NMDA antagonists are not widely used. However, magnesium, which is commonly used, and xenon show potential benefit and are discussed in the following sections.

Magnesium

Magnesium is an NMDA antagonist, blocking neuronal influx of Ca^{2+} within the ion channel. In a developmental study in mice, excitotoxic neuronal death was limited by magnesium.[67] In addition to NMDA receptor blockade, magnesium is thought to potentially have antioxidant, anticytokine, and antiplatelet effects in the setting of perinatal asphyxia.[1] Magnesium sulfate is an appealing agent because of its frequent use for tocolysis or to prevent seizures in women with pregnancy-induced hypertension. One large multicenter trial assessed outcomes of infants born to women treated with magnesium sulfate who were at imminent risk for delivery between 24 and 31 weeks' gestation. Moderate or severe cerebral palsy occurred significantly less frequently in the magnesium-treated group (1.9% vs. 3.5%; RR 0.55, 95% CI 0.32–0.95).[68]

With this promise of neuroprotection in preterm infants, there has been speculation about potential benefit in term asphyxiated infants. In a piglet model of asphyxia, however, magnesium sulfate administered 1 hour after resuscitation did not decrease the severity of delayed cerebral energy failure.[69] In addition, in a near-term fetal lamb model of asphyxia, magnesium sulfate administered before and during umbilical cord occlusion did not influence electroencephalogram responses or neuronal loss.[70] Overall, a systematic review of preclinical studies by Galinsky et al., including the two mentioned here, suggests that magnesium is unlikely to be neuroprotective.[71] Conversely, potential benefit was described by Bhat et al. in a study of term infants with severe perinatal asphyxia who received 3 doses of magnesium (250 mg/kg per dose) within 6 hours of birth and at 24-hour intervals. An abnormal neurologic examination at discharge, performed by a clinician blinded to group assignment, was found in 22% of the treatment group compared with 56% of the placebo group ($P = .04$). Although not statistically significant, a trend toward fewer abnormal findings on head computed tomography performed at 14 days of life in the treatment group was also reported.[72] This is an interesting finding and is supported by a recent clinical study in which low plasma magnesium (<0.76 mmol/L) in the first 3 days of life was associated with impaired brain metabolism as measured by magnetic resonance spectroscopy in term infants with HIE.[73] Despite these interesting observations, there is a paucity of data with long-term outcome of magnesium administration to term infants with HIE. A meta-analysis of five clinical studies, including the study by Bhat et al., demonstrated a reduction in adverse short-term outcome with no difference in mortality or seizures.[74] Clearly larger clinical studies are needed with long-term follow-up, as well as studies assessing the combined effect of magnesium with hypothermia.

Xenon

Xenon appears to have a synergistic neuroprotective effect when combined with hypothermia at doses that are likely to be well tolerated.[1] In the past xenon has been used as an inhaled anesthetic, with rapid induction and recovery secondary to poor blood solubility. It does, however, rapidly cross the blood-brain barrier, and in the brain, acts as a noncompetitive antagonist of the NMDA subtype of the glutamate receptor.[1,75] Xenon has also been shown to exhibit antiapoptotic effects.[76] There have been several preclinical studies investigating the use of xenon with hypothermia in the setting of asphyxia. In a newborn pig model, animals subjected to 45 minutes of global hypoxia-ischemia demonstrated 75% histologic (averaged regional neuropathology scores) global neuroprotection when 18 hours of 50% xenon inhalation was combined with 24 hours of hypothermia. Although regional neuroprotection was evident in all seven brain regions assessed, it was most prominent in the basal ganglia and thalamus.[77] In a neonatal rat model, the combination of xenon and hypothermia after HIE resulted in almost complete restoration of long-term functional outcomes as well as improved regional histopathology.[78] In both studies, the effect of xenon with hypothermia was additive and not synergistic—that is, each individual treatment neither augmented nor reduced the effect of the other. Furthermore, in both studies xenon was administered either shortly after the hypoxic-ischemic insult (30 minutes) or during recovery from hypoxia-ischemia. This leaves the question of whether xenon would be neuroprotective if administration was delayed but still given within 6 hours from the time of delivery, the window in which clinicians institute hypothermia to asphyxiated newborns. In a study evaluating the protective effect of xenon with hypothermia both in mixed glial-neuronal co-cultures, and in a rat pup model, xenon was found to be protective up to 6 hours after the insult at concentrations of 70% administered for 90 minutes.[76] Results of the first randomized clinical study in term newborns with HIE have not been as promising. The Total Body hypothermia plus Xenon (TOBY-Xe) trial assessed a total of 92 infants, 46 treated with cooling alone and 46 with cooling plus 30% inhaled xenon administered within 12 hours of life for a duration of 24 hours. There were no differences in biomarkers of cerebral damage, including a lactate-to-N-acetyl aspartate ratio in the thalamus and fractional anisotropy in the posterior limb of the internal capsule. This finding was thought to potentially be related to the late administration of xenon (median 10 hours), the lack of power to detect a difference in the N-acetyl aspartate ratio, or the possibility that infants in this cohort were too severely affected at enrollment.[79] One larger study of adults who had an out-of-hospital cardiac arrest and were subsequently treated with therapeutic hypothermia in addition to xenon demonstrated less white matter damage as measured by fractional anisotropy compared with those treated with hypothermia alone. There was no difference in neurologic outcome or mortality at 6 months, though the study was not designed to assess those outcomes.[80] Overall, xenon is a well-tolerated anesthetic without major respiratory or cardiovascular side effects in one small series of 14 infants treated with therapeutic hypothermia.[81] It is, however, expensive and requires delivery with a specialized ventilator that can scavenge exhaled xenon.[82] Larger clinical studies are still needed to determine the time window in which xenon could be administered with hypothermia, the dose and duration of treatment needed, as well as xenon's effect on long-term neurodevelopmental outcomes.

Erythropoietin

Erythropoietin (Epo) is a glycoprotein hormone most recognized for its role in erythropoiesis. However, it has also been shown to naturally increase during hypoxia-ischemia, along with an increase in Epo receptors. Erythropoietin is thought to provide a neuroprotective adaptive response during hypoxia-ischemia because of this effect.[1] Suggested protective mechanisms of action include antioxidant and antiinflammatory responses, induction of antiapoptotic factors, as well as decreased nitric oxide–mediated injury and susceptibility to glutamate toxicity.[75] Both stroke and hypoxic-ischemic animal models have demonstrated histologic protection with recombinant human Epo treatment.[83–86] In the neonatal rat stroke model, treated animals also performed better in most components of spatial learning and memory performance.[83]

Epo has also shown a beneficial effect in a study of term infants with moderate-severe HIE who were not treated with therapeutic hypothermia. In this study, infants were randomly assigned to receive recombinant Epo (rEpo) at either 300 U/kg or 500 U/kg every other day for 2 weeks beginning at less than 48 hours after birth. The rate of death or moderate-severe disability at 18 months was significantly reduced, occurring in 43.8% in the control group versus 24.6% in the rEpo group (RR 0.62, 95% CI 0.41–0.94). Benefit was seen in infants with moderate (P = .001) but not severe HIE (P = .227). There was no difference in primary outcome between doses used in this study and Epo was well tolerated.[87] In a multicenter phase 1 study of infants of at least 36 weeks' gestation with HIE, Epo (1000 U/kg) administered in conjunction with therapeutic hypothermia was safe and resulted in plasma concentrations that were neuroprotective in animal studies.[88] Follow-up of infants enrolled in this pharmacokinetics study between 8 and 34 months of age (mean 22 months) reported no deaths and moderate-severe developmental disability in only 1 of 22 patients available for follow-up, though this study was not designed to determine efficacy.[89] A larger phase II double-blinded trial of 50 infants treated with hypothermia and randomly assigned to either placebo or five total doses of Epo at 1000 U/kg per dose showed fewer infants treated with Epo with brain injury on MRI performed at 4 to 7 days of age and improved motor outcome at 1 year of life.[90] Larger published trials are still needed to establish efficacy; however, these early results are promising.

Gaps in Knowledge

1. Is it possible or ethical to perform more trials comparing 21% with higher concentrations of supplemental oxygen during intensive resuscitation of term infants with HIE using a uniform definition of HIE and performed in the developed world?
2. Is there a critical mean blood pressure below which cerebral perfusion becomes compromised?
3. Is there a benefit to prophylactic anticonvulsant therapy in the high-risk infant, given that around 50% of infants exhibit early seizures?[49,91,92]
4. What is the therapeutic window in which xenon may be administered along with hypothermia? What is the optimal dose and duration of treatment needed? What are the effects on long-term neurodevelopmental outcomes?
5. Larger trials of Epo administered in conjunction with hypothermia are needed to determine if it confers neuroprotection.
6. Should passive or active cooling be administered while transferring an infant to a cooling center?

REFERENCES

1. Volpe JJ. *Neurology of the Newborn*. 5th ed. Philadelphia: Saunders/Elsevier; 2008.
2. Perlman JM. Intervention strategies for neonatal hypoxic-ischemic cerebral injury. *Clin Ther*. 2006;28(9):1353–1365.
3. Shalak L, Perlman JM. Hypoxic-ischemic brain injury in the term infant-current concepts. *Early Hum Dev*. 2004;80(2):125–141.
4. Perlman JM. Summary proceedings from the neurology group on hypoxic-ischemic encephalopathy. *Pediatrics*. 2006;117(3 Pt 2):S28–S33.
5. Stola A, Perlman J. Post-resuscitation strategies to avoid ongoing injury following intrapartum hypoxia-ischemia. *Semin Fetal Neonatal Med*. 2008;13(6):424–431.
6. Wyckoff MH, Aziz K, Escobedo MB, et al. Part 13: Neonatal Resuscitation: 2015 American Heart Association Guidelines Update for Cardiopulmonary Resuscitation and Emergency Cardiovascular Care. *Circulation*. 2015;132(18 suppl 2):S543–S560.
7. Davis PG, Tan A, O'Donnell CP, Schulze A. Resuscitation of newborn infants with 100% oxygen or air: a systematic review and meta-analysis. *Lancet*. 2004;364(9442):1329–1333.
8. Tan A, Schulze A, O'Donnell CP, Davis PG. Air versus oxygen for resuscitation of infants at birth. *Cochrane Database Syst Rev*. 2005;(2):CD002273.

9. Rabi Y, Rabi D, Yee W. Room air resuscitation of the depressed newborn: a systematic review and meta-analysis. *Resuscitation*. 2007;72(3):353–363.
10. Vento M, Asensi M, Sastre J, Garcia-Sala F, Pallardo FV, Vina J. Resuscitation with room air instead of 100% oxygen prevents oxidative stress in moderately asphyxiated term neonates. *Pediatrics*. 2001;107(4):642–647.
11. Saugstad OD, Ramji S, Irani SF, et al. Resuscitation of newborn infants with 21% or 100% oxygen: follow-up at 18 to 24 months. *Pediatrics*. 2003;112(2):296–300.
12. Saugstad OD, Vento M, Ramji S, Howard D, Soll RF. Neurodevelopmental outcome of infants resuscitated with air or 100% oxygen: a systematic review and meta-analysis. *Neonatology*. 2012;102(2):98–103.
13. Klinger G, Beyene J, Shah P, Perlman M. Do hyperoxaemia and hypocapnia add to the risk of brain injury after intrapartum asphyxia? *Arch Dis Child Fetal Neonatal Ed*. 2005;90(1):F49–F52.
14. Kapadia VS, Chalak LF, DuPont TL, Rollins NK, Brion LP, Wyckoff MH. Perinatal asphyxia with hyperoxemia within the first hour of life is associated with moderate to severe hypoxic-ischemic encephalopathy. *J Pediatr*. 2013;163(4):949–954.
15. Presti AL, Kishkurno SV, Slinko SK, et al. Reoxygenation with 100% oxygen versus room air: late neuroanatomical and neurofunctional outcome in neonatal mice with hypoxic-ischemic brain injury. *Pediatr Res*. 2006;60(1):55–59.
16. Solas AB, Kutzsche S, Vinje M, Saugstad OD. Cerebral hypoxemia-ischemia and reoxygenation with 21% or 100% oxygen in newborn piglets: effects on extracellular levels of excitatory amino acids and microcirculation. *Pediatr Crit Care Med*. 2001;2(4):340–345.
17. Matsiukevich D, Randis TM, Utkina-Sosunova I, Polin RA, Ten VS. The state of systemic circulation, collapsed or preserved defines the need for hyperoxic or normoxic resuscitation in neonatal mice with hypoxia-ischemia. *Resuscitation*. 2010;81(2):224–229.
18. Gunn AJ, Bennet L, Gunning MI, Gluckman PD, Gunn TR. Cerebral hypothermia is not neuroprotective when started after postischemic seizures in fetal sheep. *Pediatr Res*. 1999;46(3):274–280.
19. Gunn AJ, Gunn TR, Gunning MI, Williams CE, Gluckman PD. Neuroprotection with prolonged head cooling started before postischemic seizures in fetal sheep. *Pediatrics*. 1998;102(5):1098–1106.
20. Gunn AJ. Cerebral hypothermia for prevention of brain injury following perinatal asphyxia. *Curr Opin Pediatr*. 2000;12(2):111–115.
21. Hellstrom-Westas L, Rosen I, Svenningsen NW. Predictive value of early continuous amplitude integrated EEG recordings on outcome after severe birth asphyxia in full term infants. *Arch Dis Child Fetal Neonatal Ed*. 1995;72(1):F34–F38.
22. al Naqeeb N, Edwards AD, Cowan FM, Azzopardi D. Assessment of neonatal encephalopathy by amplitude-integrated electroencephalography. *Pediatrics*. 1999;103(6 Pt 1):1263–1271.
23. Shalak LF, Laptook AR, Velaphi SC, Perlman JM. Amplitude-integrated electroencephalography coupled with an early neurologic examination enhances prediction of term infants at risk for persistent encephalopathy. *Pediatrics*. 2003;111(2):351–357.
24. Rosenberg AA, Jones Jr MD, Traystman RJ, Simmons MA, Molteni RA. Response of cerebral blood flow to changes in PCO2 in fetal, newborn, and adult sheep. *Am J Physiol*. 1982;242(5):H862–H866.
25. Vannucci RC, Brucklacher RM, Vannucci SJ. Effect of carbon dioxide on cerebral metabolism during hypoxia-ischemia in the immature rat. *Pediatr Res*. 1997;42(1):24–29.
26. Kaiser JR, Gauss CH, Williams DK. The effects of hypercapnia on cerebral autoregulation in ventilated very low birth weight infants. *Pediatr Res*. 2005;58(5):931–935.
27. Pappas A, Shankaran S, Laptook AR, et al. Hypocarbia and adverse outcome in neonatal hypoxic-ischemic encephalopathy. *J Pediatr*. 2011;158(5):752–758.e751.
28. Lingappan K, Kaiser JR, Srinivasan C, Gunn AJ. Relationship between PCO2 and unfavorable outcome in infants with moderate-to-severe hypoxic ischemic encephalopathy. *Pediatr Res*. 2016;80(2):204–208.
29. Nadeem M, Murray D, Boylan G, Dempsey EM, Ryan CA. Blood carbon dioxide levels and adverse outcome in neonatal hypoxic-ischemic encephalopathy. *Am J Perinatol*. 2010;27(5):361–365.
30. Wyckoff MH, Perlman JM, Laptook AR. Use of volume expansion during delivery room resuscitation in near-term and term infants. *Pediatrics*. 2005;115(4):950–955.
31. Wyckoff M, Garcia D, Margraf L, Perlman J, Laptook A. Randomized trial of volume infusion during resuscitation of asphyxiated neonatal piglets. *Pediatr Res*. 2007;61(4):415–420.
32. Jenik AG, Ceriani Cernadas JM, Gorenstein A, et al. A randomized, double-blind, placebo-controlled trial of the effects of prophylactic theophylline on renal function in term neonates with perinatal asphyxia. *Pediatrics*. 2000;105(4):E45.
33. Bhat MA, Shah ZA, Makhdoomi MS, Mufti MH. Theophylline for renal function in term neonates with perinatal asphyxia: a randomized, placebo-controlled trial. *J Pediatr*. 2006;149(2):180–184.
34. Al-Wassia H, Alshaikh B, Sauve R. Prophylactic theophylline for the prevention of severe renal dysfunction in term and post-term neonates with perinatal asphyxia: a systematic review and meta-analysis of randomized controlled trials. *J Perinatol*. 2013;33(4):271–277.
35. Vannucci RC, Mujsce DJ. Effect of glucose on perinatal hypoxic-ischemic brain damage. *Biol Neonate*. 1992;62(4):215–224.
36. Yager JY. Hypoglycemic injury to the immature brain. *Clin Perinatol*. 2002;29(4):651–674.vi.
37. Salhab WA, Wyckoff MH, Laptook AR, Perlman JM. Initial hypoglycemia and neonatal brain injury in term infants with severe fetal acidemia. *Pediatrics*. 2004;114(2):361–366.
38. Basu SK, Kaiser JR, Guffey D, et al. Hypoglycaemia and hyperglycaemia are associated with unfavourable outcome in infants with hypoxic ischaemic encephalopathy: a post hoc analysis of the CoolCap Study. *Arch Dis Child Fetal Neonatal Ed*. 2016;101(2):F149–F155.

5

39. Basu SK, Salemi JL, Gunn AJ, Kaiser JR, CoolCap Study Group. Hyperglycaemia in infants with hypoxic-ischaemic encephalopathy is associated with improved outcomes after therapeutic hypothermia: a post hoc analysis of the CoolCap Study. *Arch Dis Child Fetal Neonatal Ed.* 2016.

40. Laptook AR, Corbett RJ. The effects of temperature on hypoxic-ischemic brain injury. *Clin Perinatol.* 2002;29(4):623–649.vi.

41. Laptook A, Tyson J, Shankaran S, et al. Elevated temperature after hypoxic-ischemic encephalopathy: risk factor for adverse outcomes. *Pediatrics.* 2008;122(3):491–499.

42. Laptook AR, McDonald SA, Shankaran S, et al. Elevated temperature and 6- to 7-year outcome of neonatal encephalopathy. *Ann Neurol.* 2013;73(4):520–528.

43. Kendall GS, Kapetanakis A, Ratnavel N, Azzopardi D, Robertson NJ. Cooling on Retrieval Study G. Passive cooling for initiation of therapeutic hypothermia in neonatal encephalopathy. *Arch Dis Child Fetal Neonatal Ed.* 2010;95(6):F408–F412.

44. Takenouchi T, Cuaycong M, Ross G, Engel M, Perlman JM. Chain of brain preservation—a concept to facilitate early identification and initiation of hypothermia to infants at high risk for brain injury. *Resuscitation.* 2010;81(12):1637–1641.

45. Chaudhary R, Farrer K, Broster S, McRitchie L, Austin T. Active versus passive cooling during neonatal transport. *Pediatrics.* 2013;132(5):841–846.

46. Dzhala V, Ben-Ari Y, Khazipov R. Seizures accelerate anoxia-induced neuronal death in the neonatal rat hippocampus. *Ann Neurol.* 2000;48(4):632–640.

47. Holmes GL, Gairsa JL, Chevassus-Au-Louis N, Ben-Ari Y. Consequences of neonatal seizures in the rat: morphological and behavioral effects. *Ann Neurol.* 1998;44(6):845–857.

48. Glass HC, Glidden D, Jeremy RJ, Barkovich AJ, Ferriero DM, Miller SP. Clinical neonatal seizures are independently associated with outcome in infants at risk for hypoxic-ischemic brain injury. *J Pediatr.* 2009;155(3):318–323.

49. Gluckman PD, Wyatt JS, Azzopardi D, et al. Selective head cooling with mild systemic hypothermia after neonatal encephalopathy: multicentre randomised trial. *Lancet.* 2005;365(9460):663–670.

50. Kwon JM, Guillet R, Shankaran S, et al. Clinical seizures in neonatal hypoxic-ischemic encephalopathy have no independent impact on neurodevelopmental outcome: secondary analyses of data from the neonatal research network hypothermia trial. *J Child Neurol.* 2011;26(3):322–328.

51. Scher MS, Aso K, Beggarly ME, Hamid MY, Steppe DA, Painter MJ. Electrographic seizures in preterm and full-term neonates—clinical correlates, associated brain-lesions, and risk for neurologic sequelae. *Pediatrics.* 1993;91(1):128–134.

52. Mizrahi EM. Consensus and controversy in the clinical management of neonatal seizures. *Clin Perinatol.* 1989;16(2):485–500.

53. van Rooij LG, Hellstrom-Westas L, de Vries LS. Treatment of neonatal seizures. *Semin Fetal Neonatal Med.* 2013;18(4):209–215.

54. Barks JD, Liu YQ, Shangguan Y, Silverstein FS. Phenobarbital augments hypothermic neuroprotection. *Pediatr Res.* 2010;67(5):532–537.

55. Goldberg RN, Moscoso P, Bauer CR, et al. Use of barbiturate therapy in severe perinatal asphyxia: a randomized controlled trial. *J Pediatr.* 1986;109(5):851–856.

56. Hall RT, Hall FK, Daily DK. High-dose phenobarbital therapy in term newborn infants with severe perinatal asphyxia: a randomized, prospective study with three-year follow-up. *J Pediatr.* 1998;132(2):345–348.

57. Singh D, Kumar P, Narang A. A randomized controlled trial of phenobarbital in neonates with hypoxic ischemic encephalopathy. *J Matern Fetal Neonatal Med.* 2005;18(6):391–395.

58. Meyn Jr DF, Ness J, Ambalavanan N, Carlo WA. Prophylactic phenobarbital and whole-body cooling for neonatal hypoxic-ischemic encephalopathy. *J Pediatr.* 2010;157(2):334–336.

59. Young L, Berg M, Soll R. Prophylactic barbiturate use for the prevention of morbidity and mortality following perinatal asphyxia. *Cochrane Database Syst Rev.* 2016;(5):CD001240.

60. Shimizu K, Rajapakse N, Horiguchi T, Payne RM, Busija DW. Neuroprotection against hypoxia-ischemia in neonatal rat brain by novel superoxide dismutase mimetics. *Neurosci Lett.* 2003;346(1–2):41–44.

61. Van Bel F, Shadid M, Moison RM, et al. Effect of allopurinol on postasphyxial free radical formation, cerebral hemodynamics, and electrical brain activity. *Pediatrics.* 1998;101(2):185–193.

62. Peeters C, Hoelen D, Groenendaal F, van Bel F, Bar D. Deferoxamine, allopurinol and oxypurinol are not neuroprotective after oxygen/glucose deprivation in an organotypic hippocampal model, lacking functional endothelial cells. *Brain Res.* 2003;963(1–2):72–80.

63. Chaudhari T, McGuire W. Allopurinol for preventing mortality and morbidity in newborn infants with hypoxic-ischaemic encephalopathy. *Cochrane Database Syst Rev.* 2012;(7):CD006817.

64. Kaandorp JJ, van Bel F, Veen S, et al. Long-term neuroprotective effects of allopurinol after moderate perinatal asphyxia: follow-up of two randomised controlled trials. *Arch Dis Child Fetal Neonatal Ed.* 2012;97(3):F162–F166.

65. van der Kooij MA, Groenendaal F, Kavelaars A, Heijnen CJ, van Bel F. Combination of deferoxamine and erythropoietin: therapy for hypoxia-ischemia-induced brain injury in the neonatal rat? *Neurosci Lett.* 2009;451(2):109–113.

66. Aly H, Elmahdy H, El-Dib M, et al. Melatonin use for neuroprotection in perinatal asphyxia: a randomized controlled pilot study. *J Perinatol.* 2015;35(3):186–191.

67. Marret S, Gressens P, Gadisseux JF, Evrard P. Prevention by magnesium of excitotoxic neuronal death in the developing brain: an animal model for clinical intervention studies. *Dev Med Child Neurol.* 1995;37(6):473–484.

68. Rouse DJ, Hirtz DG, Thom E, et al. A randomized, controlled trial of magnesium sulfate for the prevention of cerebral palsy. *N Engl J Med*. 2008;359(9):895–905.
69. Penrice J, Amess PN, Punwani S, et al. Magnesium sulfate after transient hypoxia-ischemia fails to prevent delayed cerebral energy failure in the newborn piglet. *Pediatr Res*. 1997;41(3):443–447.
70. de Haan HH, Gunn AJ, Williams CE, Heymann MA, Gluckman PD. Magnesium sulfate therapy during asphyxia in near-term fetal lambs does not compromise the fetus but does not reduce cerebral injury. *Am J Obstet Gynecol*. 1997;176(1 Pt 1):18–27.
71. Galinsky R, Bennet L, Groenendaal F, et al. Magnesium is not consistently neuroprotective for perinatal hypoxia-ischemia in term-equivalent models in preclinical studies: a systematic review. *Dev Neurosci*. 2014;36(2):73–82.
72. Bhat MA, Charoo BA, Bhat JI, Ahmad SM, Ali SW, Mufti MU. Magnesium sulfate in severe perinatal asphyxia: a randomized, placebo-controlled trial. *Pediatrics*. 2009;123(5):e764–e769.
73. Chakkarapani E, Chau V, Poskitt KJ, et al. Low plasma magnesium is associated with impaired brain metabolism in neonates with hypoxic-ischaemic encephalopathy. *Acta Paediatr*. 2016;105(9): 1067–1073.
74. Tagin M, Shah PS, Lee KS. Magnesium for newborns with hypoxic-ischemic encephalopathy: a systematic review and meta-analysis. *J Perinatol*. 2013;33(9):663–669.
75. Kelen D, Robertson NJ. Experimental treatments for hypoxic ischaemic encephalopathy. *Early Hum Dev*. 2010;86(6):369–377.
76. Ma D, Hossain M, Chow A, et al. Xenon and hypothermia combine to provide neuroprotection from neonatal asphyxia. *Ann Neurol*. 2005;58(2):182–193.
77. Chakkarapani E, Dingley J, Liu X, et al. Xenon enhances hypothermic neuroprotection in asphyxiated newborn pigs. *Ann Neurol*. 2010;68(3):330–341.
78. Hobbs C, Thoresen M, Tucker A, Aquilina K, Chakkarapani E, Dingley J. Xenon and hypothermia combine additively, offering long-term functional and histopathologic neuroprotection after neonatal hypoxia/ischemia. *Stroke*. 2008;39(4):1307–1313.
79. Azzopardi D, Robertson NJ, Bainbridge A, et al. Moderate hypothermia within 6 h of birth plus inhaled xenon versus moderate hypothermia alone after birth asphyxia (TOBY-Xe): a proof-of-concept, open-label, randomised controlled trial. *Lancet Neurol*. 2015.
80. Laitio R, Hynninen M, Arola O, et al. Effect of inhaled xenon on cerebral white matter damage in comatose survivors of out-of-hospital cardiac arrest: a randomized clinical trial. *JAMA*. 2016;315(11):1120–1128.
81. Dingley J, Tooley J, Liu X, et al. Xenon ventilation during therapeutic hypothermia in neonatal encephalopathy: a feasibility study. *Pediatrics*. 2014;133(5):809–818.
82. Cilio MR, Ferriero DM. Synergistic neuroprotective therapies with hypothermia. *Semin Fetal Neonatal Med*. 2010;15(5):293–298.
83. Gonzalez FF, Abel R, Almli CR, Mu D, Wendland M, Ferriero DM. Erythropoietin sustains cognitive function and brain volume after neonatal stroke. *Dev Neurosci*. 2009;31(5):403–411.
84. Aydin A, Genc K, Akhisaroglu M, Yorukoglu K, Gokmen N, Gonullu E. Erythropoietin exerts neuroprotective effect in neonatal rat model of hypoxic-ischemic brain injury. *Brain Dev*. 2003;25(7):494–498.
85. Kellert BA, McPherson RJ, Juul SE. A comparison of high-dose recombinant erythropoietin treatment regimens in brain-injured neonatal rats. *Pediatr Res*. 2007;61(4):451–455.
86. Fan X, Heijnen CJ, van der KM, Groenendaal F, van Bel F. Beneficial effect of erythropoietin on sensorimotor function and white matter after hypoxia-ischemia in neonatal mice. *Pediatr Res*. 2011;69(1):56–61.
87. Zhu C, Kang W, Xu F, et al. Erythropoietin improved neurologic outcomes in newborns with hypoxic-ischemic encephalopathy. *Pediatrics*. 2009;124(2):e218–e226.
88. Wu YW, Bauer LA, Ballard RA, et al. Erythropoietin for neuroprotection in neonatal encephalopathy: safety and pharmacokinetics. *Pediatrics*. 2012;130(4):683–691.
89. Rogers EE, Bonifacio SL, Glass HC, et al. Erythropoietin and hypothermia for hypoxic-ischemic encephalopathy. *Pediatr Neurol*. 2014;51(5):657–662.
90. Wu YW, Mathur AM, Chang T, et al. High-dose erythropoietin and hypothermia for hypoxic-ischemic encephalopathy: a phase II trial. *Pediatrics*. 2016;137(6).
91. Shankaran S, Laptook AR, Ehrenkranz RA, et al. Whole-body hypothermia for neonates with hypoxic-ischemic encephalopathy. *N Engl J Med*. 2005;353(15):1574–1584.
92. Azzopardi DV, Strohm B, Edwards AD, et al. Moderate hypothermia to treat perinatal asphyxial encephalopathy. *N Engl J Med*. 2009;361(14):1349–1358.

5

CHAPTER 6

Focal Cerebral Infarction

Dawn Gano and Donna M. Ferriero

- Stroke is common in newborns, affecting up to 1 in 1600 live births.
- Neonatal stroke can be classified according to blood supply (venous vs. arterial), age at stroke (fetal vs. neonatal), age at diagnosis (neonatal symptomatic vs. presumed perinatal), or type of stroke (ischemic vs. hemorrhagic).
- Focal seizures in a well-appearing newborn should prompt investigation for stroke, whereas the presence of intraventricular and thalamic hemorrhage should prompt investigation for cerebral sinovenous thrombosis.
- Magnetic resonance imaging with diffusion-weighted imaging is the gold standard for diagnosis of acute stroke.
- There are multiple risk factors for neonatal stroke, including maternal inherited or acquired thrombophilic disorders, hypertensive disorders of pregnancy, birth trauma, and neonatal comorbidities, such as intracranial infection, polycythemia, and congenital heart disease.
- Treatment of neonatal stroke is largely symptomatic, including maintenance of physiologic homeostasis, and early intervention with occupational therapy, physical therapy, and speech language pathology to promote acquisition of milestones.
- Acute treatment with anticoagulation should be considered for infants with embolic ischemic stroke or cerebral sinovenous thrombosis.
- Controversies in perinatal stroke include the role of therapeutic hypothermia, optimal timing for hematologic investigation to exclude inherited prothrombotic disorders, as well as the approach to anticoagulation.

Neonatal stroke is increasingly recognized as an important cause of neurologic morbidity, including cerebral palsy, epilepsy, and behavioral disorders, as well as impaired visual function and language development.[1-8] The estimated incidence of neonatal stroke is approximately 1 in 2000 live births.[9]

Stroke in the newborn can be classified by blood supply (venous vs. arterial), age at stroke (fetal vs. neonatal), age at diagnosis (neonatal symptomatic vs. presumed perinatal/neonatal asymptomatic), or type of stroke (ischemic vs. hemorrhagic). Investigators have used a variety of terms, including "neonatal stroke, perinatal stroke," "arterial ischemic stroke," and "perinatal arterial stroke" to describe the conditions. Neonatal stroke is the broader term describing stroke occurring anytime from in utero to 28 days of life. Perinatal stroke is that which occurs at or near the time of birth. Perinatal arterial ischemic stroke (PAIS) is defined as "a group of heterogeneous conditions in which there is focal disruption of cerebral blood flow secondary to arterial or cerebral sinovenous thrombosis (CSVT) or embolization confirmed by neuroimaging or neuropathologic studies."[10] PAIS is further divided into three categories based on the timing of diagnosis: (1) *fetal ischemic stroke*, diagnosed before birth using fetal imaging or following stillbirth on the basis of neuropathologic examination, (2) *neonatal ischemic stroke*, diagnosed at birth or by the 28th postnatal day (including preterm infants), and (3) *presumed perinatal ischemic stroke* (PPIS), diagnosed in children after 28 days of life in whom the ischemic event is presumed to have occurred between the 20th week of fetal life and the 28th postnatal day.[10] This terminology does not take into account venous thrombosis without ischemic infarction or purely hemorrhagic conditions. Hemorrhagic stroke of the newborn is less well characterized with no consensus on terminology or classification.

This chapter begins with a discussion of arterial ischemic stroke, followed by cerebral sinovenous thrombosis and then hemorrhagic stroke. Fetal ischemic stroke, PPIS, and stroke in the premature infant are also discussed in the section on arterial ischemic stroke. Controversies in the investigation and management of these conditions are addressed at the end of the chapter.

Perinatal Arterial Ischemic Stroke

Arterial ischemic stroke occurs when an artery is occluded by a thrombus or an embolus resulting in ischemic injury to the brain tissue distal to the occlusion. The cascade of cellular and molecular events that occur after hypoxia-ischemia culminate in apoptotic and necrotic cell death. Because right-to-left shunts are an integral part of cardiovascular physiology during the transition from fetal circulation to neonatal circulation, paradoxical emboli appear most likely to occur among newborns, particularly in the first days of life. PAIS is often a single lesion and occurs most frequently in the anterior circulation, commonly in the left middle cerebral artery territory.[11] Bilateral strokes occur in approximately 20% of patients.

Epidemiology

The incidence of neonatal stroke is estimated to be between 1:1600 and 1:5000 live births.[9,12–14] Neonatal stroke accounts for approximately 25% of arterial strokes in the pediatric population.[4] There are no apparent differences by infant sex or racial group, although data are somewhat inconsistent between study cohorts.[9,11–14] Mortality was estimated in one study as 13.4% (8 died of hemorrhagic stroke, 9 died of arterial ischemic stroke, and 1 died of asphyxia and cerebral sinovenous thrombosis).[14]

Risk Factors

Risk factors for PAIS can be grouped according to maternal, infant, or placental origin, and there is substantial overlap among these categories. Frequently, multiple concurrent risk factors are present and, in one study, the presence of multiple risk factors before delivery significantly increased the risk of perinatal stroke.[13] Notably important is that most infants with one or more of these risk factors are entirely normal, and conversely, no risk factor is identified in many cases of neonatal stroke. Further understanding of the genetic factors that predispose newborns to stroke may help explain the cause in a proportion of newborns with no discernible etiology.

Maternal Risk Factors

Maternal acquired and inherited thrombophilias are important risk factors for perinatal stroke. Pregnancy itself is a physiologic prothrombotic and proinflammatory state for the mother and her child.[15] In a normal pregnancy, there is a marked increase in the procoagulant activity in the maternal blood characterized by elevation of factors V, VII, VIII, IX, X, XII, fibrinogen, and von Willebrand factor, which is maximal around term.[16] In addition, there is a decrease in protein S activity and an acquired activated protein C resistance, leading to less effective thrombolysis.[16] The hypercoagulable state of pregnancy is also associated with an increased risk of maternal stroke in the first 3 postpartum days compared with nonpregnant women.[17]

Antiphospholipid antibodies, including lupus anticoagulant and cardiolipin antibody, present in women with systemic lupus erythematosus or other autoimmune disorders, increase the risk for fetal loss and for ischemic perinatal stroke.[18–20] Inherited thrombophilias may be present in either the mother or her child with perinatal stroke and are further discussed in the "Infant Factors" section.

Hypertensive disorders of pregnancy, specifically eclampsia and preeclampsia, are associated with a higher risk of neonatal stroke.[13,21] The pathophysiology may be related to a high frequency of factor V Leiden mutation in women with preeclampsia and with HELLP (hemolytic anemia, elevated liver enzymes, and low platelet count) syndrome.[21]

Further maternal risk factors for perinatal stroke include a history of infertility and primiparity,[13] as well as risk factors for maternal thrombosis, such as obesity, older maternal age, family history of thromboembolic events, surgery, dehydration, shock, and prolonged bed rest.[22] Maternal cocaine or amphetamine use can lead to vasospasm and poor perfusion of the placenta, and fetal exposure in utero is a rare but important cause of ischemic perinatal stroke.[23,24]

Antepartum and Intrapartum Risk Factors

Independent risk factors that may occur during pregnancy and delivery include oligohydramnios, cord abnormality, chorioamnionitis, and prolonged rupture of membranes.[13]

Placental Risk Factors

The placenta is highly susceptible to clotting caused by the effects of stasis in this low-flow system. Thrombotic lesions are often found in the placenta of those neonates diagnosed with stroke. In a paper dedicated to the topic of the role of placental pathology in neonatal stroke,[25] Elbers described abnormal placental pathology in 10 of 12 patients with neonatal stroke (7 with arterial ischemic stroke and 5 with cerebral venous sinus thrombosis). In these patients, 50% demonstrated thromboinflammatory processes such as chorioamnionitis. A further 42% demonstrated acute catastrophic events and 25% demonstrated decreased placental reserve.

Infant Factors

A number of systemic illnesses or conditions may increase the risk of stroke in the newborn infant. Meningitis/encephalitis, polycythemia, congenital heart disease, and extracorporeal membrane oxygenation have all been reported in infants with stroke.[26–29] Additional risk factors in the infant also include birth-related trauma that may result in stretch injury of carotid or vertebral arteries, leading to dissection, thrombus formation, and subsequent stroke.

Several prothrombotic disorders have been reported in infants with stroke, including protein S, protein C, and antithrombin III deficiencies, elevated lipoprotein(a), antiphospholipid antibodies, factor V G1691A, prothrombin G20210A, methylene tetrahydrofolate reductase *(MTHFR)* gene mutations, and elevated homocysteine.[20,21,30–35] However, many of these prothrombotic disorders are seen with high frequency in the general population, and conversely, some infants with stroke have no detectable abnormality.[36] Therefore the exact role of thrombophilia in the pathophysiology of neonatal stroke remains uncertain. Mutations in the genes *COL4A1* and *COL4A2* are associated with a wide spectrum of cerebrovascular lesions in newborns, in particular hemorrhagic stroke and porencephaly (see the "Hemorrhagic Stroke" section).[37]

Congenital cardiac disease may lead to embolic stroke intracardiac thrombus formation caused by diminished flow or the presence of right-to-left shunts. Cardiac surgery,[38] atrial septostomy,[39] and the presence of catheters[40] have been shown to increase the risk of stroke in newborns.

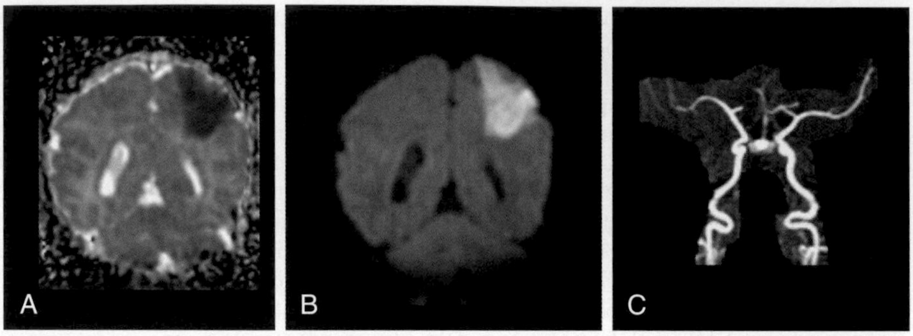

Fig. 6.1   Arterial ischemic stroke in a 2-day-old term infant presenting with focal clonic seizures at 24 hours of life. Placental pathology showed thrombotic vasculopathy and chorioamnionitis. A, Apparent diffusion coefficient map shows hypointense signal in the territory of the left middle cerebral artery posterior division. B, Corresponding hyperintensity is seen on diffusion-weighted imaging. C, Magnetic resonance angiography findings were normal.

Clinical Manifestations

The clinical manifestations of neonatal stroke depend on the timing of presentation (fetal, neonatal, or during infancy and childhood), as well as the location and extent of brain involvement.

Fetal Ischemic Stroke

Fetal ischemic stroke is diagnosed before birth using ultrasound and/or magnetic resonance imaging (MRI) or following stillbirth on neuropathology. Although fetal ischemic stroke is typically asymptomatic to the mother and child before delivery, there is a high rate of pregnancy termination, preterm delivery, and neonatal complications, including hypotonia and seizures.[41]

Neonatal Arterial Stroke

Term newborn infants with arterial stroke most commonly present with persistent focal seizures in the first hours of life.[42,43] Infants may otherwise appear well. However, a study from the International Pediatric Stroke Study found that a quarter of the babies presenting in the newborn period with PAIS actually are systemically ill.[11] Motor asymmetry, if present, is usually subtle, although the infant's general movements are frequently abnormal.[44] In the setting of concurrent global hypoxic-ischemic brain injury, signs of encephalopathy also occur, characterized by depressed level of alertness and altered feeding.[3,45]

Arterial infarcts are slightly more common in the left hemisphere than in the right hemisphere and frequently occur in the anterior circulation (Figs. 6.1 and 6.2).[11] The stroke may involve small- or large-artery territory, and multiple infarcts are present in up to 20% of cases.[4] Recent data have demonstrated that noncortical strokes in regions supplied by perforator arteries have pathogenic mechanisms similar to large-artery territory infarcts, such as hypoxia-ischemia, embolism, and infection.[46] Perforator artery strokes are frequently asymptomatic.[46]

Ischemic Stroke in the Preterm Infant

Increased use of imaging in premature infants has led to greater recognition of arterial stroke prior to term-equivalent postmenstrual age. The clinical presentation in premature infants can differ greatly from that of term infants, with less than one-third presenting with seizures or apnea.[47] Most often premature infants with stroke are identified during routine cranial ultrasound and the diagnosis of stroke is later confirmed using MRI.[47] As with term gestation infants, arterial stroke in premature newborns is more often unilateral, in the middle cerebral artery territory distribution, and left-sided. Lenticulostriate distribution is common, especially in infants born at 28 to 32 weeks' gestation.[48] Twin-to-twin

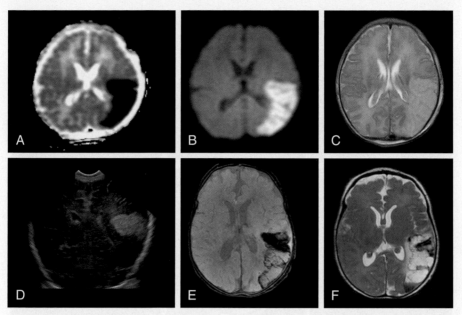

Fig. 6.2   Serial imaging of an infant treated with therapeutic hypothermia who was subsequently diagnosed with arterial ischemic stroke and later development of hemorrhagic transformation. Initial magnetic resonance imaging (MRI) obtained on day 4 of life with (A) apparent diffusion coefficient map and (B) diffusion-weighted imaging showing acute infarct of the left middle cerebral artery. C, T2-weighted MRI shows hyperintensity in the area of acute stroke consistent with vasogenic edema. D, Cranial ultrasound image obtained 3 days later for recurrent seizures showed increased echogenicity on the left, raising concern for hemorrhagic transformation. (E) Susceptibility-weighted imaging shows areas of hypointensity consistent with hemorrhage. (F) Axial T2-weighted MRI 2 weeks after the acute infarct shows evolving encephalomalacia and residual hemorrhage.

transfusion syndrome, fetal heart rate abnormalities, and hypoglycemia appear to be risk factors for preterm arterial stroke.[47,48]

Presumed Perinatal Ischemic Stroke

PPIS is diagnosed in a child older than 28 days who presents with nonacute neurologic signs or symptoms referable to focal, remote (gliosis, encephalomalacia, and/or atrophy and absent restricted diffusion) infarct(s) on neuroimaging (Fig. 6.3).[10,49] Presenting signs and symptoms include asymmetric motor development typically characterized by pathologic early hand preference or hemiplegia, as well as nonmotor delay, or seizures leading to a diagnosis of PPIS at a median age of 1 year.[50,51] PPIS may be due to either arterial (80%) or venous infarction but excludes global injuries, such as periventricular leukomalacia, basal ganglia, or watershed injury caused by hypoxic-ischemic injury.[49–51] Cases of children diagnosed with arterial PPIS reviewed retrospectively indicate that acute perinatal risk factors, such as fetal distress, emergency cesarean section, or a requirement for neonatal resuscitation, are often present.[50]

Imaging Arterial Ischemic Stroke

Magnetic resonance imaging (MRI) is the study of choice for the diagnosis and evaluation of neonatal stroke. Cranial ultrasound with transcranial Doppler may detect obliteration of normal gyral patterns, echogenicity in an arterial territory distribution, mass effect, or decrease in cerebral artery flow velocities in the affected hemisphere.[52,53] However, cranial ultrasound is less sensitive than other imaging modalities.[54,55] When possible, ultrasound should be supplemented with additional imaging, and MRI is preferable compared with computed tomography (CT). CT has the advantage of rapid acquisition and it can often be performed without sedation, but it provides less detailed anatomy than MRI and exposes the infant to ionizing radiation.

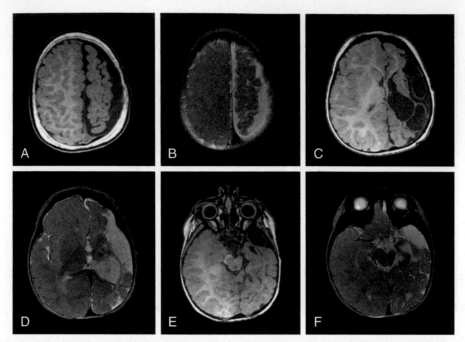

Fig. 6.3 Remote left middle cerebral artery stroke in an 11-month-old child presenting with congenital hemiparesis and early handedness. Axial T1-weighted magnetic resonance imaging (A, C, E) and T2-weighted images (B, D, F) show reduced volume of the left hemisphere and cystic encephalomalacia in the left middle cerebral artery territory. Note the diminished size of the left cerebral peduncle at the level of the midbrain, reflecting Wallerian degeneration of the left corticospinal tract (E, F).

MRI is highly sensitive to evolving injury caused by ischemia and provides the highest level of resolution to determine the location and extent of injury. Reduced water motion on diffusion-weighted imaging sequences is apparent within hours after the injury (see Figs. 6.1 and 6.2) but becomes falsely negative with pseudonormalization by approximately 7 days in newborns.[56] Conventional T1- and T2-weighted MRI sequences may be normal in the first 48 hours, making 2 to 5 days of life an ideal time to performing imaging in the infant with suspected stroke.[57] MR angiography (MRA) permits the evaluation of the intracranial and neck arterial vasculature. MRA is useful to reveal underlying vessel pathology such as dissection from birth trauma or arterial malformation. MRI and MRA are often performed with anesthesia to improve image quality by sedating the neonate to reduce motion artifact. Wrapping techniques have been developed that use vacuum devices to immobilize the unsedated neonate and improve image quality.[58] MR venogram (MRV) is warranted if there is thrombosis or suggestion of venous distribution infarct on the MRI (see later text).

In cases of PPIS, conventional T1- and T2-weighted images may reveal signs of remote infarct, including cystic encephalomalacia, gliosis, focal ventricular dilation, and Wallerian degeneration of the descending corticospinal tracts (Fig. 6.3).[49,50,59–61]

Management of Perinatal Arterial Ischemic Stroke

During the acute phase of neonatal stroke, attentive supportive care is important to minimize secondary brain injury. While there are no data from human neonatal trials, animal and adult studies support active maintenance of physiologic homeostasis, including temperature and blood glucose levels.[62,63] Expert opinion supports aggressive treatment of clinical and electrographic seizures that are frequent or prolonged.[64]

The value of antithrombotic therapy in newborns with ischemic stroke is uncertain, and guidelines or recommendations are based on clinical experience in older populations, observational or case studies, and clinical consensus. Guidelines by the American College of Chest Physicians recommend 3 months of anticoagulation with unfractionated or low-molecular-weight heparin for infants with cardioembolic arterial stroke (or cerebral venous sinus thrombosis [CSVT]) and without large territory involvement or hemorrhage.[65] Anticoagulation therapy is not suggested for noncardioembolic neonatal arterial stroke.

Long-term management of cerebral palsy involves traditional rehabilitation with passive stretching, splinting, and casting, as well as medical or surgical treatment for spasticity, including baclofen, tendon release surgery, or botulinum toxin A.[66] Constraint-induced movement therapy (CIMT), which involves restraint of the unaffected limb and frequent repetition of manual therapeutic tasks with the affected limb, is a promising treatment approach for children with hemiplegic cerebral palsy. Emerging evidence from studies using functional MRI suggests CIMT is associated with changes in cortical activation[67,68]; however, a Cochrane review concluded that there is only limited evidence of the clinical effect and suggested further trials to evaluate the efficacy of CIMT for hemiplegic children.[69] Transcranial magnetic stimulation (TMS) is a noninvasive brain stimulation and neuromodulation technique that is currently under investigation in children with neonatal stroke.[70] Preliminary data indicate safety and tolerability of contralesional inhibitory TMS with CIMT and intensive rehabilitation. Children with neonatal stroke should also be monitored through school age for subtle signs of cognitive impairment and referred for psychoeducational testing as needed.

Recent data from animal models have demonstrated that erythropoietin is a promising therapy to promote repair of injury following neonatal stroke.[71,72] Benders and colleagues have demonstrated safety and feasibility of erythropoietin for neuroprotection after PAIS,[73] and a larger randomized controlled trial is needed to determine whether treatment improves repair after PAIS and, consequently, neurodevelopmental outcomes.

Cerebral Sinovenous Thrombosis

CSVT occurs when a venous sinus, deep vein, or cortical vein is completely or partially obstructed by thrombus. CSVT may occur without associated parenchymal injury when there is incomplete occlusion of the vessel or adequate collateralization. The rate of venous infarct associated with neonatal CSVT varies between studies, but the risk for secondary hemorrhagic conversion is consistently high.[74,75] Blood is not limited to the confines of the infarct, as there is also frequent intraventricular and extraparenchymal hemorrhage.[75–77]

The anatomic distribution of infarct in CSVT occurs in predictable patterns referable to the areas drained by the affected sinus. For instance, with a straight sinus thrombosis, there may be evidence of injury to unilateral or bilateral basal ganglia and thalami, whereas with sagittal sinus thrombosis there may be evidence of injury in a parasagittal watershed distribution.[78] Hemorrhagic lesions have been reported with the following associations; thalamoventricular hemorrhage with internal cerebral vein occlusion, bilateral thalamoventricular hemorrhage with vein of Galen occlusion, striato-hippocampal hemorrhage with basal vein thrombosis, temporal lobe or cerebellar hemorrhage with transverse sinus thrombosis, or temporal lobe hemorrhage alone with vein of Labbé thrombosis.[79]

Epidemiology

The incidence of venous ischemic stroke is estimated at 2.6 to 12 per 100,000 term newborns each year.[75] Among reported cases of CSVT in pediatric patients, newborns are at highest risk.[76] Mortality estimates range from 6% to 19% depending on the study.[14,80] Male newborns appear to have an increased frequency of CSVT compared with female newborns.[74,80]

Risk Factors for CSVT

Infants with CSVT frequently have comorbid risk factors, including dehydration, cardiac defects, sepsis, or meningitis, and extracorporeal life support requirement.[74,81–83] In one study, hypoxic-ischemic encephalopathy was present in 20% of newborns diagnosed with CSVT.[75] Maternal risk factors include premature rupture of membranes, chorioamnionitis, gestational diabetes, and preeclampsia with associated endothelial dysfunction.[82] A difficult delivery with or without trauma to the skull and injury to superior sagittal sinus also increases the risk of CSVT.

Although prothrombotic disorders are present in up to two-thirds of patients with CSVT, these disorders are less common among newborns with CSVT.[84] Few abnormalities were detected in a study of 52 newborns with CSVT, including 2 infants diagnosed with *G20210A* prothrombin gene mutation, as well as 13 with *MTHFR* C677T and *A1298C* mutations.[80] Anticardiolipin antibody, lupus anticoagulant, prothrombin time, partial thromboplastin time, and fibrinogen testing should not be overlooked.

Clinical Manifestations

CSVT typically presents in the first weeks of life with nonspecific signs and symptoms, including encephalopathy, apnea, and seizures. A term infant presenting with intraventricular hemorrhage with thalamic hemorrhage and seizures is a common triad suggestive of venous sinus thrombosis.[76,80] A full fontanelle and prominent scalp veins may also be seen.

Imaging CSVT

Cranial ultrasound in the term newborns with CSVT may show intraventricular and thalamic hemorrhage.[76,77] In the hands of experienced technicians and radiologists, color Doppler ultrasound can demonstrate absent flow in the sinuses consistent with CSVT.[78] Computed tomography, magnetic resonance, or conventional angiographic venography is much more sensitive for CSVT. Most often the sagittal, transverse, or straight sinus is involved,[74,81] and in one study, the majority of newborns (80%) had multiple sinuses involved (Fig. 6.4).

Common sequelae include venous infarction with parenchymal and intraventricular hemorrhage.[76,77,81] CSVT should be suspected when infarcts are *not* confined to known vascular territories or they are bilateral and involve deep gray nuclei. Hemorrhage is frequently associated with CSVT and can be seen on MRI with susceptibility-weighted image. In one study of 67 neonates for whom full imaging data were available, an infarct or hemorrhage was present in two-thirds.[85] Serial imaging is required if a clot is present to evaluate for extension or propagation.[65,84]

Management of CSVT

Management of neonatal CSVT includes supportive care, such as management of dehydration, treatment of infection, and seizures, as well as anticoagulation. The American Heart Association recommendations suggest considering

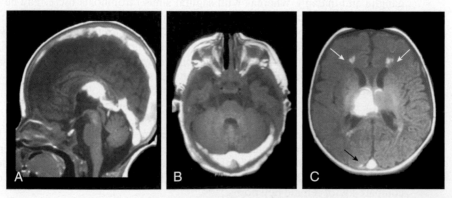

Fig. 6.4 Cerebral sinovenous thrombosis in a newborn with congenital heart disease. A, Sagittal T1-weighted magnetic resonance imaging (MRI) shows extensive thrombosis with hyperintensity in the superior sagittal sinus, straight sinus, and great cerebral vein. B, Axial T1-weighted MRI shows thrombosis of the transverse sinuses and (C) thalamic hemorrhage and bilateral watershed injury with hemorrhage *(white arrows)*. Thrombus is also seen in the superior sagittal sinus *(black arrow)*.

anticoagulation in selected newborns with severe thrombophilic disorders, multiple cerebral or systemic emboli, or when there is clinical or radiologic evidence of propagating clot.[84] The recommendations from the American College of Chest Physicians are more inclusive and suggest anticoagulation when there is not extensive intracranial hemorrhage.[65] They further recommend consideration of treatment when clot is propagating even in the presence of extensive hemorrhage. In one retrospective study, slightly more than half of the 81 newborns with CSVT were treated with anticoagulation and there were no adverse events.[85] In a prospective study of 104 neonates with CSVT, half received anticoagulation therapy with unfractionated heparin or low-molecular-weight heparin.[75] Anticoagulation was initiated at diagnosis in three-fourths of treated infants and after confirmation of thrombus propagation on serial imaging in one-fourth. In the treated group, there were no serious adverse events such as systemic hemorrhage or anticoagulant-related deaths. Fourteen newborns had significant hemorrhage before receiving anticoagulation and none experienced worsening hemorrhage with treatment. Thrombus propagation occurred in one-third of the newborns who were not treated with anticoagulation but only occurred in one treated newborn. Venous infarction was common in infants with clot propagation. Thrombus propagation was clinically silent in all but one neonate who developed worsening seizures.

For infants with CSVT who are not treated with antithrombotic therapy, imaging should be repeated to look for propagation of the thrombosis. There is no consensus regarding the timing of repeat imaging, and 5 to 7 days is a reasonable approach in a clinically stable infant. Newborns with CSVT who are treated with antithrombotic therapy should have imaging performed again at 3 months to ensure complete recanalization of the venous sinuses.[65]

Hemorrhagic Stroke

Perinatal hemorrhagic stroke has received little attention. The estimated incidence of perinatal hemorrhagic stroke was 6.2 per 100,000 live births in a population-based study.[86] Hemorrhagic stroke can be primary (Fig. 6.5) or secondary to hemorrhagic transformation of an arterial or venous ischemic infarct (see Fig. 6.2).

Clinical Features

Newborns with hemorrhagic stroke present with encephalopathy or seizures, and strokes are typically unilateral, occurring in the frontal or parietal lobes.[86,87] In one study, seizures with an apneic semiology were particularly associated with temporal lobe hemorrhage and frequently required more than one antiepileptic agent.[87]

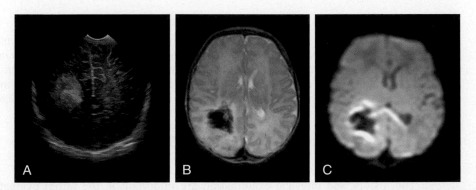

Fig. 6.5   Hemorrhagic stroke in a 3-day-old girl presenting with status epilepticus. A, Coronal ultrasound shows area of increased echogenicity in the right parieto-occipital region, corresponding with (B) axial T2-weighted magnetic resonance imaging (MRI) showing hypointense lesion consistent with hemorrhage. C, Diffusion-weighted MRI shows hyperintensity surrounding the hemorrhage and across the splenium consistent with pre-Wallerian degeneration.

Fetal distress and postterm delivery at greater than 41 weeks' gestation are independently associated with neonatal hemorrhagic stroke.[86,87] Additional risk factors include thrombocytopenia, vitamin K deficiency, and deficiency of coagulation factors; however, hemorrhagic stroke of the newborn is a rare complication of each of these.

Type IV collagen α1 and α2 (*COL4A1* and *COL4A2*) mutations are a risk factor for intracerebral hemorrhage, particularly hemorrhagic stroke occurring in utero that results in porencephaly.[37,88–90] Recently a widened phenotypic spectrum of *COL4A1* mutation–related disorders has been described.[37] In addition to porencephaly and transmantle lesions, which result in hydranencephaly or schizencephaly, mutations in *COL4A1* and *COL4A2* are also associated with systemic features, including lesions of the kidneys, eyes, heart, and skeletal muscle. Mutations in *COL4A1* and *COL4A2* are autosomal dominant and often occur de novo.[37]

Infrequently, neonatal intracranial hemorrhage is the result of a vascular malformation—namely, aneurysms and arteriovenous malformations including vein of Galen malformations. Intracranial hemorrhage related to aneurysmal rupture is often characterized by rapid neurologic deterioration and subarachnoid hemorrhage.

Hemorrhagic Stroke in Preterm Infants

Premature infants, particularly those less than 28 weeks' gestation at birth, are at risk for periventricular venous hemorrhagic infarction, which is also known as grade IV intraventricular hemorrhage using the Papile classification system.[91] The mechanism is thought to be related to mass effect from germinal matrix hemorrhage on the draining medullary veins, causing subsequent infarction and hemorrhage.[61]

Imaging Hemorrhagic Stroke

Bedside cranial ultrasound is an important tool to quickly assess for intracranial hemorrhage. Further imaging with MRI or CT is needed to better define the location of hemorrhage, and when possible, the underlying cause. While CT has excellent sensitivity for hemorrhage, MRI is preferred due to the better spatial resolution, and safety profile. Susceptibility-weighted imaging (SWI) or gradient echo (GRE) sequences can be used to demonstrate the presence of blood products and is as sensitive as CT.[93] Both MRA and MRV should be considered in the evaluation of a newborn with intracerebral hemorrhage.

Cranial ultrasound is additionally useful to noninvasively monitor the size of the hemorrhage in the acute period and should be repeated serially to evaluate for progression in the days after diagnosis of hemorrhagic stroke. Because identification of an underlying vascular malformation is difficult in the setting of acute hemorrhage, vascular imaging should be performed following resolution of the hemorrhage.

Management of Perinatal Hemorrhagic Stroke

The management of intracranial hemorrhage is supportive, including maintenance of physiologic homeostasis and correction of coagulation abnormalities. Serial imaging and sequential neurologic examination in the asymptomatic newborn is an appropriate approach. If a large lesion is present or there are signs of increased intracranial pressure or brainstem compromise, then immediate neurosurgical evaluation is necessary.

Evaluation of Newborns With Suspected Stroke

History and Physical Examination

The history and physical examination are important in the initial evaluation of an infant with suspected stroke (Table 6.1). Detailed family history, as well as evaluation of maternal medical conditions and events during pregnancy and delivery, may reveal one or more risk factors for perinatal stroke. Although the initial examination results may be normal, newborns with arterial ischemic stroke are

Table 6.1 PERTINENT CLINICAL HISTORY

Investigation	Comment
Family	Careful history may reveal one or more risk factors for perinatal stroke
Maternal	History of lupus and autoimmune disease, infertility, miscarriage(s), cocaine use
Antepartum/intrapartum	Hypertensive disorders of pregnancy, oligohydramnios, cord abnormality, chorioamnionitis
Delivery	Prolonged rupture of membranes, fetal distress, emergency cesarean section, requirement for neonatal resuscitation
Infant	Sepsis, meningitis/encephalitis, hypoxic-ischemic encephalopathy, polycythemia, congenital heart disease, extracorporeal membrane oxygenation

often systemically sick, presenting with seizures, encephalopathy, and nonfocal neurologic signs.[11] The skin should be closely examined in an infant with hemorrhagic stroke to detect cutaneous hemangioma, which may indicate hereditary hemorrhagic telangiectasia.

Differential Diagnosis

The differential diagnosis for neonatal stroke is ostensibly the same differential diagnosis for neonatal encephalopathy, a broad term defined as an alteration in level of consciousness in the newborn. Hypoxic-ischemic encephalopathy should be considered foremost with this differential diagnosis, particularly in light of the significant overlap of its symptoms and risk factors with neonatal stroke. Other considerations include any form of intracranial hemorrhage (including intraventricular, subarachnoid, subdural, and intraparenchymal hemorrhage), sepsis, and central nervous system infection (encephalitis or meningitis), which may similarly present with altered mental status and seizures. Metabolic encephalopathy, whether the result of inherited or acquired causes, must also be considered. Hypoglycemia and electrolyte derangements (sodium, calcium, and magnesium) are treatable causes of neonatal seizures and thus should be ruled out. Inherited inborn errors of metabolism, while rare, collectively comprise an important class of conditions to consider with this differential diagnosis, as prompt diagnosis may lead to a specific treatment. Uncommonly structural masses, such as congenital vascular malformations and brain tumors, may present in the neonate with symptoms of encephalopathy and seizure.

Approach to Investigations (Table 6.2)

Neuroimaging

Cranial ultrasound is a helpful initial imaging study to quickly evaluate for hemorrhage at the bedside. Further imaging with MRI, including diffusion-weighted imaging sequences, is recommended if available (see Table 6.2). CT should be reserved for use when MRI is not available or is infeasible because of clinical instability. The addition of vascular studies should be considered. In the presence of multifocal lesions with reduced diffusion, MRA of the neck and intracranial arteries should be obtained to evaluate for a proximal thromboembolic source including dissection. In infants suspected to have CSVT based on Doppler studies, intraventricular hemorrhage and/or thalamic hemorrhage, or an acute venous infarct, MRV with gadolinium should also be considered. If intraparenchymal hemorrhage is present, both MRA and MRV imaging should be obtained when possible to evaluate for vascular malformation and CSVT.

Laboratory Investigations

Initial laboratory evaluation should include studies that are routinely performed in an infant with seizures or encephalopathy, such as complete blood cell count with differential, electrolytes (including calcium and magnesium), glucose levels,

Table 6.2 INVESTIGATIONS IN NEONATAL STROKE

Investigation	Comment
Imaging	
Magnetic resonance imaging (MRI)	MRI with diffusion-weighted imaging is the imaging study of choice. Consider additional vascular imaging with magnetic resonance angiography and/or magnetic resonance venography.
Computed tomography	Use low-ionization radiation protocol if performed.
Cranial ultrasound	Quickly identifies intracranial hemorrhage at the bedside. Limited utility in ischemic stroke unless performed by highly experienced technician.
Laboratory evaluation	
Complete blood cell count with differential	Polycythemia, leukocytosis, thrombocytopenia.
Serum electrolytes and glucose	
Prothrombin time with international normalized ratio (PT/INR)	
Partial thromboplastin time (PTT)	

Thrombophilia evaluation
  Protein S/C activity
  Antithrombin III activity
  Activated protein C resistance
  Lipoprotein(a)
  Homocysteine
  Factor V Leiden
  Prothrombin G20210A
  Antiphospholipid antibody testing
	Thrombophilia evaluation can be performed in the mother and child in the acute and convalescent periods.

Other	
Electroencephalography	Can be tailored to nature and timing of insult.
Placental pathology	
Echocardiography	Evaluate for structural cardiac disease, cardioembolic source.

prothrombin time with international normalized ratio, partial thromboplastin time, as well as cultures for infection. Once ischemic stroke is confirmed by imaging, the infant and mother can be evaluated for thrombophilia, although the results are unlikely to change management.[94] The hypercoagulable workup may be deferred from the acute setting, where values are often reflective of the pregnancy state rather than intrinsic abnormalities of the neonate. In the acute period, the mother should be tested for antiphospholipid antibodies and anticardiolipin antibodies if she has a history of thromboembolism or recurrent miscarriage. Further testing of the infant can be obtained as part of outpatient follow-up and may include antithrombin III, protein C, protein S, activated protein C resistance, factor V Leiden mutation, prothrombin gene mutation (*G20210A*), and antiphospholipid antibodies. Transthoracic echocardiography should be performed in infants with abnormal cardiac examination results or suspected embolic infarct to exclude underlying cardiac disease. For infants with parenchymal hemorrhage or suspected stroke in utero with resultant porencephaly, ophthalmology consultation to check for retinal evidence of vasculopathy and *COL4A* gene testing are recommended.

Electroencephalography

Recurrent focal seizure is the most common initial presentation of neonatal stroke.[43] An electroencephalogram (EEG) is essential to evaluate for subclinical seizures, especially after administration of antiseizure medication, which may lead to electroclinical dissociation.[95] EEG can also identify background abnormalities, which indicate poor neuromotor prognosis.[3,95] EEG abnormalities, including focal attenuation, epileptiform discharges, and/or focal seizures, are typically transient and present only during the first days to weeks after the injury.[96]

Placental Pathology

Pathologic examination of the placenta may identify lesions to support a pathogenic mechanism, such as a thromboinflammatory process, stressful intrauterine environment, or catastrophic event.[25]

Neurologic Outcome

Neurodevelopmental outcome following neonatal stroke varies considerably in the published literature, reflecting heterogeneity in the extent and location of injury, variable duration of follow-up, and differences in outcome measures. Most studies suggest high risk for neurodevelopmental disability, including cerebral palsy, epilepsy, and behavioral disorders, as well as impaired visual function and language development.[1–8,97,98] In one population-based study, 68% of children who presented in the neonatal period and 94% of children with delayed presentation were diagnosed with one or more disability.[8]

Despite high rates of neurologic disabilities, many studies show that children who survive after neonatal stroke have good functional outcomes, which may in part reflect the inherent plasticity of the developing brain. Studies using functional MRI have shown bilateral or right-sided activation of language area homologs in children with a history of left-hemisphere perinatal stroke.[99,100] A recent study of resting-state functional connectivity in children with neonatal stroke supports the hypothesis of plasticity by demonstrating that connectivity values in areas of injury were better correlated with simulated values of a healthy brain than those of an injured brain.[101]

Neuromotor Outcome

Perinatal stroke is a common cause of hemiplegic cerebral palsy. Among children with motor impairment caused by neonatal stroke, approximately two-thirds present after 3 months of age.[102] Functional motor impairment is present in up to 30% to 40% of children examined after 12 months of age, and 30% have some asymmetry of tone without definite hemiplegia.[1,3,8] The risk of motor impairment is approximately twice as high in children who present after the neonatal period, which may reflect ascertainment bias because many of these children are diagnosed following evaluation of pathologic early handedness or evolving cerebral palsy.[8,49] The great majority of children with neonatal ischemic stroke achieve independent walking, especially in cases of unilateral stroke.[103]

The prediction of neuromotor outcome based on early clinical, EEG, and imaging features is important for providing prognostic information to families and facilitating rehabilitation. Furthermore, accurate early tools for predicting outcome may ultimately help identify patients for specific therapeutic interventions. Stroke size and location are helpful in predicting neuromotor outcome. Infants with larger stroke size have a higher risk of hemiplegia, especially when there is injury to the motor cortex, basal ganglia, and posterior limb of the internal capsule.[1,3,8] Children with injury to only the cortex, the basal ganglia, or the posterior limb of the internal capsule have a good chance of normal neuromotor outcome.[1,3] Neuromotor outcome is also highly correlated with the length and volume of diffusion changes along the descending corticospinal tracts.[59,104] Early abnormal EEG background may also be helpful in predicting hemiparesis, with 93% sensitivity and 100% specificity in one study.[1]

Neonatal Seizures and Epilepsy

The incidence of epilepsy after neonatal stroke is variable and likely depends on the nature of the lesion, as well as the timing and duration of long-term follow-up. Published rates of epilepsy after age 6 months range widely, from 0% to 67%.[6,8,96,105,106] In one study of 64 children with neonatal stroke and at least 6 months of follow-up, 67% developed seizures at a median age of 16 months.[106] Most children were seizure-free with or without medication.[106]

Neurobehavioral Outcome

Cognitive outcome in children with PAIS or CSVT is variable but often impaired. Some studies report "language delay" in up to 25% to 30% of children.[8,49] In a study of preschool children, average scores on the mental development index of the Bayley

Scales of Infant Development (normative mean 100 and standard deviation 15) at age 24 months were in the low 90s (range 50s–120s).[5] In school-age children, language development and intelligence quotient were lower in infants with unilateral hemispheric neonatal stroke than in age-matched peers.[107] Interestingly, the laterality of the lesion did not appear to be an important factor in language development. The presence of seizures beyond the neonatal period was associated with worse outcome in this study.

In one population-based study, behavioral abnormalities were diagnosed by a physician in 11% of children who presented with stroke in the neonatal period and 35% of children with delayed presentation.[8] Another study, which used the Achenbach Child Behavior Checklist, found no evidence of clinically significant behavioral or emotional problems in children and adolescents with neonatal stroke, even when the frontal lobe was involved.[108] However, children with more extensive and bilateral injury may be at higher risk for behavioral and emotional dysfunction.

Visual Function

Impairment of acuity, visual fields, or stereopsis was present in approximately 30% of school-age children with a history of perinatal stroke in one study.[2] There was no relationship between injury to the optic radiations or visual cortex and visual impairment, but larger middle cerebral artery lesions were more often associated with visual field deficits. Other studies have shown that children presenting with congenital hemiplegia have a higher incidence of visual field defects.[109,110]

Stroke Recurrence

The rate of stroke recurrence following perinatal stroke is much lower than for childhood or adult stroke, which suggests that long-term prophylaxis is probably unwarranted in most cases. There were no recurrences in a population-based study that identified 40 children with perinatal stroke.[8] Most of the symptomatic recurrences (including extracerebral venous thrombosis) seen in a prospective cohort of 215 children occurred in the context of congenital or acquired systemic illness including congenital heart disease.[35]

Controversies in Neonatal Stroke

Hematologic Investigations

There is no consensus regarding the appropriate timing of the hypercoagulable workup in perinatal ischemic stroke. The approach to hematologic investigations in this patient population is typically determined institutionally. Because values in the acute period are thought to reflect the pregnancy state rather than intrinsic abnormalities of the newborn, the utility of performing the hypercoagulable workup acutely in the newborn with stroke is unclear. In many centers, testing for hypercoagulability is often deferred until the infant is at least 3 months of age. The practice at our center is to refer all infants with PAIS for outpatient consultation with a hematologist. In the absence of a family history suggestive of thrombophilic disorders, families are given the option to obtain additional testing after counseling on the very low likelihood of the test results changing management or outcome.

Therapeutic Hypothermia for Neonatal Stroke

The risk factors and clinical signs associated with hypoxic-ischemic encephalopathy overlap with those of perinatal stroke. One prospective cohort of 124 encephalopathic newborns showed that 6 (5%) had evidence of acute stroke on imaging.[45] Whether therapeutic hypothermia ameliorates the progression and extent of permanent injury caused by stroke—for example, by preserving the penumbra—is not known. Among encephalopathic newborns who were subsequently found to have PAIS, one study showed a decreased frequency of seizures in newborns treated with hypothermia for HIE (0/5 cooled neonates had seizures vs. 7/10 neonates who were not cooled had seizures).[111] Future research should focus on the impact of therapeutic hypothermia initiated after the diagnosis of acute ischemic stroke in newborns, whether it leads to reduced extent of injury on follow-up imaging, and improved long-term neurologic outcomes.

Anticoagulation for CSVT

Guidelines by the American College of Chest Physicians recommend 3 months of anticoagulation with unfractionated or low-molecular-weight heparin for infants with cardioembolic arterial stroke or CSVT and without large-territory involvement or hemorrhage.[65] However, the implementation of these guidelines varies across institutions, and often the decision to treat with anticoagulation is made on a case-by-case basis contingent on evidence of thrombus propagation. It is not presently clear whether earlier treatment with anticoagulation at initial diagnosis of CSVT leads to improved outcomes. Although outcome appears to be worse among newborns with clot extension, likely mediated by development of a venous infarction, this may reflect an ascertainment bias in light of the fact that clot propagation is typically asymptomatic in the neonatal period. A randomized controlled trial of anticoagulation in neonatal CSVT is needed to determine whether use or timing of anticoagulation leads to improved outcomes.

The optimal timing of repeat imaging in newborns with CSVT to monitor for clot progression is also unclear. In an infant who is clinically stable, follow-up imaging approximately 1 week after diagnosis with CSVT is a reasonable approach. Additional studies are needed to identify which newborns are at highest risk for thrombus propagation, which may enable earlier diagnosis and treatment and ultimately lead to improved outcomes.

REFERENCES

1. Mercuri E, Barnett A, Rutherford M, et al. Neonatal cerebral infarction and neuromotor outcome at school age. *Pediatrics*. 2004;113:95–100.
2. Mercuri E, Anker S, Guzzetta A, et al. Neonatal cerebral infarction and visual function at school age. *Arch Dis Child Fetal Neonatal Ed*. 2003;88:F487–F491.
3. Mercuri E, Rutherford M, Cowan F, et al. Early prognostic indicators of outcome in infants with neonatal cerebral infarction: a clinical, electroencephalogram, and magnetic resonance imaging study. *Pediatrics*. 1999;103:39–46.
4. deVeber GA, MacGregor D, Curtis R, et al. Neurologic outcome in survivors of childhood arterial ischemic stroke and sinovenous thrombosis. *J Child Neurol*. 2000;15:316–324.
5. McLinden A, Baird AD, Westmacott R, et al. Early cognitive outcome after neonatal stroke. *J Child Neurol*. 2007;22:1111–1116.
6. Sran SK, Baumann RJ. Outcome of neonatal strokes. *Am J Dis Child*. 1988;142:1086–1088.
7. Sreenan C, Bhargava R, Robertson CM. Cerebral infarction in the term newborn: clinical presentation and long-term outcome. *J Pediatr*. 2000;137:351–355.
8. Lee J, Croen LA, Lindan C, et al. Predictors of outcome in perinatal arterial stroke: a population-based study. *Ann Neurol*. 2005;58:303–308.
9. Schulzke S, Weber P, Luetschg J, Fahnenstich H. Incidence and diagnosis of unilateral arterial cerebral infarction in newborn infants. *J Perinat Med*. 2005;33:170–175.
10. Raju TN, Nelson KB, Ferriero D, et al. Ischemic perinatal stroke: summary of a workshop sponsored by the National Institute of Child Health and Human Development and the National Institute of Neurological Disorders and Stroke. *Pediatrics*. 2007;120:609–616.
11. Kirton A, Armstrong-Wells J, Chang T, et al. Symptomatic neonatal arterial ischemic stroke: the international pediatric stroke study. *Pediatrics*. 2011;128:e1402–e1410.
12. Laugesaar R, Kolk A, Tomberg T, et al. Acutely and retrospectively diagnosed perinatal stroke: a population-based study. *Stroke*. 2007;38:2234–2240.
13. Lee J, Croen LA, Backstrand KH, et al. Maternal and infant characteristics associated with perinatal arterial stroke in the infant. *JAMA*. 2005;293:723–729.
14. Govaert P, Ramenghi L, Taal R, Dudink J, Lequin M. Diagnosis of perinatal stroke II: mechanisms and clinical phenotypes. *Acta Paediatr*. 2009;98(11):1720–1726.
15. Arkel YS, Ku DH. Thrombophilia and pregnancy: review of the literature and some original data. *Clin Appl Thromb Hemost*. 2001;7:259–268.
16. Brenner B. Haemostatic changes in pregnancy. *Thromb Res*. 2004;114(5–6):409–414.
17. Nelson KB. Perinatal ischemic stroke. *Stroke*. 2007;38(suppl 2):742–745.
18. Silver RK, MacGregor SN, Pasternak JF, et al. Fetal stroke associated with elevated maternal anticardiolipin antibodies. *Obstet Gynecol*. 1992;80:497–499.

19. Akanli LF, Trasi SS, Thuraisamy K, et al. Neonatal middle cerebral artery infarction: association with elevated maternal anticardiolipin antibodies. *Am J Perinatol.* 1998;15:399–402.

20. Gunther G, Junker R, Strater R, et al. Symptomatic ischemic stroke in full-term neonates: role of acquired and genetic prothrombotic risk factors. *Stroke.* 2000;31:2437–2441.

21. Rigo J, Nagy B, Fintor L, et al. Maternal and neonatal outcome of preeclamptic pregnancies: the potential roles of factor V Leiden mutation and 5,10 methylenetetrahydrofolate reductase. *Hypertens Pregnancy.* 2000;19:163–172.

22. Hague WM, Dekker GA. Risk factors for thrombosis in pregnancy. *Best Pract Res Clin Haematol.* 2003;16:197–210.

23. Chasnoff IJ, Bussey ME, Savich R, et al. Perinatal cerebral infarction and maternal cocaine use. *J Pediatr.* 1986;108:456–459.

24. Heier LA, Carpanzano CR, Mast J, et al. Maternal cocaine abuse: the spectrum of radiologic abnormalities in the neonatal CNS. *AJNR Am J Neuroradiol.* 1991;12:951–956.

25. Elbers J, Viero S, MacGregor D, et al. Placental pathology in neonatal stroke. *Pediatrics.* 2011;127:e722–e729.

26. Ment LR, Ehrenkranz RA, Duncan CC. Bacterial meningitis as an etiology of perinatal cerebral infarction. *Pediatr Neurol.* 1986;2:276–279.

27. Amit M, Camfield PR. Neonatal polycythemia causing multiple cerebral infarcts. *Arch Neurol.* 1980;37:109–110.

28. Jarjour IT, Ahdab-Barmada M. Cerebrovascular lesions in infants and children dying after extracorporeal membrane oxygenation. *Pediatr Neurol.* 1994;10:13–19.

29. Pellicer A, Cabanas F, Garcia-Alix A, et al. Stroke in neonates with cardiac right-to-left shunt. *Brain Dev.* 1992;14:381–385.

30. Brenner B, Fishman A, Goldsher D, et al. Cerebral thrombosis in a newborn with a congenital deficiency of antithrombin III. *Am J Hematol.* 1988;27:209–211.

31. Hogeveen M, Blom HJ, Van Amerongen M, et al. Hyperhomocysteinemia as risk factor for ischemic and hemorrhagic stroke in newborn infants. *J Pediatr.* 2002;141:429–431.

32. Garoufi AJ, Prassouli AA, Attilakos AV, et al. Homozygous MTHFR C677T gene mutation and recurrent stroke in an infant. *Pediatr Neurol.* 2006;35:49–51.

33. Curry CJ, Bhullar S, Holmes J, et al. Risk factors for perinatal arterial stroke: a study of 60 mother–child pairs. *Pediatr Neurol.* 2007;37:99–107.

34. Lynch JK, Han CJ, Nee LE, et al. Prothrombotic factors in children with stroke or porencephaly. *Pediatrics.* 2005;116:447–453.

35. Kurnik K, Kosch A, Strater R, et al. Recurrent thromboembolism in infants and children suffering from symptomatic neonatal arterial stroke: a prospective follow-up study. *Stroke.* 2003;34:2887–2892.

36. Miller SP, Wu YW, Lee J, et al. Candidate gene polymorphisms do not differ between newborns with stroke and normal controls. *Stroke.* 2006;37:2678–2683.

37. Meuwissen MEC Halley DJJ, Smit LS, et al. The expanding phenotype of COL4A1 and COL4A2 mutations: clinical data on 13 newly identified families and a review of the literature. *Genet Med.* 2015;17(11):843–853.

38. Chen J, Zimmerman RA, Jarvik GP, et al. Perioperative stroke in infants undergoing open heart operations for congenital heart disease. *Ann Thorac Surg.* 2009;88(3):823–829.

39. Mukherjee D, Lindsay M, Zhang Y, et al. Analysis of 8681 neonates with transposition of the great arteries: outcomes with and without Rashkind balloon atrial septostomy. *Cardiol Young.* 2010;20(4):373–380.

40. Schmidt B, Andrew M. Neonatal thrombosis: report of a prospective Canadian and international registry. *Pediatrics.* 1995;96(5 Pt 1):939–943.

41. Ozduman K, Pober BR, Barnes P, et al. Fetal stroke. *Pediatr Neurol.* 2004;30:151–162.

42. Levy SR, Abroms IF, Marshall PC, et al. Seizures and cerebral infarction in the full-term newborn. *Ann Neurol.* 1985;17:366–370.

43. Clancy R, Malin S, Laraque D, et al. Focal motor seizures heralding stroke in full-term neonates. *Am J Dis Child.* 1985;139:601–606.

44. Guzzetta A, Mercuri E, Rapisardi G, et al. General movements detect early signs of hemiplegia in term infants with neonatal cerebral infarction. *Neuropediatrics.* 2003;34:61–66.

45. Ramaswamy V, Miller SP, Barkovich AJ, et al. Perinatal stroke in term infants with neonatal encephalopathy. *Neurology.* 2004;62:2088–2091.

46. Ecury-Goossen GM, Raets MM, Lequin M, et al. Risk factors, clinical presentation, and neuroimaging findings of neonatal perforator stroke. *Stroke.* 2013;44:2115–2120.

47. Benders MJ, Groenendaal F, Uiterwaal CS, et al. Maternal and infant characteristics associated with perinatal arterial stroke in the preterm infant. *Stroke.* 2007;38:1759–1765.

48. de Vries LS, Groenendaal F, Eken P, et al. Infarcts in the vascular distribution of the middle cerebral artery in preterm and fullterm infants. *Neuropediatrics.* 1997;28:88–96.

49. Golomb MR, MacGregor DL, Domi T, et al. Presumed pre- or perinatal arterial ischemic stroke: risk factors and outcomes. *Ann Neurol.* 2001;50:163–168.

50. Kirton A, Shroff M, Pontigon AM, et al. Risk factors and presentations of periventricular venous infarction vs. arterial presumed perinatal ischemic stroke. *Arch Neurol.* 2010;67:842–848.

51. Takanashi J, Tada H, Barkovich AJ, et al. Magnetic resonance imaging confirms periventricular venous infarction in a term-born child with congenital hemiplegia. *Dev Med Child Neurol.* 2005;47:706–708.

52. Hernanz-Schulman M, Cohen W, Genieser NB. Sonography of cerebral infarction in infancy. *AJR Am J Roentgenol.* 1988;150:897–902.

53. Messer J, Haddad J, Casanova R. Transcranial Doppler evaluation of cerebral infarction in the neonate. *Neuropediatrics*. 1991;22:147–151.
54. Golomb MR, Dick PT, MacGregor DL, et al. Cranial ultrasonography has a low sensitivity for detecting arterial ischemic stroke in term neonates. *J Child Neurol*. 2003;18:98–103.
55. Cowan F, Mercuri E, Groenendaal F, et al. Does cranial ultrasound imaging identify arterial cerebral infarction in term neonates? *Arch Dis Child Fetal Neonatal Ed*. 2005;90:F252–F256.
56. Mader I, Schoning M, Klose U, et al. Neonatal cerebral infarction diagnosed by diffusion-weighted MRI: pseudonormalization occurs early. *Stroke*. 2002;33:1142–1145.
57. Kuker W, Mohrle S, Mader I, et al. MRI for the management of neonatal cerebral infarctions: importance of timing. *Childs Nerv Syst*. 2004;20:742–748.
58. Mathur AM, Neil JJ, McKinstry RC, Inder TE. Transport, monitoring, and successful brain MR imaging in unsedated neonates. *Pediatr Radiol*. 2008;38(3):260–264.
59. De Vries LS, Van der Grond J, Van Haastert IC, et al. Prediction of outcome in new-born infants with arterial ischaemic stroke using diffusion-weighted magnetic resonance imaging. *Neuropediatrics*. 2005;36:12–20.
60. Groenendaal F, Benders MJ, de Vries LS. Pre-Wallerian degeneration in the neonatal brain following perinatal cerebral hypoxia–ischemia demonstrated with MRI. *Semin Perinatol*. 2006;30:146–150.
61. Kirton A, Deveber G, Pontigon AM, et al. Presumed perinatal ischemic stroke: vascular classification predicts outcomes. *Ann Neurol*. 2008;63:436–443.
62. Baird TA, Parsons MW, Phanh T, et al. Persistent poststroke hyperglycemia is independently associated with infarct expansion and worse clinical outcome. *Stroke*. 2003;34:2208–2214.
63. Vannucci RC, Mujsce DJ. Effect of glucose on perinatal hypoxic–ischemic brain damage. *Biol Neonate*. 1992;62:215–224.
64. Clancy RR. Prolonged electroencephalogram monitoring for seizures and their treatment. *Clin Perinatol*. 2006;33:649–665, vi.
65. Monagle P, Chalmers E, Chan A, et al. Antithrombotic therapy in neonates and children: american college of chest physicians evidence-based clinical practice guidelines (8th edition). *Chest*. 2008;133(suppl 6):S887–S968.
66. Jones MW, Morgan E, Shelton JE. Primary care of the child with cerebral palsy: a review of systems (part II). *J Pediatr Health Care*. 2007;21:226–237.
67. Juenger H, Linder-Lucht M, Walther M, et al. Cortical neuromodulation by constraint-induced movement therapy in congenital hemiparesis: an FMRI study. *Neuropediatrics*. 2007;38:130–136.
68. Sutcliffe TL, Gaetz WC, Logan WJ, et al. Cortical reorganization after modified constraint-induced movement therapy in pediatric hemiplegic cerebral palsy. *J Child Neurol*. 2007;22:1281–1287.
69. Hoare BJ, Wasiak J, Imms C, et al. Constraint-induced movement therapy in the treatment of the upper limb in children with hemiplegic cerebral palsy. *Cochrane Database Syst Rev*. 2007;(2):CD004149.
70. Rajapakse T, Kirton A. Non-invasive brain stimulation in children: applications and future directions. *Transl Neurosci*. 2013;4:217–233.
71. Gonzalez FF, Larpthaveesarp A, McQuillen P, et al. Erythropoietin increases neurogenesis and oligodendrogliosis of subventricular zone precursor cells after neonatal stroke. *Stroke*. 2013;44:753–758.
72. Gonzalez FF, Abel R, Almli CR, et al. Erythropoietin sustains cognitive function and brain volume after neonatal stroke. *Dev Neurosci*. 2009;31:403–411.
73. Benders MJ, van der Aa NE, Roks M, et al. Feasibility and safety of erythropoietin for neuroprotection after perinatal arterial ischemic stroke. *J Pediatr*. 2014;164:481–486.e1–e2.
74. de Veber G, Andrew M, Adams C, et al. Cerebral sinovenous thrombosis in children. *N Engl J Med*. 2001;345:417–423.
75. Moharir MD, Shroff M, Pontigon AM, et al. A prospective outcome study of neonatal cerebral sinovenous thrombosis. *J Child Neurol*. 2011;26(9):1137–1144.
76. Roland EH, Flodmark O, Hill A. Thalamic hemorrhage with intraventricular hemorrhage in the full-term newborn. *Pediatrics*. 1990;85:737–742.
77. Wu YW, Hamrick SE, Miller SP, et al. Intraventricular hemorrhage in term neonates caused by sinovenous thrombosis. *Ann Neurol*. 2003;54:123–126.
78. Govaert P. Sonographic stroke templates. *Semin Fetal Neonatal Med*. 2009;14(5):284–298.
79. Govaert P, Ramenghi L, Taal R, de Vries L, Deveber G. Diagnosis of perinatal stroke I: definitions, differential diagnosis and registration. *Acta Paediatr*. 2009;98(10):1556–1567.
80. Berfelo FJ, Kersbergen KJ, van Ommen CH, et al. Neonatal cerebral sinovenous thrombosis from symptom to outcome. *Stroke*. 2010;41(7):1382–1388.
81. Fitzgerald KC, Williams LS, Garg BP, et al. Cerebral sinovenous thrombosis in the neonate. *Arch Neurol*. 2006;63:405–409.
82. Wu YW, Miller SP, Chin K, et al. Multiple risk factors in neonatal sinovenous thrombosis. *Neurology*. 2002;59:438–440.
83. Fitzgerald KC, Golomb MR. Neonatal arterial ischemic stroke and sinovenous thrombosis associated with meningitis. *J Child Neurol*. 2007;22:818–822.
84. Roach ES, Golomb MR, Adams R, et al. Management of stroke in infants and children: a scientific statement from a special writing group of the american heart association stroke council and the council on cardiovascular disease in the young. *Stroke*. 2008;39(9):2644–2691.
85. Jordan LC, Rafay MF, Smith SE, et al. Antithrombotic treatment in neonatal cerebral sinovenous thrombosis: results of the International Pediatric Stroke Study. *J Pediatr*. 2010;156(5):704–710, 710.e701–710.e702.
86. Armstrong-Wells J, Johnston CS, Wu YW, et al. Prevalence and predictors of perinatal hemorrhagic stroke: results from the Kaiser pediatric stroke study. *Pediatrics*. 2009;123:823–828.

87. Brouwer AJ, Groenendaal F, Koopman C, Nievelstein RJ, Han SK, de Vries LS. Intracranial hemorrhage in full-term newborns: a hospital-based cohort study. *Neuroradiology*. 2010;52(6):567–576.
88. Gould DB, Phalan FC, Breedveld GJ, et al. Mutations in Col4a1 cause perinatal cerebral hemorrhage and porencephaly. *Science*. 2005;308:1167–1171.
89. Breedveld G, de Coo IF, Lequin MH, et al. Novel mutations in three families confirm a major role of COL4A1 in hereditary porencephaly. *J Med Genet*. 2006;43:490–495.
90. de Vries LS, Koopman C, Groenendaal F, et al. COL4A1 mutation in two preterm siblings with antenatal onset of parenchymal hemorrhage. *Ann Neurol*. 2009;65:12–18.
91. Papile LA, Burstein J, Burstein R, Koffer H. Incidence and evolution of subependymal and intraventricular hemorrhage: a study of infants with birth weights less than 1500 gm. *J Pediatr*. 1978;92:529–534.
92. Deleted in review.
93. Tong KA, Ashwal S, Obenaus A, Nickerson JP, Kido D, Haacke EM. Susceptibility-weighted MR imaging: a review of clinical applications in children. *AJNR Am J Neuroradiol*. 2008;29(1):9–17.
94. Chalmers EA. Perinatal stroke: risk factors and management. *Br J Haematol*. 2005;130:333–343.
95. Weiner SP, Painter MJ, Geva D, et al. Neonatal seizures: electroclinical dissociation. *Pediatr Neurol*. 1991;7:363–368.
96. Koelfen W, Freund M, Varnholt V. Neonatal stroke involving the middle cerebral artery in term infants: clinical presentation, EEG and imaging studies, and outcome. *Dev Med Child Neurol*. 1995;37:204–212.
97. Trauner DA, Chase C, Walker P, et al. Neurologic profiles of infants and children after perinatal stroke. *Pediatr Neurol*. 1993;9:383–386.
98. Wulfeck BB, Trauner DA, Tallal PA. Neurologic, cognitive, and linguistic features of infants after early stroke. *Pediatr Neurol*. 1991;7:266–269.
99. Tillema JM, Byars AW, Jacola LM, et al. Cortical reorganization of language functioning following perinatal left MCA stroke. *Brain Lang*. 2008;105:99–111.
100. Jacola LM, Schapiro MB, Schmithorst VJ, et al. Functional magnetic resonance imaging reveals atypical language organization in children following perinatal left middle cerebral artery stroke. *Neuropediatrics*. 2006;37:46–52.
101. Adhikari MH, Beharelle AR, Griffa A, et al. Computational modeling of resting-state activity demonstrates markers of normalcy in children with prenatal or perinatal stroke. *J Neurosci*. 2015;35:8914–8924.
102. Wu YW, March WM, Croen LA, et al. Perinatal stroke in children with motor impairment: a population-based study. *Pediatrics*. 2004;114:612–619.
103. Golomb MR, deVeber GA, MacGregor DL, et al. Independent walking after neonatal arterial ischemic stroke and sinovenous thrombosis. *J Child Neurol*. 2003;18:530–536.
104. Kirton A, Shroff M, Visvanathan T, et al. Quantified corticospinal tract diffusion restriction predicts neonatal stroke outcome. *Stroke*. 2007;38:974–980.
105. Estan J, Hope P. Unilateral neonatal cerebral infarction in full term infants. *Arch Dis Child Fetal Neonatal Ed*. 1997;76:F88–F93.
106. Golomb MR, Garg BP, Carvalho KS, et al. Perinatal stroke and the risk of developing childhood epilepsy. *J Pediatr*. 2007;151:409–413.e2.
107. Hetherington R, Tuff L, Anderson P, et al. Short-term intellectual outcome after arterial ischemic stroke and sinovenous thrombosis in childhood and infancy. *J Child Neurol*. 2005;20:553–559.
108. Trauner DA, Nass R, Ballantyne A. Behavioural profiles of children and adolescents after pre- or perinatal unilateral brain damage. *Brain*. 2001;124:995–1002.
109. Mercuri E, Spano M, Bruccini G, et al. Visual outcome in children with congenital hemiplegia: correlation with MRI findings. *Neuropediatrics*. 1996;27:184–188.
110. Guzzetta A, Fazzi B, Mercuri E, et al. Visual function in children with hemiplegia in the first years of life. *Dev Med Child Neurol*. 2001;43:321–329.
111. Harbert MJ, Tam EW, Glass HC, et al. Hypothermia is correlated with seizure absence in perinatal stroke. *J Child Neurol*. 2011;26(9):1126–1130.

CHAPTER 7

Diagnosis and Management of Acute Seizures in Neonates

Francesco Pisani and Carlotta Spagnoli

- Seizures are the most common manifestation of acute neurologic dysfunction in newborns. Neurophysiological monitoring (with cEEG or, if unavailable, aEEG) is recommended for correct diagnosis.
- After EEG confirmation, management is based upon diagnostic work-up and the choice of the optimal therapy according to the clinical scenario (acute symptomatic origin versus suspected genetic origin).
- Prognosis seems to be mostly related to etiology, and whether seizures may aggravate the underlying brain injury/disfunction is still debated.
- The introduction of new, more effective, anti-seizure drugs and their combined use with neuroprotective agents may improve the outcome of these newborns in the next future.

Neonatal seizures represent a frequent clinical sign of a central nervous system (CNS) disorder in newborns. The vast majority (85%) of seizures are of acute symptomatic origin and need to be distinguished from neonatal-onset epilepsies and neonatal-onset epileptic encephalopathy, mainly of genetic origin[1] (as discussed later in the chapter). Acute symptomatic neonatal seizures may indicate a potentially treatable etiology, such as metabolic derangements (i.e., glucose or electrolyte abnormalities) or the presence of an acquired brain injury or dysfunction, or they can be secondary to neonatal encephalopathy and hypoxic-ischemic encephalopathy, structural brain injuries (i.e., ischemic/hemorrhagic stroke), or CNS/systemic infections,[2] with prognostic implications for both mortality and subsequent neurologic outcome.

The importance of acute symptomatic seizures also derives from their epidemiologic relevance (the estimated incidence being between 1% and 3.5% in full-term newborns and even higher in preterm infants).[3] Moreover, they require complex acute medical decision making regarding treatment strategies, which are mandatory because of a potential risk of additive detrimental effects of seizures on the neonatal brain, as suggested by experimental models yet not clearly elucidated in humans.[4]

Diagnosis

Classifications

Various clinical classifications of seizures have been proposed in the literature (Table 7.1).[5–7] Clinical classifications of seizures are based mainly on the description of their motor manifestations (focal clonic, multifocal clonic, tonic, myoclonic, and subtle). "Subtle" seizures are described as such because their signs may be difficult to recognize; the signs include abnormal eye movements, automatisms (e.g., tongue protrusion or lip smacking, swimming/pedaling/boxing movements), or autonomic phenomena (e.g., apnea, tachycardia, tachypnea, flushing).

Focal Clonic Seizures

Focal clonic seizures are repetitive, rhythmic contractions of specific muscle groups. Clonic movements typically show a rate of repetition of 1 to 3 Hz with decreasing

Table 7.1 CLASSIFICATION OF NEONATAL SEIZURES BY DIFFERENT AUTHORS

Author (Year)	Type	Characterization	Ictal EEG Discharges	
			Common	**Uncommon**
Volpe (1989)[6]	Subtle	Ocular, oro-buccal-lingual movements, autonomic, repetitive stereotyped movements (i.e., pedaling, boxing, swimming)	Variable/inconsistent	
	Clonic			
	• Focal	Repetitive rhythmic jerking	+	
	• Multifocal		+	
	Tonic			
	• Focal	Stiffening, decerebrate posturing	+	
	• Generalized			+
	Myoclonic			
	• Focal/multifocal	Rapid, isolated jerks		+
	• Generalized		+	
Lombroso (1996)[7]	Subtle, minimal, fragmentary	Paroxysmal, stereotyped, periodic. Mostly in newborns with severe CNS insult	Good or variable ictal correlation. Interictal background patterns usually abnormal. Absence of EEG ictal discharge does not necessarily rule out seizures	
	Clonic			
	• Unifocal	Migrating form limb to limb, alternate side. Rare. Jacksonian march exceptional.	Consistent	
	• Multifocal			
	• Hemiconvulsive			
	Tonic			
	• Focal	Stereotyped, often accompanied by autonomic changes. Symmetric tonic postures	Frequently abnormal background. δ/α/β discharges. No ictal EEG correlate, abnormal background	
	• Generalized	Abrupt tonic limb abduction/adduction or extension/flexion → epileptic spasms		
	Myoclonic	Erratic, fragmentary or more generalized myoclonic jerks often associated with tonic spasms/multifocal tonic or clonic patterns/mixed seizure types	EEG discharges usually (not invariably) present. Burst-suppression pattern	

Mizrahi and Kellaway (1987, 1998)[5,7a]		Pathophysiology
Focal clonic	Rhythmic muscle contractions. Unifocal/multifocal, Synchronous/asynchronous, Not suppressed by restraint.	Epileptic
Focal tonic	Sustained posturing, tonic eye deviation Not provoked, not suppressed by restraint	Epileptic
Myoclonic	Random, single rapid muscle contraction • Generalized • Focal • Fragmentary • May be provoked by stimulation	Epileptic/nonepileptic
Spasms	Flexor/extensor May occur in clusters Not provoked, not suppressed by restraint	Epileptic
Generalized tonic	Sustained symmetric posturing, may be stimulus-sensitive, may be suppressed by restraint	Nonepileptic
Motor automatisms	Ocular, oro-bucco-lingual, progression movements of limbs May be provoked or intensified by external stimuli and suppressed by restraint	Nonepileptic
Electrographic	None	Epileptic

CNS, Central nervous system; EEG, electroencephalogram.

frequency and increasing amplitude with the passing of time and with increasing size of the involved muscle groups. They have a consistent electrocardiographic (EEG) correlate. Compared with paroxysmal nonepileptic phenomena such as clonus or tremor, they tend to be slower and more rhythmic. Most importantly, they cannot be stopped by restraint of the involved body part. They can be unifocal or multifocal, alternate between involved sites, or be simultaneous but asynchronous, different from what is usually observed in older age groups.

Focal Tonic Seizures

Focal tonic seizures are characterized by sustained asymmetric posturing of the limbs or trunk or by tonic deviation of the eyes. They are typically associated with focal EEG discharges.

Myoclonic Jerks

Myoclonic jerks in newborns can be either epileptic or nonepileptic in origin. The movements have a brief, jerky, shocklike appearance. Speed is influenced by the size of the muscle group involved. They can involve different districts and be fragmentary, focal, or multifocal. They can be isolated or repetitive, in this case with a slow, erratic, or irregular rate of recurrence (differentiating them from clonic events). Some forms of myoclonic jerks may occur with consistent EEG seizure discharges, although some do not. Finally, they can be spontaneous or provoked by stimulation.

Autonomic Signs

Autonomic changes such as alterations in heart rate, respiration rate, and blood pressure; flushing' salivation; or pupil dilatation[5,8] have been described in seizures, although they are rarely isolated and typically associated with motor phenomena.

Spasms

Epileptic spasms may occur in neonates. Although they are not seen in neonates with seizure symptomatic of acute events such as hypoxic-ischemic encephalopathy (HIE) or stroke, they are the main seizure type in Ohtahara syndrome (see later text). They mainly involve truncal and upper limb muscle groups and can be divided into extensor, flexor, or mixed types.

Subclinical Seizures

Seizures may present without overt clinical manifestations, especially in critically ill infants.[9,10] This phenomenon is possibly linked to the involvement of non-eloquent areas[11] or rather to the involvement of nonmotor areas.[2] It might also be that, in some instances, the high figures of electrographic-only seizures are secondary to ascertainment methods such as the duration of monitoring; the use of a multiple-camera approach compared with a single camera synchronized to the EEG was associated with improved detection of subtle facial motor components to seizures.[12] On the other hand, it is interesting to note that exclusively electrographic neonatal status epilepticus (NSE) seems to be exceptional, as we found that in our cohort of preterm newborns, in all cases NSE became clinically evident at some point.[13]

Definition of Seizures

Based on the high rate of subclinical seizures, the need for differential diagnosis with various paroxysmal nonepileptic phenomena and the unreliability of clinical diagnosis of seizures even by experienced personnel,[14] a definition of seizures based only on clinical grounds is considered inaccurate. Therefore the current definition of neonatal seizures is based on EEG criteria. A seizure is defined as a sudden, repetitive, stereotyped episode of abnormal electrographic activity with peak-to-peak amplitude of at least 2 µV, a minimum duration of 10 seconds, and evolution with a clear beginning, middle, and end, with or without a clinical correlate.[15] Conventionally, seizures need to be separated by at least 10 seconds to be considered as distinct, even if this cutoff has not been based on physiologic considerations.[16]

Definition of Neonatal Status Epilepticus

NSE has been variably defined in the literature.[17] Its most widely accepted definition is continuous seizures lasting for more than 30 minutes or seizure present for at least 50% of the recording time, with no return to the baseline neurologic condition.[18] Alternative operational definitions with a shorter time cutoff have also been proposed,[16] even if a specific threshold has yet to be found. For this reason, the literature has also referred to "seizure burden" to indicate the percentage of the EEG recording with ictal activity.[19]

Controversies in Definition and Classification of Seizures

The current EEG definition of seizures poses some issues related to its applications to seizure types characteristically shorter than 10 seconds in duration, such as myoclonic seizures and spasms.

Myoclonic seizures are considered truly epileptic in origin if they are time-locked to an epileptic discharge on EEG that precedes the motor event (as detected on the electromyogram trace) by typically 20 to 40 msec.[20] The gold standard for the confirmation of the epileptic nature of myoclonic phenomena is represented by back-averaging.[20]

Similarly, in the case of epileptic spasms, which are rare but possible in newborns, the "diamond-shaped" potential on the electromyograph (typical duration of 1–2 seconds) correlates with typical, although variable, EEG discharges.[21] In addition, newborns typically have more than one seizure type.[12,13,22,23]

Differential Diagnosis

For electrographic discharges, the two main differential diagnoses are seizures with artifacts and those with brief rhythmic discharges. A wide range of artifacts of both biologic and environmental origin can be detected, especially in the high–background noise situation of neonatal intensive care units (NICUs). A description of such artifacts and the methods used to discriminate them from real electrographic discharges is beyond the scope of this chapter. Brief rhythmic discharges are, by definition, electrographic discharges shorter than the duration required for an EEG definition of seizures. They have been associated with the occurrence of seizures and with background EEG abnormalities.[24]

Clinically the main differential diagnosis for seizures is with paroxysmal nonepileptic motor phenomena, which can be either physiologic or abnormal. There is a wide range of paroxysmal nonepileptic motor phenomena that occur in newborns, including tremor and jitteriness, benign neonatal sleep myoclonus, startle reflex, ocular movement disorders (i.e., paroxysmal tonic upgaze and downgaze, opsoclonus), paroxysmal dystonia, bilateral tonic stiffening, and hyperekplexia. The occurrence of these events is facilitated by the immaturity of corticospinal tracts in newborns.

A number of features can assist in the differential diagnosis versus epileptic events in some, although not all, of these phenomena. These include stimulus sensitivity (e.g., different stimuli, especially auditory, for startle reflex; crying and stress for tremors and jitteriness; sudden visual stimuli or movement for paroxysmal tonic up/downgaze; rocking or repetitive auditory stimuli for benign neonatal sleep myoclonus), habituation (present in startle reflex but absent in hyperekplexia), and association with behavioral states (benign neonatal sleep myoclonus occurs only during sleep, mainly in quiet sleep, and stops with arousal). Holding the affected limbs can differentiate some paroxysmal motor phenomena from epileptic ones: gentle restraint stops physiologic tremor and may exacerbate benign neonatal sleep myoclonus, while it does not modify epileptic events. Paroxysmal nonepileptic events can be situational—for example, paroxysmal dystonic events in Sandifer syndrome are brought on by feeding.[25,26] The use of polygraphic video-EEG recording is often crucial for correct diagnosis in many of these conditions and is considered a cornerstone for the discrimination between true epileptic seizures and, for example, brainstem release phenomena.[5] However, seizures originating from subcortical regions or from deep, mesial cortical areas and not propagating to the cortical surface may not be detected by surface EEG electrodes and remain an open issue.[27]

Diagnostic Tools and Monitoring

When seizures are suspected because of the presence of risk factors (i.e., fetal distress, CNS infection, HIE, preterm birth, intracranial hemorrhage, cardiac surgery) or because of suspicious clinical events, a video-EEG recording is necessary for correct interpretation of clinical phenomena to avoid the prescription of unnecessary anticonvulsant therapy. Based on the high rate of electrographic-only seizures[9,14] (which would otherwise go unrecognized), initiation of video-EEG monitoring is recommended[19] and should be continued for a period of 24 hours after seizure cessation according to the American Clinical Neurophysiology Society.[28,29] When the indication for EEG is the differential diagnosis of a clinical event, its duration should primarily depend on the ability to record multiple typical clinical events.[29]

Once seizures have been diagnosed, prolonged or continuous monitoring is necessary to correctly estimate the seizure burden, to monitor the efficacy of anticonvulsant medications, and to assist in differential diagnosis with the uncoupling phenomenon. Monitoring is also recommended during and after drug discontinuation[29] and during therapeutic hypothermia and rewarming in newborns with HIE,[30,31] given the risk of seizure occurrence in this population.[29]

Furthermore, conventional EEG provides relevant information for prognosis based on background activity.[29] Correct evaluation of background activity requires the recording of wakefulness and active and quiet sleep, usually corresponding to at least 1 hour of recording, which might need to be prolonged in case of disruption of sleep rhythms—for example, after the acute phase of encephalopathy.[29]

An alternative strategy for brain function monitoring is represented by amplitude-integrated EEG (aEEG).[30] aEEG is an EEG-based bedside brain monitoring instrument commonly used in NICUs. Current practice implies use mainly by neonatologists and nurses.[33] It displays one or two channels of EEG data after filtering, rectification, and smoothing on a semilogarithmic scale,[34] enabling a reduction in the time needed both for electrode placement and diagnostic interpretation. It is especially used in the context of neonatal HIE for infants undergoing therapeutic hypothermia. Studies confirm the reliability in assessing background activity and degree of HIE with good correlation with outcome.[35] Nevertheless, aEEG is characterized by poor reliability if reported by unexperienced personnel compared with continuous EEG, especially for seizures monitoring.[32] aEEG filters out most of the slow activity and uses a time-compressed scale and a limited set of electrodes, with a potential risk of underdiagnosis, especially for seizures arising outside the centrotemporal regions or seizures of short duration. This might be a relevant issue in preterm newborns, as some studies report a higher prevalence of seizures from the frontal[10] or occipital regions,[10,36] especially under 29 weeks of gestational age (WGA).[36] Whereas conventional EEG is characterized by high sensitivity, reliance on aEEG alone might be misleading in preterm infants because seizures tend to propagate less.[36,37] A risk of overdiagnosis also exists, because the long monitoring periods and the high background noise typical of ICUs might facilitate the occurrence of false-positive findings secondary to artifacts.[16,38,39] Therefore for the diagnosis of seizures, aEEG is considered a screening tool.[16,29] Consequently, evaluation of the raw EEG trace on the digital aEEG devices is often required and recommended to recognize and quantify seizures as it allows higher sensitivity and specificity.[40,41] Table 7.2 briefly summarizes the main aims of cEEG monitoring in newborns with suspected seizures or at risk of seizures.

Table 7.2   ROLE OF CONVENTIONAL EEG MONITORING

Neonatal Seizures (Suspected/Confirmed)	High-Risk Newborn
Differential diagnosis (including verification of aEEG patterns)	Evaluation of background activity
Diagnosis of NSE	Diagnosis of associated seizures or NSE (especially electrographic-only)
Treatment assessment	Prognostication (with serial recordings)
Diagnosis of uncoupling	Detection of focal cerebral injury

aEEG, Amplitude-integrated electroencephalography; NSE, neonatal status epilepticus.

EEG Characteristics of Neonatal Seizures

Seizures typically last between 1 and 5 minutes and most last less than 3 minutes.[15,19,37,42] Seizure duration has been reported to be longer in full-term newborns owing to a higher incidence of NSE.[43] These data, based on the use of standard cEEG,[11] were later confirmed by continuous EEG monitoring, although NSE (seizures lasting 30–40 minutes) were also frequent.[14,44–46]

Considering the onset focus and the region involved at the time of the maximal spread, seizures are divided into localized or lateralized or unifocal, multifocal, and bilateral independent.[16] A focal onset is present in the majority of cases, especially in full-term newborns, whereas the onset in preterm newborns can be either regional[47] or focal.[37] In the majority of cases, seizure onset is from the centrotemporal[19,48,49] or vertex region.[19] However, the presence of multiple independent areas of discharge at seizure onset is not unusual in the newborn period.[50] Typical features of seizures in newborns include migration (defined as a change of seizure focus within one hemisphere) and shifting (defined as a change of focus from one hemisphere to the other, termed "flip-flop" when discharges finally shift back to the original hemisphere[49] of ictal discharges).[37] According to some authors the spread of discharges is mainly ipsilateral for seizures with a focal onset and contralateral or bilateral for regional-onset seizures.[47] Description of the seizure spread might enable improved correlation with evolving clinical signs in term infants,[51] even though previous reports failed to clearly describe such correlation in preterm newborns.[37] In addition, the spread to the contralateral hemisphere has been associated with outcome.[50] Ictal discharges in newborns tend to be characterized as follows: focal spike/sharp wave discharges, focal low-frequency discharges, focal rhythmic discharges, and multifocal discharges.[52] Repetitive spikes, sharp waves, stereotyped wave complexes, and α, θ, or δ discharges are also frequent.[53] Different patterns can be associated in single patients in one-third of cases.[50] It is also possible to record different seizures occurring simultaneously over different areas of both hemispheres.[8] Spike potentials often show slower rate and longer duration in neonates ("burn-out spikes") compared with older patients.[54] During the ictal discharge, delta and sharp waves are among the most frequent findings in both full-term and preterm infants.[47] Evolution of discharges during the seizure usually consists of a decrease in frequency and an increase in amplitude.[37] The ability to generate well-formed spikes at high discharge rates tends to improve with increasing conceptional age (CA) but is impaired in case of severe brain injury.[55] Nonetheless, in severely affected neonates seizures might lack a clear field and pattern of evolution, with a prevalence of low amplitude and slow frequency.[2] In these patients, seizures also tend to be prolonged[56] and to remain confined to one single EEG channel or to alternatively change hemispheres.[39]

The impact on brain physiology or on subsequent outcome of different ictal patterns is still unknown,[16] although α discharges have been associated with worse prognosis.[57] No correlation between seizure characteristics and etiology has been reported.[37,47] Furthermore, there is no clear association between clinical semiology and characteristics of EEG discharges.[53] However, in a cohort of preterm newborns Okumura and colleagues found that the duration of seizures was relatively shorter when motor phenomena were present compared with apneic or electrographic-only seizures.[37] There is a tendency for neonates with severely abnormal background to present with electrographic-only seizures.[47,49]

Standard EEG Versus Long-Term or Continuous Monitoring

Continuous conventional long-term EEG monitoring (cEEG) is now considered the gold standard for seizures diagnosis.[31]

Controversies in Monitoring

- Electrographic-only seizures: Owing to the high incidence of subclinical seizures and the caveats for clinically based differential diagnosis of seizures, continuous electroencephalographic (cEEG) monitoring is required.[29]
- Identification of high-risk newborns: Infants with acute brain insult, including HIE and stroke, and/or suspected seizures on clinical observation, or neonates with encephalopathy of unknown origin.[29,58]

- Higher seizure burden period in full-term versus preterm newborns: The onset of electrographically confirmed seizures tends to be earlier in full-term than preterm newborns.[22,50] As recently shown by Lynch and colleagues, in full-terms infants with HIE the seizure burden tends to be maximal at a mean of 22.7 hours of life, and the last seizure is recorded at a mean of 55.5 hours.[44]
- Seizures in preterm newborns: Among preterm infants, seizures occur in the first 48 hours after birth in approximately 10% of infants born below 29 weeks CA and in 50% of infants born at 30 weeks or later.[59]

Prolonged EEG monitoring in full-term newborns is recommended in the context of encephalopathy, including HIE, during hypothermia and rewarming, and in neonates with suspected seizures, while in preterm infants it is based on gestational age and on the existence of specific risk factors, based mainly on the major etiologic role of intraventricular hemorrhage and its complications.[60] The optimal duration and timing of monitoring in other etiologic groups are less clearly defined.

Management

Investigations and Etiologies

Seizures may have many different underlying etiological factors. A list of the main diagnostic investigations that might be required in the diagnostic workup of the newborn with seizures is reported in Table 7.3. Some causes of seizures have been diminishing—for instance, transient metabolic disorders and neonatal traumatic lesions, infections—owing to the marked advances in neonatal care, whereas other etiologies, such as stroke and genetic etiologies, are growing in number and are likely due to improved early recognition with widespread use of prolonged video-EEG in the NICU and more sophisticated testing. Overall, the past few years have seen a major improvement in recognition and definite diagnosis and a reduction of the number of newborns with seizures of unknown etiology.

HIE still represents the major cause of seizures in neonates,[7,61–63] especially in term infants. Usually seizure onset is between 6 and 24 hours after birth. Seizures are usually short and isolated at onset and progressively become more frequent and prolonged, mainly between the 12th and the 24th hours of life, and are often resistant to antiseizure therapy.[45] The advent of hypothermia as the standard of care for newborns with HIE has partially changed the profile of seizures in these newborns. First, the typical time evolution found in normothermic newborns with HIE[45] seems to be absent in newborns treated with hypothermia, where no consistent pattern can be recognized.[64] The postnatal age of first recorded electrographic seizure is found to be similar in cooled and normothermic newborns by some authors[66] and to be later by others (in the first 48 hours in 76% of cases).[65] The use of hypothermia as standard of care has led to a significant reduction of seizure burden in cooled neonates with moderate HIE, possibly contributing to improved outcome.[66]

Table 7.3 DIAGNOSTIC APPROACH TO NEONATAL SEIZURES

History (identification of newborn at high risk for neonatal seizures)	Family history, pregnancy history; delivery history; feeding history; clinical characteristics of the events
Physical examination	Physical examination (dysmorphic features) Neurologic examination (signs of encephalopathy) Fundus oculi examination.
Investigations	*First-line investigations:* complete blood cell count; glycemia; arterial pH; calcemia, electrolytes, urea and creatinine; urine microscopy and culture; blood lactate and pyruvate; ammonemia; blood culture; lumbar puncture including CSF lactate, CSF cells and protein, prolonged video-EEG, head ultrasounds *Second-line investigations:* screen for congenital infections; blood, urinary and cerebrospinal amino acids evaluation; urine organic acids; plasma acyl-carnitines; urine sulfite; Very long chain fatty acids; urinary organic acids, MRI, genetic testing.

CSF, Cerebrospinal fluid; *EEG,* electroencephalograpy; *MRI,* magnetic resonance imaging.

Glass et al., who used continuous EEG monitoring, detected seizures in approximately 50% of newborns in the majority of cases during the cooling period.[66] Interestingly, early EEG background was the best predictor of seizure occurrence, even superior to the clinical signs of encephalopathy.[66] Therapeutic hypothermia has been found to be associated with a lower incidence of seizures in the first 6 months of life after discharge (16% vs. 53%), although the short follow-up likely limits the significance of these findings.[67] The rewarming period is also considered at risk of breakthrough seizures in this population, although there are few data to support this assumption.[68] The association between the occurrence of seizures and the presence of brain injury, already found in noncooled neonates with HIE, has been confirmed in cooled neonates. Moderate to severe brain injury (as detected by magnetic resonance imaging [MRI] performed at a median of 5 days of age) is more common in newborns with seizures than in those without (irrespective of the presence or absence of a clinical correlate to discharges) and is universal in the subgroup with status epilepticus. Seizures are also more likely to occur later and to be resistant to phenobarbital load in the more severely affected newborns.[69] The transient metabolic disorders that can be associated (hypoglycemia, hypocalcemia, hyponatremia) can be responsible for the refractoriness of the seizures. Novel therapeutic neuroprotective strategies (preventive, rescue, and repair) in association with hypothermia are being developed, aiming to obtain a better outcome, particularly in the severe cases in which rescue cannot currently be achieved.[70]

Intracranial hemorrhages represent another important cause of seizures in neonatal age, and intraventricular hemorrhage of grade III or IV is the most frequent etiology in preterm newborns. Almost 90% of intracranial bleeding develops within the first 3 days of life, with an incidence higher in the early gestational ages. Strokes are frequently reported in newborns with seizures (10%–18% of seizures),[63,71] especially in recent years, probably owing to our better ability to diagnose them with improved neuroimaging techniques. Strokes should be suspected in newborns with (1) focal or multifocal clonic seizures that begin at 12 hours to 3 days of life, (2) normal or almost normal interictal neurologic examination findings, (3) normal Apgar scores at birth, and (4) with no evidence of encephalopathy. Subarachnoid and subdural hemorrhages are rare and are often due to obstetric trauma and occasionally can lead to seizures; however, they have a good prognosis.[72] CNS infections such as meningitis and/or encephalitis are responsible for 3% to 9% of neonatal seizures,[62,73] particularly from viruses of the TORCH (toxoplasmosis; other [congenital syphilis and viruses], rubella, cytomegalovirus, and herpes) complex, whereas bacterial agents are more likely to be involved are group B *Streptococcus, Listeria,* and *Escherichia coli.*[73] Herpes simplex viruses usually determine a diffuse brain damage with a specific EEG pattern (diffuse slow background with periodic complexes, sharp and slow waves over the frontal and temporal regions, which, nevertheless, are only present in 50% of cases).[74] A lumbar puncture should be performed in any neonate with seizures and signs of infection. Cerebral malformations can be responsible for 3% to 9% of the epileptic seizures in the first days of life.[62,63,71] Most have a genetic basis and are associated with an adverse outcome. Seizures are also observed in 2% to 11% of infants with neonatal abstinence syndrome, together with tremors, irritability, excessive crying, and diarrhea.[75] The spectrum of abstinence syndrome has changed because in the 1970s it was generally secondary to the use of opioids, whereas more recently an increased use of multiple opioids has been observed to be complicated by the abuse of several other licit and illicit substances.[75]

Among the transient metabolic alterations, hypoglycemia, particularly when glycemia is less than 40 mg/dL, is one of the most common causes of seizures; it can be either isolated or more frequently is associated with congenital metabolic defects of glucose metabolism or fatty acid β-oxidation or with pancreatic lesions, causing early-onset, prolonged and severe convulsions, and high mortality and morbidity.[76] Another common condition is early hypocalcemia occurring between the second and the third day of life, or the late form at the end of the first week or the beginning of the second week. This condition can be controlled by calcium and today is easy to cure. Hyponatremia/hypernatremia are uncommon etiologies that can result from inappropriate secretion of antidiuretic hormone, congenital adrenal dysfunction, or inappropriate management of intravenous fluids. Neonatal hypernatremia can be seen in breastfed infants with excessive weight loss,[61] dehydration, and poor feeding. Electrolyte abnormalities may be caused by HIE, intracranial hemorrhage, or meningitis.[73]

Seizures during the neonatal period caused by inherited metabolic diseases (IMDs) are rare and they can provoked by several mechanisms: cerebral energy failure, toxic effects of metabolites, neurotransmitter modification–associated brain malformations, and vitamin defects.[76] A suspicion of IMD must arise when the newborn is severely encephalopathic and shows a severe disorganization of the EEG background activity, early onset of several seizure types (sometimes within the first hour of life, sometimes beginning antenatally), myoclonic seizures that are usually drug-resistant, and sometimes with suggestive MRI findings[71] (such as signs of brain atrophy or of hypoxic-ischemic injury in the absence of a hypoxic insult at delivery).[77] Other neurologic signs such as abnormal movements, tremor, hyperexcitability, hypotonia, and chronic hiccup (nonketotic hyperglycinemia) can also be associated.[76] This clinical scenario should alert the physician to an IMD, and the infant should be immediately evaluated with analysis of known biomarkers[78]; an early dietary restriction or supplementation of vitamin trials should be started, even before establishing a definitive diagnosis that might require time, because it is important in those treatable conditions to avoid permanent brain damage. The causes more often identified are nonketotic hyperglycinemia, pyridoxine-dependent epilepsy, pyridoxamine 5′-phosphate oxidase deficiency, sulfite oxidase deficiency, molybdenum cofactor deficiency, glucose transporter type 1 deficiency, congenital lack of glutamate transporter, and mitochondrial disorders.[76]

Infants with brain malformations can rarely present with neonatal seizures because they usually will develop seizures in the postneonatal period. Most are related to cortical migration disorders such as lissencephaly, pachygyria, polymicrogyria, cortical dysplasia, schizencephaly, and heterotopia. Some of these disorders may be seen in congenital infection or in IMD and there is increasing evidence of a genetic basis in the majority.[79] The prognosis is generally poor.

Neonatal epilepsy syndromes are rare and their genetically molecular mechanisms are being better delineated owing to the recent advances in genetics. They may vary in their clinical findings from a benign condition to neonatal-onset epileptic encephalopathies characterized by the association of epilepsy and cognitive deficit.

There are also epileptic syndromes with onset during the neonatal period.[1,80] These are benign familial neonatal epilepsy, early myoclonic encephalopathy, and early epileptic neonatal encephalopathy, although more etiology-specific syndromes have being recognized in the past few years.

Neonatal seizures are a critical clinical condition often sustained by an acute brain injury; the most common etiologies are HIE, intracranial hemorrhage, and ischemic stroke. However, in a few cases the etiology still remains unknown even despite progresses in neuroimaging techniques and in the genetic analysis methodologies. In the most severe clinical scenarios, including the early-onset neonatal epilepsies and epileptic encephalopathies, repeated genetic testing may identify new mutations even later in life, possibly suggesting interesting diagnostic and therapeutic perspective. In other cases, a second brain MRI later in life with higher resolution properties may discover small causative structural lesions.

Therapy

Based on the unavailability of strong evidence-based data from clinical studies, existing guidance for the pharmacologic management of seizures in the neonate is currently scanty. In fact, the majority of papers on the management of seizures are retrospective chart reviews or case reports, and the low number of participants reduces the generalizability of results. Only three randomized controlled trials (RCTs) have been published so far.[85–87]

The World Health Organization elaborated a guideline for neonatal seizures in 2011,[88] and a proposal for seizure management in low-income countries was published in 2007.[89] Flow-charts and protocols have been published in various review articles.[90,91]

The strong recommendation of the use of phenobarbital as the first-line drug in seizures, despite very low-quality evidence,[88] derives from the availability of RCT studies and from longstanding, widespread use in clinical practice. Although the reported efficacy of phenytoin is not significantly different from that of phenobarbital, the former is usually administered as a second-line treatment rather than as a first-line one owing to the risk of side effects and unease of use, its link to poorly predictable blood concentrations, and difficulties in titration. The suggested third-line treatment is usually represented by benzodiazepines, notably midazolam. However, advocated treatment strategies after phenobarbital or phenytoin failure are based on very low-quality evidence. Adjusted dosing regimens for lidocaine have been reported to be associated with a lower rate of cardiac adverse events than previously reported.[92] Lidocaine has been included in a small RCT comparing it with benzodiazepines.[87]

Recommendations from treatment guidelines are partially reflected by clinical practice. According to hospital-based studies, phenobarbital is the most common initial loading dose and the most used medication, with no differences between preterm and full-term newborns and no dosage changes based on gestational age. However, the second most commonly prescribed medication was levetiracetam, while phenytoin was the least likely to be prescribed.[93] The increasing use of levetiracetam is motivated by the availability of intravenous and enteral preparations and reassuring data on its safety and efficacy,[94] even though it represents an off-label prescription and data on its effectiveness are still limited and of poor quality (RCTs are not available).

Efficacy and Safety of Antiseizure Medications for Seizures

The response rate to first-line anticonvulsant medications used for the treatment of acute symptomatic seizures is suboptimal.[88] No clear-cut differences in response seem to exist between preterm and full-term newborns,[95] even if some age or etiology dependency might exist. For example, the administration of lidocaine determined a lower response rate in preterm newborns compared with full-term newborns.[96]

Concern has been raised about the possible long-term detrimental side effects of anticonvulsant medications, especially phenobarbital. However, the only clinical data are translated from the negative effects on intelligence quotient (IQ) reported in cohorts of children with febrile seizures,[97] although experimental data on animal models seem to confirm an association between phenobarbital administration in the neonatal period and neuronal apoptosis in the developing rat brain[98] and an interference with maturation of synaptic connections.[99,100] Described long-term effects in animals (exposed to very high loading doses of phenobarbital) include schizophrenia-like behavioral abnormalities and impaired learning, memory, and social interaction.[101] A retrospective clinical study of infants receiving phenobarbital for seizures (adjusted for the number of electrographic seizures and gestational age) and evaluating the effect of cumulative exposure to levetiracetam and phenobarbital found a greater association with worse Bayley Scales of Infant Development cognitive and motor scores with phenobarbital compared with levetiracetam and a higher rate of cerebral palsy in the group treated with phenobarbital but not with levetiracetam.[102] In immature animal models, doses of phenytoin higher than the usual loading dose in humans have been experimentally associated with apoptosis and synaptic disruption.[98,100] Data for levetiracetam are controversial, showing both a possible neuroprotective effect and detrimental effects (apoptosis, increased brain injury).[103,104]

Phenobarbital and Phenytoin

The two RCTs comparing phenobarbital and phenytoin report the following percentages of response: 43% of responders to phenobarbital as first-line treatment compared with 45% with phenytoin; nonresponders had similar results once switched to the alternative medication (total response of 57% in those receiving phenytoin as second-line treatment versus 62% in those receiving phenobarbital as second-line treatment).[85] The second open-label, cross-over study[86] found a 14.5% response with phenytoin as first-line treatment, increasing to 80% when switched to phenobarbital as second-line treatment, while the second arm had a 72.2% response with pheno-barbital, increasing to 96.3% with phenytoin. However, these studies have relevant limitations, including a clinically based diagnosis of seizures and the absence of EEG monitoring, that might have resulted in underestimation of the seizure burden or even a potential for misdiagnosis.

Pharmacokinetic data in newborns are better known for phenobarbital compared with other medications,[105] as they have been investigated in various papers. Neither weight nor gestational age seems to significantly influence dose-related blood levels. However, infants of less than 30 weeks' gestational age or weighing less than 1500 g might need lower doses to achieve the same blood levels.[106] As protein levels are lower in newborns than in older ages, the free fraction of drugs is expected to be higher and might be altered by organ dysfunction, leading to toxic side effects, especially respiratory and cardiovascular.[106]

Difficulties in the management of phenytoin (independent of gestational age) consist of the need for frequent monitoring of blood levels, erratic absorption when administered enterally, the need for frequent dose administration (every 6–8 hours), and ongoing metabolism changes in infancy.[107]

Midazolam

Low-quality evidence from clinical studies limited by methodologic issues, including study design and sample size, report a highly variable efficacy of midazolam used as a second- or third-line agent (0%–100%).[108–111]

Lidocaine

The reported efficacy of lidocaine varies between approximately 10% and 78%.[96,112,113] Interestingly, a recent retrospective cohort study of 413 newborns found an increasing response rate when given as third-line as opposed to second-line treatment (67.6% vs. 21.4% in term newborns and 40.7% vs. 16.4% in preterm newborns), possibly highlighting the importance of the timing of treatment.[96]

In the past, cardiotoxic concentrations were found in the majority of neonates receiving lidocaine with standard lidocaine infusion, with the risk of cardiac adverse events increasing with concentrations higher than 9 mg/L.[112] Therefore new dosing regimens were proposed, with resultant improved tolerability.[96]

Levetiracetam

Available clinical studies on levetiracetam (mainly as second- or third-line treatment) have a weak design, limiting the value of data on efficacy. There are no RCTs; studies are mainly retrospective (only two prospective studies have been published to date[114,115]) or case reports. The reported effectiveness is variable, ranging from 35% to 86%,[116,117] although differences (and potential biases) in study design, timing, and method of ascertainment of response limit the quality of the evidence. Additionally, the mechanism of action is not fully known. Because of the increased volume of distribution in neonates, it might be possible that newborns require higher loading doses; however, elimination half-life seems to be longer than in older patients owing to the immaturity of renal function.[118] Clearance of levetiracetam in preterm infants is lower than in older children (half-life: 9 hours compared with 5–7 hours).[119] Safety-wise, its use has not been associated with severe or life-threatening adverse events.

Topiramate

There are few studies on the use of topiramate in newborns.[120–122] Its use is limited by the unavailability of a formulation for intravenous use.[123] Hypothermia increases its half-life and concentrations.[124] The data on efficacy and safety of the main anti-convulsant medications used in newborns are summarized in Table 7.4.

Antiepileptic Drug Treatment Duration and Discontinuation

The crescendo-decrescendo pattern and self-limited nature of acute symptomatic seizures, the potential detrimental effect of anticonvulsants on neurodevelopmental

Table 7.4 MOST USED ANTICONVULSANT MEDICATIONS FOR SEIZURES THERAPY

Anticonvulsant Drug	Current Place in Treatment Protocols	Efficacy (%)	Adverse Effects	Effects of Hypothermia
Phenobarbital	First-line	43–50	Clinical: CNS depression and respiratory depression Experimental: neuronal apoptosis, altered long-term behavior, learning, memory, and social interaction (animal data)	Minimal. No dose adjustments required.
Phenytoin	Second-line	45	Clinical: hypotension, CNS depression Experimental: apoptosis and synaptic disruption (animal data)	Possible clearance decrease, increased risk of bradycardia
Midazolam	Second-line	0–100	Clinical: well tolerated; no serious adverse effects Experimental: possible neuronal apoptosis	Increased risk of cardiac depression.
Lidocaine	Second-/third-line	10–78	Clinical: cardiac toxicity	Risk of arrhythmia. Need for modified dosing.
Levetiracetam	Emerging second-/third-line	Limited data; 35–86	Clinical: well tolerated Experimental: controversial (animal data)	Likely unaffected.
Topiramate	Emerging	Limited data (case series)	Clinical: no increase in risk of death, short-term detrimental effects, or gross brain pathology	Increased half-life and concentration

Modified from Donovan MD, Griffin BT, Kharoshankaya L, et al. Pharmacotherapy for neonatal seizures: current knowledge and future perspectives. *Drugs.* 2016;76:647–661; and El-Dib M, Soul JS. The use of phenobarbital and other anti-seizure drugs in newborns. *Semin Fetal Neonatal Med.* 2017;22:321–327.

outcome, and the risks associated with indiscriminate treatment are important considerations in the pharmacologic management of seizures. Nevertheless, there is no clear guidance on when to discontinue medication and on factors determining this decision. The duration of anticonvulsant therapy largely depends on the etiology.[125]

Hypothermia

Therapeutic hypothermia is the current standard of care in neonatal HIE. It may alter pharmacodynamics and pharmacokinetics of anticonvulsant medications, with a further, clinically significant increase of this effect in case of multiorgan dysfunction.[126] However, aside from cases with renal/hepatic dysfunction, maximum phenobarbital concentrations are unchanged[127] as pharmacokinetic changes do not reach statistical significance. Pharmacokinetic data for phenytoin are extrapolated from pediatric populations as they are not available in newborns. Of note, it is possible that hypothermia will lead to prolonged clearance of phenytoin with increased risk of bradycardia.[128] For lidocaine, posology is reduced to 70% of what is normally prescribed in normothermia to avoid cardiotoxicity.[127] Conversely, the rewarming phase might be associated with accelerated metabolism of anticonvulsant drugs.[126]

Controversies in Therapy

"Newborn-Tailored" Pharmacotherapy

Despite our knowledge on the ontogeny of ion channels and neurotransmitter receptors in the immature brain,[129] a pilot clinical study administering the antidiuretic bumetanide (an inhibitor of the Na^+-K^+-$2Cl^-$ cotransporter [NKCC] highly expressed in the immature brain) as an add-on to phenobarbital was terminated because of an increased risk of hearing loss and the lack of evidence of an improvement in seizure control.[130] Therefore, although anticonvulsant medications developed for older children and adults do not show adequate efficacy in newborns, in the meantime no specific therapies are available.

Age-Appropriate Antiseizure Therapies

A great deal of interest is also being focused on the real need for a differential approach in seizure therapy in preterm versus full-term newborns. The potential need for age-dependent prescription strategies is based on the changes in pharmacokinetics, hepatic and renal function, and developmental processes in the CNS with increasing gestational age. However, no RCT studies are available for seizure therapy exclusively in preterm infants. Efficacy and safety of most antiseizure drugs are ill known in the newborn population—particularly, but not only, in preterm infants.[131]

Timing of Therapy Administration

Very few data exist regarding the time window for decision making in the acute management of seizures, and even the definition of status epilepticus is still controversial.[17] Few therapy flow charts provide advice on when to check for efficacy, repeat loading doses, or skip to second- or third-line medications.[90,132]

However, in the context of acute symptomatic seizures, given their self-limiting course, the time frame in which a medication is administered is expected to create a possible bias in the evaluation of efficacy[123] and should be taken into account in future studies.

Predictors of Response to Antiseizure Medications

In the context of seizures, factors associated with or predictive of response or lack of response to therapy have been seldom investigated. Background EEG and seizure type (electroclinical versus electrographic-only) were found as the only statistically significant predictors of response to phenobarbital; moderate to severe abnormal EEG findings and electrographic-only seizures were associated with lack of response.[133]

Electrographic-Only Seizures

An additional controversy concerns the treatment of electrographic-only (subclinical) seizures. Experimental data show a contribution to neonatal brain injury,[134,135] whereas in human newborns one small study showed lower seizure burden and better neurodevelopmental outcome at 18 to 24 months among patients treated for EEG-proven seizures compared with those treated only in case of clinical seizures.[136]

Synergistic Effects of Hypothermia and Anticonvulsant Medications

Preclinical studies seem to suggest the existence of a synergism with topiramate,[137–139] whereas dose-dependent association with apoptosis has been found with levetiracetam.[140] Phenobarbital has been considered a potentially harmful drug,[141] even if animal data have also suggested a possible neuroprotective effect in association with hypothermia.[142]

Conclusions

Most seizures in neonates occur as a response to an acute symptomatic event; the predominant etiologies are HIE, hemorrhage, or stroke. However, a substantial proportion of neonates with neonatal-onset epilepsies associated with structural brain malformations and/or of genetic origin are increasingly recognized.

A prompt and accurate diagnosis of seizures with electrographic confirmation is necessary to discriminate epileptic from nonepileptic paroxysmal movements often seen in the newborns. Video-EEG monitoring plays an important role for diagnosis and evaluation of efficacy of antiseizure medications. It has greatly contributed to the knowledge of seizure semiology and of neonatal ictal EEG features that are now fundamental to address instances deriving from the expanding laboratory, instrumental, and genetic techniques.

There are no worldwide accepted therapeutic protocols for the treatment of neonatal seizures, and first-line antiseizure drugs are only partially effective. Many drugs are used off-label and only a few RCTs are available, so further studies are warranted to optimize seizure control. Moreover, no specific drugs are indicated for the different gestational ages, despite some interesting perspectives opening up in the treatment of seizures of genetic origin. Prognosis seems to be related mostly to the etiology, and whether seizures may aggravate the underlying brain injury/dysfunction is still debated. Hopefully, in the near future a wider field of application of therapeutic hypothermia, the introduction of new antiseizure drugs more effective in the neonatal brain, and their combined use with neuroprotective or antioxidant agents might change the natural course of the affected newborns.

REFERENCES

1. Shellhaas RA, Wusthoff CJ, Tsuchida TN, et al. Neonatal Seizure Registry. Profile of neonatal epilepsies: characteristics of a prospective US cohort. *Neurology*. 2017;89:893–899.
2. Shellhaas R. *Clinical features, evaluation, and diagnosis of neonatal seizures*. UpToDate; 2017. Internet: https://www.uptodate.com/contents/clinical-features-evaluation-and-diagnosis-of-neonatal-seizures. [accessed 25.08.17]
3. Glass HC, Wirrell E. Controversies in neonatal seizure management. *J Child Neurol*. 2009;24: 591–599.
4. Holmes GL. What is more harmful, seizures or epileptic EEG abnormalities? Is there any clinical data? *Epileptic Disord*. 2014;16:S12–S22.
5. Mizrahi EM, Kellaway P. Characterization and classification of neonatal seizures. *Neurology*. 1987;37:1837–1844.
6. Volpe JJ. Neonatal seizures: current concepts and revised classification. *Pediatrics*. 1989;84:422–428.
7. Lombroso CT. Neonatal seizures: historic note and present controversies. *Epilepsia*. 1996;37(S3): 5–13.
7a. Mizrahi EM, Kellaway P. *Diagnosis and Management of Neonatal Seizures*. Lippincott-Raven, Philadelphia: Lippincott Williams & Wilkins; 1998, p.181.
8. Watanabe K, Hara K, Miyazaki S, et al. Electroclinical studies of seizures in the newborn. *Folia Psychiatr Neurol Jpn*. 1977;31:383–392.
9. Clancy RR, Legido A, Lewis D. Occult neonatal seizures. *Epilepsia*. 1988;29:256–261.
10. Lloyd RO, O'Toole JM, Pavlidis E. Electrographic seizures during the early postnatal period in preterm infants. *J Pediatr*. 2017;187:18–25.e2.
11. Boylan GB, Stevenson NJ, Vanhatalo S. Monitoring neonatal seizures. *Semin Fetal Neonatal Med*. 2013;18:202–208.
12. Pisani F, Pavlidis E, Cattani L, et al. Optimizing detection rate and characterization of subtle paroxysmal neonatal abnormal facial movements with multi-camera video-electroencephalogram recordings. *Neuropediatrics*. 2016;47:169–174.
13. Pisani F, Facini C, Pelosi A, et al. Neonatal seizures in preterm newborns: A predictive model for outcome. *Eur J Paediatr Neurol*. 2016;20:243–251.
14. Murray DM, Boylan GB, Ali I, et al. Defining the gap between electrographic seizure burden, clinical expression and staff recognition of neonatal seizures. *Arch Dis Child Fetal Neonatal Ed*. 2008;93:F187–F191.
15. Clancy RR, Legido A. The exact ictal and interictal duration of electroencephalographic neonatal seizures. *Epilepsia*. 1987;28:537–541.
16. Abend NS, Wusthoff CJ. Neonatal seizures and status epilepticus. *J Clin Neurophysiol*. 2012;29:441–448.
17. Pavlidis E, Spagnoli C, Pelosi A, et al. Neonatal status epilepticus: differences between preterm and term newborns. *Eur J Paediatr Neurol*. 2015;19:314–319.
18. Commission on classification and terminology of the international league against epilepsy. proposal for revised classification of epilepsies and epileptic syndromes. *Epilepsia*. 1989;30:389–399.
19. Shellhaas RA, Clancy RR. Characterization of neonatal seizures by conventional EEG and single-channel EEG. *Clin Neurophysiol*. 2007;118:2156–2161.
20. Tassinari CA, Rubboli G, Shibasaki H. Neurophysiology of positive and negative myoclonus. *Electroencephalogr Clin Neurophysiol*. 1998;107:181–195.
21. Fusco L, Vigevano F. Ictal clinical electroencephalographic findings of spasms in West syndrome. *Epilepsia*. 1993;34:671–678.
22. Pisani F, Cerminara C, Fusco C, Sisti L. Neonatal status epilepticus vs recurrent neonatal seizures: clinical findings and outcome. *Neurology*. 2007;69:2177–2185.
23. Pisani F, Sisti L, Seri S. A scoring system for early prognostic assessment after neonatal seizures. *Pediatrics*. 2009;124:e580–e587.
24. Alix JJ, Ponnusamy A, Hart AR. Brief rhythmic discharges in neonates: a marker for seizures. *Epileptic Disord*. 2015;17:349.

25. Orivoli S, Facini C, Pisani F. Paroxysmal nonepileptic motor phenomena in newborn. *Brain Dev.* 2015;37:833–839.
26. Facini C, Spagnoli C, Pisani F. Epileptic and non-epileptic paroxysmal motor phenomena in newborns. *J Matern Fetal Neonatal Med.* 2016;29:3652–3659.
27. Scher MS. Controversies regarding neonatal seizure recognition. *Epileptic Disord.* 2002;4:139–158.
28. Chang T, Tsuchida TN. Conventional (continuous) EEG monitoring in the NICU. *Curr Pediatr Rev.* 2014;10:2–10.
29. Shellhaas RA, Chang T, Tsuchida T, et al. The American clinical neurophysiology society's guideline on continuous electroencephalography monitoring in neonates. *J Clin Neurophysiol.* 2011;28:611–617.
30. Battin M, Bennet L, Gunn AJ. Rebound seizures during rewarming. *Pediatrics.* 2004;114:1369.
31. Glass HC, Wusthoff CJ, Shellhaas RA, et al. Risk factors for EEG seizures in neonates treated with hypothermia: a multicenter cohort study. *Neurology.* 2014;82:1239–1244.
32. Cilio MR. EEG and the newborn. *J Ped Neurol.* 2009;7:25–49.
33. Boylan G, Burgoyne L, Moore C, et al. An international survey of EEG use in the neonatal intensive care unit. *Acta Paediatr.* 2010;99:1150–1155.
34. de Vries LS, Toet MC. Amplitude integrated electroencephalography in the full-term newborn. *Clin Perinatol.* 2006;33:619–632.
35. de Vries LS, Hellström-Westas L. Role of cerebral function monitoring in the newborn. *Arch Dis Child Fetal Neonatal Ed.* 2005;90:F201–F207.
36. Janačkova S, Boyd S, Yozawitz E, et al. Electroencephalographic characteristics of epileptic seizures in preterm neonates. *Clin Neurophysiol.* 2016;127:2721–2727.
37. Okumura A, Hayakawa F, Kato T, et al. Ictal electroencephalographic findings of neonatal seizures in preterm infants. *Brain Dev.* 2008;30:261–268.
38. Shah DK, Boylan GB, Rennie JM. Monitoring of seizures in the newborn. *Arch Dis Child Fetal Neonatal Ed.* 2012;97:F65–F69.
39. McCoy B, Hahn CD. Continuous EEG monitoring in the neonatal intensive care unit. *J Clin Neurophysiol.* 2013;30:106–114.
40. Shah DK, Mackay MT, Lavery S, et al. Accuracy of bedside electroencephalographic monitoring in comparison with simultaneous continuous conventional electroencephalography for seizure detection in term infants. *Pediatrics.* 2008;121:1146–1154.
41. Zimbric MR, Sharpe CM, Albright KC, Nespeca MP. Three-channel electroencephalogram montage in neonatal seizure detection and quantification. *Pediatr Neurol.* 2011;44:31–34.
42. Scher MS, Aso K, Beggarly ME, et al. Electrographic seizures in preterm and full-term neonates: clinical correlates, associated brain lesions, and risk for neurologic sequelae. *Pediatrics.* 1993;91:128–134.
43. Scher MS, Hamid MY, Steppe DA, et al. Ictal and interictal electrographic seizure durations in preterm and term neonates. *Epilepsia.* 1993;34:284–288.
44. Lynch NE, Stevenson NJ, Livingstone V, et al. The temporal evolution of electrographic seizure burden in neonatal hypoxic ischemic encephalopathy. *Epilepsia.* 2012;53:549–557.
45. Low E, Boylan GB, Mathieson SR, et al. Cooling and seizure burden in term neonates: an observational study. *Arch Dis Child Fetal Neonatal Ed.* 2012;97:F267–F272.
46. McBride MC, Laroia N, Guillet R. Electrographic seizures in neonates correlate with poor neurodevelopmental outcome. *Neurology.* 2000;55:506–513.
47. Patrizi S, Holmes GL, Orzalesi M, Allemand F. Neonatal seizures: characteristics of EEG ictal activity in preterm and fullterm infants. *Brain Dev.* 2003;25:427–437.
48. Tekgul H, Bourgeois BF, Gauvreau K, Bergin AM. Electroencephalography in neonatal seizures: comparison of a reduced and a full 10/20 montage. *Pediatr Neurol.* 2005;32:155–161.
49. Nagarajan L, Ghosh S, Palumbo L. Ictal electroencephalograms in neonatal seizures: characteristics and associations. *Pediatr Neurol.* 2011;45:11–16.
50. Pisani F, Copioli C, Di Gioia C, Turco E, Sisti L. Neonatal seizures: relation of ictal video-electroencephalography (EEG) findings with neurodevelopmental outcome. *J Child Neurol.* 2008;23:394–398.
51. Wusthoff CJ. Diagnosing neonatal seizures and status epilepticus. *J Clin Neurophysiol.* 2013;30:115–121.
52. Rowe JC, Holmes GL, Hafford J, et al. Prognostic value of the electroencephalogram in term and preterm infants following neonatal seizures. *Electroencephalogr Clin Neurophysiol.* 1985;60:183–196.
53. Watanabe K. Neurophysiological aspects of neonatal seizures. *Brain Dev.* 2014;36:363–371.
54. Rose AL, Lombroso CT. A study of clinical, pathological, and electroencephalographic features in 137 full-term babies with a long-term follow-up. *Pediatrics.* 1970;45:404–425.
55. Engel RC, ed. *Abnormal electroencephalogram in the neonatal period.* Springfield, IL: Charles C Thomas; 1975.
56. Kellaway P, Hrachovy RA. Electroencephalography. In: Swaiman KF, Wright FS, eds. *The practice of pediatric neurology.* St. Louis: CV Mosby; 1982:96–114.
57. Knauss TA, Carlson CB. Neonatal paroxysmal monorhythmic alpha activity. *Arch Neurol.* 1978;35:104–107.
58. Nash KB, Bonifacio SL, Glass HC, et al. Video-EEG monitoring in newborns with hypoxic-ischemic encephalopathy treated with hypothermia. *Neurology.* 2011;76:556–562.
59. Pisani F, Barilli AL, Sisti L, Bevilacqua G, Seri S. Preterm infants with video-EEG confirmed seizures: outcome at 30 months of age. *Brain Dev.* 2008;30:20–30.

60. Lamblin MD, André M, Auzoux M, et al. Indications of electroencephalogram in the newborn. *Arch Pediatr*. 2004;11:829–833.
61. Volpe JJ. Neonatal seizures. In: *Neurology of the newborn*. Philadelphia: WB Saunders; 2008: 203–237.
62. Tekgul H, Gauvreau K, Soul J, et al. The current etiologic profile and neurodevelopmental outcome of seizures in term newborn infants. *Pediatrics*. 2006;117:1270–1280.
63. Glass HC, Shellhaas RA, Wusthoff CJ, et al. Neonatal Seizure Registry Study Group. Contemporary profile of seizures in neonates: a prospective cohort study. *J Pediatr*. 2016;174:98–103.e1.
64. Lynch NE, Stevenson NJ, Livingstone V, et al. The temporal characteristics of seizures in neonatal hypoxic ischemic encephalopathy treated with hypothermia. *Seizure*. 2015;33:60–65.
65. Wusthoff CJ, Dlugos DJ, Gutierrez-Colina A, et al. Electrographic seizures during therapeutic hypothermia for neonatal hypoxic-ischemic encephalopathy. *J Child Neurol*. 2011;26:724–728.
66. Glass HC, Wusthoff CJ, Shellhaas RA, et al. Risk factors for EEG seizures in neonates treated with hypothermia: a multicenter cohort study. *Neurology*. 2014;82:1239–1244.
67. Ghosh S, Tran L, Shuster JJ, Zupanc ML. Therapeutic hypothermia for neonatal hypoxic ischemic encephalopathy is associated with short-term reduction of seizures after discharge from the neonatal intensive care unit. *Childs Nerv Syst*. 2017;33(2):329–335.
68. Kendall GS, Mathieson S, Meek J, Rennie JM. Recooling for rebound seizures after rewarming in neonatal encephalopathy. *Pediatrics*. 2012;130(2):e451–e455.
69. Glass HC, Nash KB, Bonifacio SL, et al. Seizures and magnetic resonance imaging-detected brain injury in newborns cooled for hypoxic-ischemic encephalopathy. *J Pediatr*. 2011;159:731–735.e1.
70. Seltzer LE, Scher MS. Neonatal seizures in the era of therapeutic hypothermia: keeping it cool. *Neurology*. 2014;82(14):1200–1201.
71. Weeke LC, Groenendaal F, Toet MC, et al. The aetiology of neonatal seizures and the diagnostic contribution of neonatal cerebral magnetic resonance imaging. *Dev Med Child Neurol*. 2015;57:248–256.
72. Vasudevan C, Levene M. Epidemiology and aetiology of neonatal seizures. *Semin Fetal Neonatal Med*. 2013;18:185–191.
73. Zupanc ML. Neonatal seizures. *Pediatr Clin N Am*. 2004;51:961–978.
74. Illis LS, Taylor FM. The electro encephalogram in herpes simplex encephalitis. *Lancet*. 1982;1:718–726.
75. Kocherlakota P. Neonatal abstinence syndrome. *Pediatrics*. 2014;134:e547–e561.
76. Dulac O, Plecko B, Gataullina S, Wolf NI. Occasional seizures, epilepsy, and inborn errors of metabolism. *Lancet Neurol*. 2014;13:727–739.
77. Ficicioglu C, Bearden D. Isolated neonatal seizures: when to suspect inborn errors of metabolism. *Pediatr Neurol*. 2011;45:283–291.
78. Van Hove JL, Lohr NJ. Metabolic and monogenic causes of seizures in neonates and young infants. *Mol Genet Metab*. 2011;104:214–230.
79. Yang Y, Muzny DM, Reid JG, et al. Clinical whole-exome sequencing for the diagnosis of mendelian disorders. *N Engl J Med*. 2013;369:1502–1511.
80. Berg AT, Berkovic SF, Brodie MJ, et al. Revised terminology and concepts for organization of seizures and epilepsies: report of the ILAE Commission on Classification and Terminology, 2005–2009. *Epilepsia*. 2010;51:676–685.
81. Deleted in review.
82. Deleted in review.
83. Deleted in review.
84. Deleted in review.
85. Painter MJ, Scher MS, Stein AD, et al. Phenobarbital compared with phenytoin for the treatment of neonatal seizures. *N Engl J Med*. 1999;341:485–489.
86. Pathak G, Upadhyay A, Pathak U, Chawla D, Goel SP. Phenobarbitone versus phenytoin for treatment of neonatal seizures: an open-label randomized controlled trial. *Indian Pediatr*. 2013;50:753–757.
87. Boylan GB, Rennie JM, Chorley G, et al. Second-line anticonvulsant treatment of neonatal seizures: a video-EEG monitoring study. *Neurology*. 2004;62:486–488.
88. *Guidelines on Neonatal Seizures*. Geneva: World Health Organization; 2011.
89. Co JP, Elia M, Engel J Jr, et al. Proposal of an algorithm for diagnosis and treatment of neonatal seizures in developing countries. *Epilepsia*. 2007;48:1158–1164.
90. Hart AR, Pilling EL, Alix JJ. Neonatal seizures—part 2: aetiology of acute symptomatic seizures, treatments and the neonatal epilepsy syndromes. *Arch Dis Child Educ Pract Ed*. 2015;100:226–232.
91. Slaughter LA, Patel AD, Slaughter JL. Pharmacological treatment of neonatal seizures: a systematic review. *J Child Neurol*. 2013;28:351–364.
92. Weeke LC, Schalkwijk S, Toet MC, et al. Lidocaine-associated cardiac events in newborns with seizures: incidence, symptoms and contributing factors. *Neonatology*. 2015;108:130–136.
93. Glass HC, Kan J, Bonifacio SL, Ferriero DM. Neonatal seizures: treatment practices among term and preterm infants. *Pediatr Neurol*. 2012;46:111–115.
94. Mikati MA, Jiang YH, Carboni M, et al. Quinidine in the treatment of KCNT1-positive epilepsies. *Ann Neurol*. 2015;78:995–999.
95. Glass HC, Shellhaas RA, Tsuchida TN, et al. Neonatal Seizure Registry study group. Seizures in preterm neonates: a multicenter observational cohort study. *Pediatr Neurol*. 2017;72:19–24.
96. Weeke LC, Toet MC, van Rooij LG, et al. Lidocaine response rate in aEEG-confirmed neonatal seizures: retrospective study of 413 full-term and preterm infants. *Epilepsia*. 2016;57:233–242.

7

97. Farwell JR, Lee YJ, Hirtz DG, et al. Phenobarbital for febrile seizures—effects on intelligence and on seizure recurrence. *N Engl J Med*. 1990;322:364–369.
98. Bittigau P, Sifringer M, Genz K, et al. Antiepileptic drugs and apoptotic neurodegeneration in the developing brain. *Proc Natl Acad Sci USA*. 2002;99:15089–15094.
99. Kim J-S, Kondratyev A, Tomita Y, Gale K. Neurodevelopmental impact of antiepileptic drugs and seizures in the immature brain. *Epilepsia*. 2007;48:19–26.
100. Forcelli PA, Janssen MJ, Vicini S, Gale K. Neonatal exposure to antiepileptic drugs disrupts striatal synaptic development. *Ann Neurol*. 2012;72:363–372.
101. Kaushal S, Tamer Z, Opoku F, Forcelli PA. Anticonvulsant drug-induced cell death in the developing white matter of the rodent brain. *Epilepsia*. 2016;57:727–734.
102. Maitre NL, Smolinsky C, Slaughter JC, Stark AR. Adverse neurodevelopmental outcomes after exposure to phenobarbital and levetiracetam for the treatment of neonatal seizures. *J Perinatol*. 2013;33(11):841–846.
103. Strasser K, Lueckemann L, Kluever V, et al. Dose-dependent effects of levetiracetam after hypoxia and hypothermia in the neonatal mouse brain. *Brain Res*. 2016;1646:116.e24.
104. Komur M, Okuyaz C, Celik Y, et al. Neuroprotective effect of levetiracetam on hypoxic ischemic brain injury in neonatal rats. *Childs Nerv Syst*. 2014;30:1001.e9.
105. Pacifici GM. Clinical pharmacology of phenobarbital in neonates: effects, metabolism and pharmacokinetics. *Current Pediatric Reviews*. 2016;12:48–54.
106. Oztekin O, Kalay S, Tezel G, Akcakus M, Oygur N. Can we safely administer the recommended dose of phenobarbital in very low birth weight infants? *Childs Nerv Syst*. 2013;29:1353–1357.
107. Hellström-Westas L, Boylan G, Agren J. Systematic review of neonatal seizure management strategies provides guidance on anti-epileptic treatment. *Acta Paediatr*. 2015;104:123.e9.
108. Shany E, Benzaqen O, Watemberg N. Comparison of continuous drip of midazolam or lidocaine in the treatment of intractable neonatal seizures. *J Child Neurol*. 2007;22:255–259.
109. Castro Conde JR, Hernández Borges AA, Doménech Martínez E, González Campo C, Perera Soler R. Midazolam in neonatal seizures with no response to phenobarbital. *Neurology*. 2005;64:876–879.
110. Sirsi D, Nangia S, LaMothe J, Kosofsky BE, Solomon GE. Successful management of refractory neonatal seizures with midazolam. *J Child Neurol*. 2008;23:706–709.
111. van Leuven K, Groenendaal F, Toet MC, et al. Midazolam and amplitude-integrated EEG in asphyxiated full-term neonates. *Acta Paediatr*. 2004;93:1221–1227.
112. Malingré MM, Van Rooij LG, Rademaker CM, et al. Development of an optimal lidocaine infusion strategy for neonatal seizures. *Eur J Pediatr*. 2006;165:598–604.
113. Lundqvist M, Ågren J, Hellström-Westas L, Flink R, Wickström R. Efficacy and safety of lidocaine for treatment of neonatal seizures. *Acta Paediatr*. 2013;102:863–867.
114. Füwentsches A, Bussmann C, Ramantani G, et al. Levetiracetam in the treatment of neonatal seizures: a pilot study. *Seizure*. 2010;19:185–189.
115. Ramantani G, Ikonomidou C, Walter B, Rating D, Dinger J. Levetiracetam: safety and efficacy in neonatal seizures. *Eur J Paediatr Neurol*. 2011;15:1–7.
116. Abend NS, Gutierrez-Colina AM, Monk HM, Dlugos DJ, Clancy RR. Levetiracetam for treatment of neonatal seizures. *J Child Neurol*. 2011;26:465–470.
117. Khan O, Chang E, Cipriani C, Wright C, Crisp E, Kirmani B. Use of intravenous levetiracetam for management of acute seizures in neonates. *Pediatr Neurol*. 2011;44:265–269.
118. Hamano S, Sugiyama N, Yamashita S, et al. Intravenous lidocaine for status epilepticus during childhood. *Dev Med Child Neurol*. 2006;48:220–222.
119. Merhar SL, Schibler KR, Sherwin CM, et al. Pharmacokinetics of levetiracetam in neonates with seizures. *J Pediatr*. 2011;159:152–154.e3.
120. Glass HC, Poulin C, Shevell MI. Topiramate for the treatment of neonatal seizures. *Pediatr Neurol*. 2011;44:439–442.
121. Kundak AA, Okumuş N, Dilli D, Erol S, Zenciroğlu A. Topiramate use in the neonatal period. *Pediatr Neurol*. 2012;46:410.
122. Riesgo R, Winckler MI, Ohlweiler L, et al. Treatment of refractory neonatal seizures with topiramate. *Neuropediatrics*. 2012;43:353–356.
123. El-Dib M, Soul JS. The use of phenobarbital and other anti-seizure drugs in newborns. *Semin Fetal Neonatal Med*. 2017;22:321–327.
124. Filippi L, la Marca G, Fiorini P, et al. Topiramate concentrations in neonates treated with prolonged whole body hypothermia for hypoxic ischemic encephalopathy. *Epilepsia*. 2009;50:2355.e61.
125. Fitzgerald MP, Kessler SK. Abend seizures. Early discontinuation of antiseizure medications in neonates with hypoxic-ischemic encephalopathy. *Epilepsia*. 2017;58:1047–1053.
126. Zhou J, Poloyac SM. The effect of therapeutic hypothermia on drug metabolism and response: cellular mechanisms to organ function. *Expert Opin Drug Metab Toxicol*. 2011;7:803–816.
127. van den Broek MP, Groenendaal F, Toet MC, et al. Pharmacokinetics and clinical efficacy of phenobarbital in asphyxiated newborns treated with hypothermia: a thermopharmacological approach. *Clin Pharmacokinet*. 2012;51:671–679.
128. Bhagat H, Bithal PK, Chouhan RS, Arora R. Is phenytoin administration safe in a hypothermic child? *J Clin Neurosci*. 2006;13:953–955.
129. Ben-Ari Y. Basic developmental rules and their implications for epilepsy in the immature brain. *Epileptic Disord*. 2006;8(2):91–102.

130. Pressler RM, Boylan GB, Marlow N, et al. Neonatal seizure treatment with Medication Off-patent (NEMO) consortium.. Bumetanide for the treatment of seizures in newborn babies with hypoxic ischaemic encephalopathy (NEMO): an open-label, dose finding, and feasibility phase 1/2 trial. *Lancet Neurol.* 2015;14:469–477.

131. Donovan MD, Griffin BT, Kharoshankaya L, Cryan JF, Boylan GB. Pharmacotherapy for neonatal seizures: current knowledge and future perspectives. *Drugs.* 2016;76:647–661.

132. Harris ML, Malloy KM, Lawson SN, Rose RS, Buss WF, Mietzsch U. Standardized treatment of neonatal status epilepticus improves outcome. *J Child Neurol.* 2016;31:1546–1554.

133. Spagnoli C, Seri S, Pavlidis E, Mazzotta S, Pelosi A, Pisani F. Phenobarbital for neonatal seizures: response rate and predictors of refractoriness. *Neuropediatrics.* 2016;47:318–326.

134. Wasterlain CG. Recurrent seizures in the developing brain are harmful. *Epilepsia.* 1997;38:728–734.

135. Stafstrom CE, Chronopoulos A, Thurber S, Thompson JL, Holmes GL. Age dependent cognitive and behavioral deficits after kainic acid seizures. *Epilepsia.* 1993;34:420–432.

136. Srinivasakumar P, Zempel J, Trivedi S, et al. Treating EEG seizures in hypoxic ischemic encephalopathy: a randomized controlled trial. *Pediatrics.* 2015;136:e1302–e1309.

137. Follett PL, Deng W, Dai W, et al. Glutamate receptor-mediated oligodendrocyte toxicity in periventricular leukomalacia: a protective role for topiramate. *J Neurosci.* 2004;24:4412–4420.

138. Schubert S, Brandl U, Brodhun M, et al. Neuroprotective effects of topiramate after hypoxia-ischemia in newborn piglets. *Brain Res.* 2005;1058:129–136.

139. Liu Y, Barks JD, Xu G, Silverstein FS. Topiramate extends the therapeutic window for hypothermia-mediated neuroprotection after stroke in neonatal rats. *Stroke.* 2004;35:1460–1465.

140. Strasser K, Lueckemann L, Kluever V, et al. Dose-dependent effects of levetiracetam after hypoxia and hypothermia in the neonatal mouse brain. *Brain Res.* 2016;1646:116–124.

141. Cilio MR, Ferriero DM. Synergistic neuroprotective therapies with hypothermia. *Semin Fetal Neonatal Med.* 2010;15:293–298.

142. Barks JD, Liu YQ, Shangguan Y, Silverstein FS. Phenobarbital augments hypothermic neuroprotection. *Pediatr Res.* 2010;67:532–537.

7

CHAPTER 8

Neonatal-Onset Epilepsies: Early Diagnosis and Targeted Treatment

Maria Roberta Cilio and Tristan T. Sands

- Long-term video-EEG monitoring and advances in neuroimaging and genetic analysis have led to a major transformation in our understanding of epilepsies presenting in the neonatal period.

- Older terms, such as Ohtahara syndrome and early myoclonic encephalopathy, are being parsed into new distinct genetic epilepsies, making possible the first attempts at precision medicine on the basis of etiology.

- Benign familial epilepsies and severe sporadic epilepsies in neonates can be caused by different variants in the same genes (e.g., KCNQ2 and SCN2A).

- Seizures in neonatal epilepsies due to variants in KCNQ2/3 and SCN2A have been showed to respond to sodium channel blockers (e.g., carbamazepine).

- Targeted therapeutic approaches have identified drugs, such as quinidine, that may be able to target the channel dysfunction induced by a genetic mutation (such as variants in KCNT1 in epilepsy of infancy with migrating focal seizures).

- A precision medicine paradigm in the nursery entails early recognition of genetic epilepsy, as well as moving beyond the monolithic concept of "neonatal seizures" and one-size-fits-all treatment protocols for seizures in neonates.

CASE HISTORY

A female neonate with unremarkable prenatal course was born at 38 weeks' gestation by uncomplicated spontaneous vaginal delivery to a 38-year-old G2P2 mother. Apgar scores were 9 and 9 at 1 and 5 minutes, respectively. On the second day of life, the mother noticed three episodes of brief rightward head turning. The child was otherwise doing well and was already "breastfeeding like a champ." A fourth event was witnessed by the nurse, who suspected it to be a seizure and initiated a transfer to the intensive care nursery. There, additional paroxysmal episodes characterized by asymmetric limb stiffening, accompanied by oxygen desaturation to the 70s, were noted. The child was given a load of 20 mg/kg intravenous phenobarbital and video-electroencephalography (EEG) was ordered. Laboratory studies performed on cerebrospinal fluid (CSF), serum, and urine revealed no abnormal metabolic findings and raised no concern for infection; the result of magnetic resonance imaging (MRI) of the brain was negative. Following a second 20 mg/kg load of phenobarbital, there was a temporary cessation of the events but the infant was notably more sedated and no longer able to breastfeed. While treated with maintenance phenobarbital, the episodes recurred

Continued

CASE HISTORY—cont'd

the next day; the phenobarbital level was 42 µg/mL. Video-EEG confirmed the events to be electroclinical seizures, consisting of asymmetric tonic posturing of the upper and lower limbs to the left or to the right, often accompanied by cyanosis and at times followed by bilateral, asynchronous clonic limb jerking, each lasting 1 to 2 minutes. Electrographically, seizures were characterized by low-voltage fast activity followed by focal spikes and waves over the central and temporal regions. Seizure onset alternated between the left and right hemispheres, corresponding to the variable lateralization of the clinical events. The EEG was essentially normal between the frequent seizures. The electroclinical presentation led the consulting neurologist to revisit the family history. Initial family history had been negative for seizures, but asking again with the maternal grandmother present elicited a history of seizures in the mother during the neonatal period. A diagnosis of benign familial neonatal epilepsy was made, phenobarbital was discontinued, and oral carbamazepine was started at 10 mg/kg per day with immediate cessation of seizures. Feeding resumed over the next couple of days; as the sedating effects of phenobarbital wore off, seizures did not recur and the child was discharged home. An epilepsy gene panel returned a pathogenic stop-gain variant in the *KCNQ2* gene 1 week later. Subsequent testing demonstrated the same variant in the child's mother.

This case illustrates the challenges and potential rewards of parsing neonatal epilepsies from among more common acute symptomatic causes of seizures in the nursery. The role of video-EEG is highlighted, not only for determining the presence of seizures, but also for providing clues to the underlying etiology. Carbamazepine is not a medication typically used to treat seizures in neonates. The application of targeted treatment for genetic epilepsy stands in contrast to a protocol-driven one-size-fits-all approach to "neonatal seizures."

The New Chapter of Neonatal Epilepsies

The past decade has witnessed a major transformation in our understanding of epilepsies presenting in the neonatal period as a result of two advances. First, the implementation of long-term video-EEG monitoring in the nursery provided an opportunity for neurologists to be more involved in the clinical evaluation of newborns with seizures. A result of this experience was the rejection of the notion that seizure phenomenology in neonates is essentially different from that in older children and adults.[1] Second, advances in neuroimaging and metabolic testing, together with readily available sophisticated genetic analysis, has allowed for the identification of an increasing proportion of epilepsies presenting in the nursery from among the large number of newborns with seizures resulting from acute brain injury.[2] The consequence of these developments has been an appreciation of the nuanced differences among patients previously combined under broad umbrella syndromes—Ohtahara syndrome and early myoclonic encephalopathy (EME)—thus allowing for the recognition of new distinct electroclinical phenotypes reflecting discrete etiologic entities (e.g., *STXBP1* encephalopathy, *KCNQ2* encephalopathy, glycine encephalopathy). Indeed, Ohtahara syndrome and EME were first described in 1976 and 1978,[3] respectively, when neuroimaging was in its infancy and gene sequencing was being developed. Differentiating neonates with epilepsy from neonates with acute symptomatic seizures has prompted controversy about treatment: does one size fit all?[4]

Parsing of the old syndromes into the neonatal epilepsies has made possible the first attempts at precision medicine on the basis of etiology. We provide an overview of the types of genetic epilepsies present in newborns and then discuss three genes in which there is some evidence for emerging targeted therapeutics.[5]

Landscape of the Neonatal Epilepsies

Genetic epilepsies may be conceptualized in a number of ways, including by genetic mechanism, inheritance pattern, pathophysiology, associated features, and outcomes. Generally, neonatal epilepsies with known genetic etiologies affect either dominant or recessive genes and the pathogenic variants either are inherited or occur de novo, in

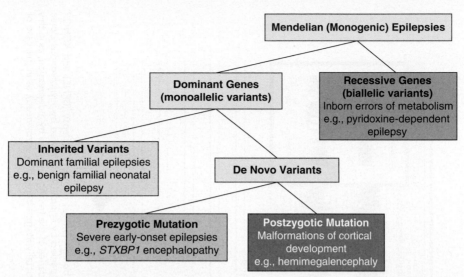

Fig. 8.1 Landscape of the Mendelian epilepsies. Monogenic epilepsies may result from biallelic or monoallelic genetic variants. This variant may be inherited or de novo. The de novo variant may occur before fertilization or in somatic cells at any point in postzygotic development, resulting in mosaicism. Broad categories of epilepsies resulting from each mechanism are given with a neonatal example.

which case the mutation may occur either before fertilization or during postzygotic development (Fig. 8.1). This dichotomous scheme is useful, as the resultant groupings tend to share certain clinical features. For example, recessive genes associated with epilepsy often give rise to metabolic disorders in which the complete lack of an enzyme or critical cofactor results in a severe, often progressive, condition (e.g., sulfite oxidase deficiency). Heterozygous de novo mutation in dominant epilepsy genes tends to cause severe epilepsies characterized by intractable seizures and encephalopathy (e.g. *STXBP1*). Malformations of cortical development arise from similar de novo genetic variants (e.g., *PAFAH1B1*, associated with lissencephaly) but can also result from postzygotic gene mutation affecting a subset of cortical cells[6] (e.g., *PIK3CA* in hemimegalencephaly). Inherited variants in dominant genes are responsible for dominant familial epilepsies.

KCNQ2/3-Associated Neonatal Epilepsies

Benign familial neonatal epilepsy (BFNE) is a rare autosomal dominant condition with incomplete penetrance and good neurodevelopmental outcome that presents with clusters of seizures in the first days of life and remits after weeks or months.[7] A recent multicenter prospective study suggested that BFNE cases may represent about 3% of neonates with seizures.[8] The seizures are characteristic, consisting of asymmetric tonic posturing evolving to unilateral or asynchronous bilateral clonic jerking, often accompanied by apnea and desaturation (Fig. 8.2). Seizures shift laterality variably and are short, typically lasting 1 to 2 minutes, but may occur as frequently as 20 to 30 times a day.[7] A distinctive pattern can be seen on amplitude-integrated EEG (Fig. 8.2B).[8a] BFNE was termed "benign" to reflect the fact that in most affected individuals, seizures are limited to the first year of life and neurologic development is normal. Nevertheless, seizures may be difficult to control in the neonatal period and some patients present with status epilepticus.[9] Recent studies have shown that up to 25% of patients with BFNE develop epilepsy later in life, the risk of which correlates with the number of seizures in the neonatal period.[10]

In more than 80% of cases BFNE is associated with pathogenic variants in *KCNQ2* or *KCNQ3*, which encode $K_v7.2$ and $K_v7.3$, voltage-gated ion channel subunits mediating a subthreshold potassium current important in limiting neuronal excitability.[11] While inherited alterations in *KCNQ2* are responsible for the vast majority of BFNE cases,[10,11] de novo variants in *KCNQ2* may result in profound neonatal encephalopathy with severe, frequent, intractable seizures, termed KCNQ2 encephalopathy.[12–14] Seizures in *KCNQ2* encephalopathy are of the same type as those of BFNE[14]; however, in contrast to BFNE, the interictal EEG is severely abnormal and the neurologic

8

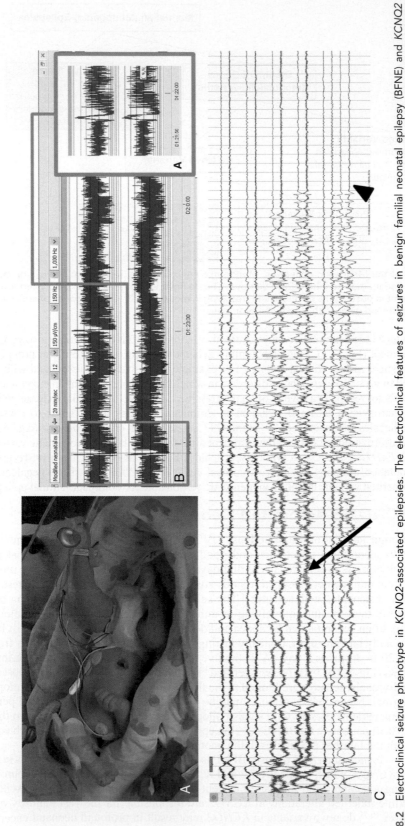

Fig. 8.2 Electroclinical seizure phenotype in *KCNQ2*-associated epilepsies. The electroclinical features of seizures in benign familial neonatal epilepsy (BFNE) and *KCNQ2* encephalopathy are shared between the two conditions. Clinically, seizures consist of asymmetric tonic posturing accompanied by apnea (A), followed by asynchronous clonic jerking, as in this case of BFNE. Amplitude-integrated EEG (B) shows a paroxysmal elevation of the upper and lower boundaries of the tracing followed by a depression, as in this case of *KCNQ2* encephalopathy. Conventional ictal EEG (C) shows increased fast activity at seizure onset (*arrow*) and postictal voltage attenuation (*arrowhead*), as in this case of *KCNQ2* encephalopathy. (B, Courtesy Ana Vilan.)

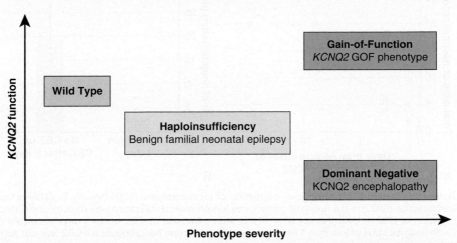

8

Fig. 8.3 *KCNQ2* genotype-phenotype spectrum. *KCNQ2* loss-of-function mutation can give rise to benign or severe carbamazepine-responsive epilepsy phenotypes, correlating with the strength of the mutation. Gain-of-function *(GOF)* variants also cause a severe phenotype but without epilepsy. Generally, the severe phenotypes result from de novo genetic variants, whereas the mild phenotype is inherited.

examination is often notable for hypotonia, paucity of spontaneous movements, no visual fixation, and altered reactivity. Whereas mutations that lead to BFNE result in mild reductions in potassium current,[15] de novo mutations responsible for KCNQ2 encephalopathy represent more profound loss-of-function alterations, acting through a dominant negative effect.[16,17] Gain-of-function variants (R201H and R201C) have also been reported to cause KCNQ2 encephalopathy,[18] but careful analysis of the electroclinical characteristics revealed a separate gain-of-function phenotype that lacks seizures in the neonatal period and is characterized instead by irregular breathing patterns, exaggerated startle responses, and nonepileptic myoclonus.[19] The association of a given gene, such as *KCNQ2*, with both benign and severe phenotypes is a recurring theme for channelopathies, epilepsies associated with genes encoding ion channels.[4] Fig. 8.3 depicts the spectrum of *KCNQ2* phenotypes by underlying genotype.

The possibility for a targeted therapeutic approach for KCNQ2 encephalopathy has been suggested for retigabine/ezogabine, a drug that specifically augments current through the K_v7 channels.[20] According to parental report, there was some improvement in mental status and development in six patients, four of whom experienced a seizure reduction, although seizure freedom was not achieved.[21] Serious adverse effects, including skin and retinal pigmentation leading to visual loss, were reported with long-term treatment, and the production of retigabine/ezogabine was discontinued as of June 2017. Interestingly, clinical observation in patients with KCNQ2 encephalopathy has suggested that sodium channel blockers are particularly effective.[14] Seizure freedom was reported with carbamazepine (CBZ) in six patients and with phenytoin in five patients.[22] Therefore sodium channel blockers appear to represent a very effective therapy for *KCNQ*-associated seizures, and this is now considered an established precision medicine treatment.[5] Interestingly, although retigabine/ezogabine had a more pertinent mechanism of action, it seemed to be less effective in KCNQ2 encephalopathy than sodium channel blockers.

Recently a multicenter study of 19 cases described treatment responses in BFNE and demonstrated rapid seizure cessation in all 17 neonates treated with low-dose (10 mg/kg per day) oral CBZ, regardless of when in the course it was initiated.[9] In contrast, response to other agents was poor (e.g., no response to phenobarbital in 12 of 14 cases). Early treatment with CBZ reduced the length of hospitalization (Fig. 8.4). These reports on the use of CBZ for *KCNQ2*-associated epilepsies constitute the best evidence for the response of a genetic epilepsy to a specific therapeutic agent (Table 8.1). It is unclear why sodium channel blockade would be particularly effective in countering potassium channel loss of function, but sodium channels are bound together with K_v7 potassium channels at the axonal initial segment and nodes of Ranvier, locations critical for action potential generation and maintenance, suggesting localized functional interaction (Fig. 8.5B).[23]

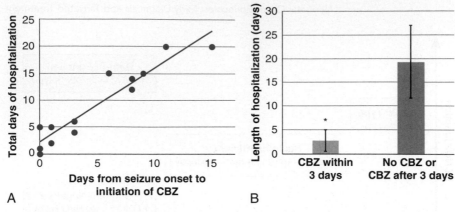

A

B

Fig. 8.4 A, Length of hospitalization by time to initiation of carbamazepine (CBZ) therapy. In patients treated with CBZ or oxcarbazepine (OXC) in the neonatal period, the length of hospitalization was directly correlated with the timing of initiation of CBZ or OXC therapy (P < .01). B, Administration of CBZ within 3 days of seizure onset was associated with hospital stays of less than 1 week compared with longer hospitalization if CBZ was not administered or if initiated after 3 days (P < .01).

Table 8.1 RESPONSE OF SEIZURES TO TREATMENT IN NEONATAL EPILEPSIES[a]

Gene	Phenotype	Effective Treatment
KCNQ3	Benign (familial) neonatal epilepsy[9]	Carbamazepine
KCNQ2	Benign (familial) neonatal epilepsy[9]	Carbamazepine
		Possibly phenytoin, oxcarbazepine
	KCNQ2 encephalopathy[21,22]	Carbamazepine, phenytoin,
		Possibly ezogabine, topiramate
KCNT1	Epilepsy of infancy with migrating focal seizures[27–29]	Possibly quinidine
SCN2A	Benign (familial) neonatal-infantile epilepsy[44]	Possibly phenytoin, oxcarbazepine
	Early infantile epilepsies with encephalopathy[39–42]	Phenytoin (super therapeutic), Carbamazepine
		Possibly mexiletine, lidocaine

[a]Epilepsies associated with genetic variants in KCNQ2 and SCN2A are generally responsive to sodium channel blockade, with the evidence for a given agent in a particular epilepsy varying by what has been reported to date. Importantly, however, at the variant level there may be differing propensities to respond to treatment.
[b]No patient with KCNT1-associated epilepsy treated with quinidine in the literature presented before 6 weeks of life.

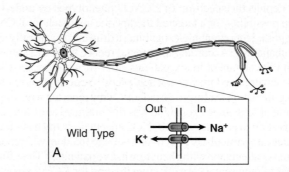

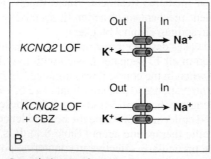

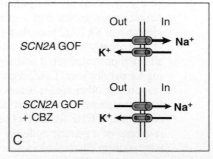

Fig. 8.5 Speculative mechanism of sodium channel blockade in neonatal epilepsies associated with genetic variants in KCNQ2 and SCN2A. Panel A shows the wild-type condition. Loss of function in KCNQ2 (KCNQ2 LOF) in panel B and gain of function in SCN2A (SCN2A GOF) in panel C create an imbalance in hyperpolarizing potassium and depolarizing sodium currents, respectively, leading to hyperexcitability. Sodium channel blockade—for example, with carbamazepine (CBZ)—restores this balance by reducing sodium currents in both conditions. K+, Potassium ion; Na+, sodium ion.

Epilepsy of Infancy With Migrating Focal Seizures Associated With *KCNT1*

Epilepsy of infancy with migrating focal seizures (EIMFS) (formerly known as malignant migrating partial seizures in infancy [MMPSI]) presents in early infancy, often in the neonatal period, with medically intractable seizures and severe developmental regression. Seizures migrate from one focus to another and multiple seizures can evolve simultaneously, giving the condition its name (Fig. 8.6). The most common cause of EIMFS is de novo gain-of-function mutation of *KCNT1*, encoding a sodium-activated potassium channel. The channel, known as SLACK (sequence like a calcium activated potassium channel), mediates the slow hyperpolarization that accompanies repetitive neuronal firing. The pathologic mutations increase the current amplitude through increased cooperativity between individual channels.[24] Remarkably, mutations of the same gene account for some cases of autosomal dominant nocturnal frontal lobe epilepsy (ADNFLE), a familial condition that presents in later childhood.[25] The mutations of *KCNT1* resulting in EIMFS have been shown to lead to higher increases in conductance compared with those associated with ADNFLE, indicating a bimodal genotype-phenotype correlation.[26]

The discovery that the class I antiarrhythmic drug quinidine can reverse this increased conductance in vitro[26] led rapidly to clinical application in a patient with an *R428Q* mutation with reported efficacy.[27] Although some publications have suggested a significant reduction of seizure frequency in patients with *KCNT1*-associated epilepsy,[27,28] treatment failures have also been reported.[28,29] Interestingly, across the

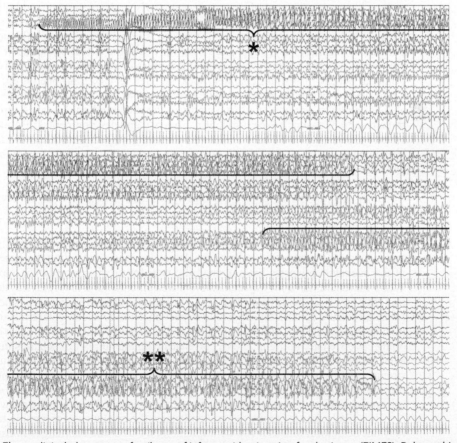

Fig. 8.6 Electroclinical phenotype of epilepsy of infancy with migrating focal seizures (EIMFS). Polygraphic ictal tracing (electroencephalogram [EEG], pneumogram, electrocardiogram) from a patient with EIMFS showing the independent evolution of an initial seizure *(asterisk)* in the left inferior parietoposterior temporal region best appreciated, which is eclipsed by a second independent seizure *(double asterisks)* in the right inferior frontoanterior temporal region. The signature feature of EIMFS is the presence of multiple independently evolving seizures on EEG, giving an impression of migration from one location to another. Gain 10 μV/mm; high-frequency filter, 70 Hz; paper speed 15 mm/sec.

patients described by Mikati et al.[28] there was a dissociation with regard to in vitro efficacy of quinidine on potassium current and clinical responsiveness, as the *K629N* mutation of the responsive patient demonstrated the least effective inhibition in vitro to quinidine. The determinants of responsiveness to quinidine remain unclear, but may include genotype, phenotype, age at the time of treatment, dose, route of administration (oral vs. intravenous vs. intrathecal), and pharmacokinetics.

SCN2A-Associated Neonatal Epilepsies

Benign familial neonatal-infantile epilepsy (BFNIE) is an autosomal dominant benign epilepsy of the early infancy with a high degree of penetrance, associated with variants in *SCN2A*[30–32] This benign form of familial epilepsy has a variable age of onset and typically presents in infancy or in the neonatal period in different individuals of a same family, ranging from 2 days and 6 months of life.[33] Seizures resemble those described in *KCNQ2*-associated epilepsy, consisting of focal onset of tonic and clonic movements, often in clusters. The interictal EEG is normal or shows occasional focal spikes.[30,31] Seizures abate within the first 2 years of life with low risk of recurrence and neurodevelopmental outcomes are good. However, as observed in BFNE, seizures in this condition can be difficult to treat and medical refractoriness may be observed.[33]

Analogous to the situation with *KCNQ2*, de novo missense variants in the *SCN2A* gene are associated with severe developmental phenotypes in the setting of refractory epilepsy presenting in the first few months of life, sometimes accompanied by a hyperkinetic movement disorder.[34–39] *SCN2A* encodes Nav1.2, a major voltage-gated sodium channel in the central nervous system early in development, and both benign and severe epilepsies are associated with gain-of-function mutations. Nav1.2 resides at the axon hillock of excitatory neurons, where it is critically poised to influence action potential firing. Nav1.2 is supplanted over time to some extent by Nav1.6 (*SCN8A*), which may account for the limited temporal expression of *SCN2A*-associated epilepsy. Potential benefit of sodium channel blockers, such as CBZ and phenytoin, in managing the seizures in *SCN2A*-associated epilepsy has been suggested.[5,38–42] Sodium channel blockers are predicted to counteract the increased conductance through the mutant sodium channels (see Fig. 8.5C). Epilepsy and developmental disability associated with variants in *SCN2A* are now appreciated to span a spectrum and later presentations are associated with loss-of-function, rather than gain-of-function mutation, and appear less likely to respond to sodium channel blockade.[39,43]

The Promise and the Challenge of Precision Medicine in the Nursery

The early identification of neonates presenting with genetic epilepsies has significant therapeutic and prognostic implications. Advances in understanding the genetic basis of the neonatal epilepsies have opened the way for precision medicine approaches. While we remain far from the realization of this potential, the first forays in this direction have now been made (see Table 8.1). The promise of such approaches is not merely for better seizure control, but a positive impact on neurodevelopmental trajectories and modification of the risk of future epilepsy. It was recently shown that the risk of developing epilepsy later in life in BFNE correlates with the number of seizures in the neonatal period.[10] Whether the increased seizure frequency and later epilepsy result from a stronger predisposition in these patients or the seizures themselves play a contributory role in epileptogenesis is unknown, but the discovery of the potent response of BFNE seizures to CBZ provides an opportunity to intervene and determine the answers.

It is likely that for many genetic epilepsies the existence of a specific treatment may not be helpful unless it can be implemented early. The challenges in early diagnosis for implementation of targeted therapy are multiple. The first challenge lies in recognizing the presence of a genetic epilepsy from among the larger number of newborns with seizures resulting from acute brain injury. The second challenge is identifying the specific phenotype, if possible. In some cases, such as BFNE, familiarity with a specific epilepsy phenotype can allow treatment even before the return of genetic test results. The final challenge is flexibility in the use of novel treatments as they are identified. Individually, neonatal epilepsies are rare. Randomized trials to demonstrate the efficacy of specific therapeutics for neonatal epilepsies associated with a certain gene, let alone for functional classes of mutation affecting a given gene, are unlikely. Rather, the novel therapeutic approaches discussed previously were either the result of (1) serendipitous clinical observation or (2) rationally devised directed therapy with in vitro validation.

An essential key to meeting these challenges will be disposing of the monolithic notion of "neonatal seizures." Treating seizures in neonates as a single entity has the unfortunate effect of obscuring seizures as heterogeneous manifestations of specific disease etiologies. Indeed, the notion of a one-size-fits-all protocol for the treatment of seizures in neonates is founded on this concept. The medical treatment of neonatal seizures has remained substantially unchanged for decades. Precision medicine will be possible in the nursery only if we can move beyond one-size-fits-all treatment protocols for neonatal seizures and embrace therapeutic approaches stratified on the basis of etiology.

REFERENCES

1. Berg AT, Berkovic SF, Brodie MJ, et al. Revised terminology and concepts for organization of seizures and epilepsies: report of the ILAE Commission on classification and terminology, 2005–2009. *Epilepsia*. 2010;51(4):676–685.
2. Sands TT, Choi H. Genetic testing in pediatric epilepsy. *Curr Neurol Neurosci Rep*. 2017;17(5):45.
3. Bureau M, Genton P, Dravet C, et al. *Epileptic Syndromes in Infancy, Childhood and Adolescence*. Montrouge, France: John Libbey Eurotext; 2012.
4. Sands TT, McDonough TL. Recent advances in neonatal seizures. *Curr Neurol Neurosci Rep*. 2016;16(10):92.
5. Reif PS, Tsai MH, Helbig I, Rosenow F, Klein KM. Precision medicine in genetic epilepsies: break of dawn? *Expert Rev Neurother*. 2017;17(4):381–392.
6. Poduri A, Evrony GD, Cai X, Walsh CA. Somatic mutation, genomic variation, and neurological disease. *Science*. 2013;341(6141):1237758.
7. Cilio MR, Sands TT. Genetics of epilepsy. In: *Swaiman's Pediatric Neurology*. 6th ed. Elsevier; 2017.
8. Glass HC, Shellhaas RA, Wusthoff CJ, et al. Contemporary profile of seizures in neonates: a Prospective Cohort Study. *J Pediatr*. 2016.
8a. Vilan A, Mendes Ribeiro J, Striano P, et al. A distinctive ictal amplitude-integrated electroencephalography pattern in newborns with neonatal epilepsy associated with KCNQ2 mutations. *Neonatology*. 2017;112(4):387–393.
9. Sands TT, Balestri M, Bellini G, et al. Rapid and safe response to low-dose carbamazepine in neonatal epilepsy. *Epilepsia*. 2016;57(12):2019–2030.
10. Grinton BE, Heron SE, Pelekanos JT, et al. Familial neonatal seizures in 36 families: clinical and genetic features correlate with outcome. *Epilepsia*. 2015;56(7):1071–1080.
11. Zara F, Specchio N, Striano P, et al. Genetic testing in benign familial epilepsies of the first year of life: clinical and diagnostic significance. *Epilepsia*. 2013;54(3):425–436.
12. Weckhuysen S, Mandelstam S, Suls A, et al. KCNQ2 encephalopathy: emerging phenotype of a neonatal epileptic encephalopathy. *Ann Neurol*. 2012;71(1):15–25.
13. Weckhuysen S, Ivanovic V, Hendrickx R, et al. Extending the KCNQ2 encephalopathy spectrum: clinical and neuroimaging findings in 17 patients. *Neurology*. 2013;81(19):1697–1703.
14. Numis AL, Angriman M, Sullivan JE, et al. KCNQ2 encephalopathy: delineation of the electroclinical phenotype and treatment response. *Neurology*. 2014;82(4):368–370.
15. Schroeder BC, Kubisch C, Stein V, Jentsch TJ. Moderate loss of function of cyclic-AMP-modulated KCNQ2/KCNQ3 K$^+$ channels causes epilepsy. *Nature*. 1998;396(6712):687–690.
16. Miceli F, Soldovieri MV, Ambrosino P, et al. Genotype-phenotype correlations in neonatal epilepsies caused by mutations in the voltage sensor of K(v)7.2 potassium channel subunits. *Proc Natl Acad Sci U S A*. 2013;110(11):4386–4391.
17. Orhan G, Bock M, Schepers D, et al. Dominant-negative effects of KCNQ2 mutations are associated with epileptic encephalopathy. *Ann Neurol*. 2014;75(3):382–394.
18. Miceli F, Soldovieri MV, Ambrosino P, et al. Early-Onset epileptic encephalopathy caused by gain-of-function mutations in the voltage sensor of Kv7.2 and Kv7.3 potassium channel subunits. *J Neurosci*. 2015;35(9):3782–3793.
19. Mulkey SB, Ben-Zeev B, Nicolai J, et al. Neonatal nonepileptic myoclonus is a prominent clinical feature of KCNQ2 gain-of-function variants R201C and R201H. *Epilepsia*. 2017;58(3):436–445.
20. Barrese V, Miceli F, Soldovieri MV, et al. Neuronal potassium channel openers in the management of epilepsy: role and potential of retigabine. *Clin Pharmacol*. 2010;2:225–236.
21. Millichap JJ, Park KL, Tsuchida T, et al. KCNQ2 encephalopathy: features, mutational hot spots, and ezogabine treatment of 11 patients. *Neurol Genet*. 2016;2(5):e96.
22. Pisano T, Numis AL, Heavin SB, et al. Early and effective treatment of KCNQ2 encephalopathy. *Epilepsia*. 2015;56(5):685–691.

23. Pan Z, Kao T, Horvath Z, et al. A common ankyrin-G-based mechanism retains KCNQ and NaV channels at electrically active domains of the axon. *J Neurosci*. 2006;26(10):2599–2613.

24. Kim GE, Kronengold J, Barcia G, et al. Human slack potassium channel mutations increase positive cooperativity between individual channels. *Cell Rep*. 2014;9(5):1661–1672.

25. Heron SE, Smith KR, Bahlo M, et al. Missense mutations in the sodium-gated potassium channel gene KCNT1 cause severe autosomal dominant nocturnal frontal lobe epilepsy. *Nat Genet*. 44(11): 1188–1190.

26. Milligan CJ, Li M, Gazina EV, et al. KCNT1 gain of function in 2 epilepsy phenotypes is reversed by quinidine. *Ann Neurol*. 2014;75(4):581–590.

27. Bearden D, Strong A, Ehnot J, DiGiovine M, Dlugos D, Goldberg EM. Targeted treatment of migrating partial seizures of infancy with quinidine. *Ann Neurol*. 2014;76(3):457–461.

28. Mikati MA, Jiang YH, Carboni M, et al. Quinidine in the treatment of KCNT1-positive epilepsies. *Ann Neurol*. 2015;78(6):995–999.

29. Chong PF, Nakamura R, Saitsu H, Matsumoto N, Kira R. Ineffective quinidine therapy in early onset epileptic encephalopathy with KCNT1 mutation. *Ann Neurol*. 2016;79(3):502–503.

30. Heron SE, Crossland KM, Andermann E, et al. Sodium-channel defects in benign familial neonatal-infantile seizures. *Lancet*. 2002;360(9336):851–852.

31. Herlenius E, Heron SE, Grinton BE, et al. SCN2A mutations and benign familial neonatal-infantile seizures: the phenotypic spectrum. *Epilepsia*. 2007;48(6):1138–1142.

32. Berkovic SF, Heron SE, Giordano L, et al. Benign familial neonatal-infantile seizures: characterization of a new sodium channelopathy. *Ann Neurol*. 2004;55(4):550–557.

33. DiMauro S, Hirano M. Mitochondrial DNA deletion syndromes. In: Pagon RA, Adam MP, Ardinger HH, et al, eds. *GeneReviews(®)*. Seattle, WA: University of Washington, Seattle; 1993.

34. Hackenberg A, Baumer A, Sticht H, et al. Infantile epileptic encephalopathy, transient choreoathetotic movements, and hypersomnia due to a De Novo missense mutation in the SCN2A gene. *Neuropediatrics*. 2014;45(4):261–264.

35. Ogiwara I, Ito K, Sawaishi Y, et al. De novo mutations of voltage-gated sodium channel alphaII gene SCN2A in intractable epilepsies. *Neurology*. 2009;73(13):1046–1053.

36. Matalon D, Goldberg E, Medne L, Marsh ED. Confirming an expanded spectrum of SCN2A mutations: a case series. *Epileptic Disord.*16(1):13–18.

37. Touma M, Joshi M, Connolly MC, et al. Whole genome sequencing identifies SCN2A mutation in monozygotic twins with Ohtahara syndrome and unique neuropathologic findings. *Epilepsia*. 2013;54(5):e81–e85.

38. Nakamura K, Kato M, Osaka H, et al. Clinical spectrum of SCN2A mutations expanding to Ohtahara syndrome. *Neurology*. 2013;81(11):992–998.

39. Wolff M, Johannesen KM, Hedrich UB, et al. Genetic and phenotypic heterogeneity suggest therapeutic implications in SCN2A-related disorders. *Brain*. 2017;140(5):1316–1336.

40. Howell KB, McMahon JM, Carvill GL, et al. SCN2A encephalopathy: a major cause of epilepsy of infancy with migrating focal seizures. *Neurology*. 2015;85(11):958–966.

41. Foster LA, Johnson MR, MacDonald JT, et al. Infantile epileptic encephalopathy associated with SCN2A mutation responsive to oral mexiletine. *Pediatr Neurol*. 2017;66:108–111.

42. Dilena R, Striano P, Gennaro E, et al. Efficacy of sodium channel blockers in SCN2A early infantile epileptic encephalopathy. *Brain Dev*. 2017;39(4):345–348.

43. Sanders SJ, Murtha MT, Gupta AR, et al. De novo mutations revealed by whole-exome sequencing are strongly associated with autism. *Nature*. 2012;485(7397):237–241.

44. Wolff M, Casse-Perrot C, Dravet C. Severe myoclonic epilepsy of infants (Dravet syndrome): natural history and neuropsychological findings. *Epilepsia*. 2006;47(suppl 2):45–48.

CHAPTER 9

Glucose and Perinatal Brain Injury— Questions and Controversies

Jerome Y. Yager

- Neonatal hypoglycemia remains a common though frequently overlooked complication of the newborn.
- In the term, otherwise normal newborn, brain injury requires prolonged episodes of glucose values below 1.1 mmol/L.
- High levels of sensitivity for hypoglycemia must be maintained in newborns with complex histories of diabetic mothers, growth restriction, fetal inflammation, or hypoxia-ischemia.
- In infants with prolonged or intractable hypoglycemia, insulin-secreting tumors, pituitary abnormalities, or metabolic disorders must be sought.

Hypoglycemia remains a common though controversial problem of the newborn infant.[1-3] Such controversy persists around issues related in the first place, to definition and subsequent diagnosis,[4] the relevance of "asymptomatic" versus "symptomatic" hypoglycemia, incidence rates, underlying pathophysiology, treatment, and of course, neurodevelopmental outcome. Importantly, contributing to the persistence of neonatal hypoglycemia as a cause of morbidity in the newborn is the increasing prevalence of both type 1 and type 2 diabetes worldwide and diagnosis in younger women of childbearing age.[5,6] Confounding these issues are improved obstetric and neonatal intensive care, which have allowed for the survival of low-birth-weight infants, with their attendant complications of prematurity and lack of nutritional stores, respiratory distress, altered metabolism, and higher risks of disorders such as hypoxia-ischemia, seizures, and sepsis.

The adult acts as a completely independent being with respect to nutritional requirements. The fetus, on the other hand, is fully dependent on the mother and the placental transfer of glucose and its other nutritional requirements. The newborn exists in the transition phase between these two states of complete dependence and independence. For normal cerebral development and consequent function to proceed, an adequate amount of metabolizable substrate must be supplied to the brain during the perinatal period. Glucose is the primary energy substrate for both the adult and newborn brain under physiologic conditions. However, other organic substrates are capable of supplementing glucose during conditions whereby the normal balance of supply and demand for energy production are superseded.[7-9]

At birth, the previously consistent supply of maternal glucose is abruptly terminated. Immediately after birth, hepatic glycogen stores are broken down to maintain adequate nutritional support. Glucose-6-phosphatase is the rate-limiting enzyme for this to occur; it is expressed at low levels in the newborn, increasing to adult values within the first few days of life.[10] To rapidly adapt, an endocrine stress response involving insulin and glucagon drives hepatic glycogenolysis, lipolysis, and fatty acid oxidation that generate lactate and ketone bodies as alternative fuels important in maintaining cerebral energy metabolism. Estimated rates of glucose metabolism in the 1-day-old newborns are threefold greater than older newborns and infants.[11] Moreover, measured rates of glucose oxidation suggest that only ~70% of the energy needs of the brain are met through the metabolism of glucose. Hence, the newborn is adapted for using ketone bodies, which can be 5- to 40-fold greater than the adult, and lactate, which contributes significantly in the first few hours of life.

Despite the obvious importance of glucose for cerebral energy utilization, particularly during the complex transition from fetal to newborn life, questions remain regarding the role of hypoglycemia per se to brain damage and neurodevelopmental outcome. It is, therefore, the intent of this chapter to provide the reader with a general review of glucose metabolism and its alternate substrates to the newborn brain and to describe the recognized derangements associated with hypoglycemia. Finally, we review clinical aspects of hypoglycemia and present case examples that exemplify neonatal hypoglycemia, highlighting questions and controversies around this still complex issue.

Glucose Metabolism in the Fetus and Newborn

In most species studied, including humans, glucose serves as the primary organic fuel for energy production under physiologic circumstances.[9,12] In the fetus, a linear relationship has been observed between the glucose level in the mother and that of the fetus.[13–16] At term birth, blood glucose concentrations in the newborn are at about 80% to 90% of those of the mother.[17] This linear relationship has been seen during all states of maternal euglycemia, hyperglycemia, and hypoglycemia and is important in that it implies at least a one-to-one relationship between maternal and fetal glucose needs.

At the time of birth, glucose concentrations in the term healthy newborn fall within the first hour of life, then recover and become more stable by 3 hours of age, and gradually increase for at least the first 96 hours, when infants receive exogenous nutrition.[17–21] In preparation for birth, a doubling of the glycogen stores occurs from 36 weeks' gestation to term. At birth, plasma insulin levels fall, together with a marked surge in glucagon levels, leading to a mobilization of glycogen stores, which are rapidly depleted within the first 12 to 24 hours of life.[22,23] Glucagon levels remain elevated through the first week of life. Subsequent glucose concentrations in the normal newborn depend on feeding practices. Although some studies have suggested feeding intervals to be a major determinant of blood glucose concentrations,[24] others have not found this to be the case.[21] Irrespective, "low" blood glucose concentrations in appropriately fed normal term infants are very rare.

Preterm Infants

It is a generally held belief that blood glucose concentrations in the preterm infant are lower than those of the term infant. Although recent studies suggest that this is not likely the case, given more recent policies of early feeding and intravenous glucose supplementation,[24] the theoretical risks certainly apply. In this regard, the preterm infant has not as yet had the opportunity afforded the term infant to build up glycogen stores, typically occurring in the last 4 weeks of gestation. Moreover, the rate-limiting enzyme for glyconeogenesis is significantly lower in the preterm compared with the term infant[10]; hence the ability to break down even these limited stores of glycogen are restricted. The capability of the preterm to mount a response with alternate substrates may also be impaired. Hawdon et al.[24] compared 156 term infants with 62 preterm infants and found that although blood glucose concentrations were not statistically different, preterm infants were unable to mount a significant ketone body response at the lower end of the blood glucose values. Others have found preterm infants to variably mount an inadequate glycemic response to glucagons, suggesting features of insulin resistance.[25]

Intrauterine Growth Restriction

Clearly, intrauterine growth restriction (IUGR), occurring as the fetus is exposed to an environment when nutrition is restricted either because of placental insufficiency or maternal lack of nutrition, predisposes the newborn to hypoglycemia. Previous reports have indicated a higher prevalence of hypoglycemia in the small infant compared with those within the normal weight range.[26,27] Other reports are more controversial; some suggest similar glucose concentrations in small-for-gestation age (SGA) versus appropriate-for-gestation age (AGA) infants,[17,28] again likely the result of more aggressive nutritional management. Still others continue to show differences between the two weight groups with SGA infants displaying lower glucose concentrations compared with AGA infants.[29] In either case, infants with IUGR display altered metabolic profiles that include reduced glycogen stores, limited oxidation of free fatty acids, and functional hyperinsulinism.[22] Combined with a relatively larger brain size, one can see the predisposition of these infants to neurologic injury from a hypoglycemic insult.

Cerebral Metabolism of Glucose

The ontogeny of regional changes in cerebral glucose utilization (CGU) has important implications regarding the sensitivity of the immature brain to hypoglycemia. Using the 2-deoxyglucose (2-DG) technique, regional cerebral glucose utilization (rCGU) in the perinatal animal has been shown to be high in brainstem gray matter structures, declining in a caudal to rostral fashion toward the cerebral cortex.[30] Using positron emission tomography (PET) scanning with fluorine 18–2-DG ([^{18}F]–2-DG) as the isotope, Chugani et al.[31–33] and others[34–36] measured rCGU in humans from birth through adulthood. In infants 5 weeks of age, rCGU was highest in the sensorimotor cortex, thalamus, midbrain-brainstem, and cerebellar vermis. By 3 months of age, maximal glucose utilization had shifted to the parietal, temporal, and occipital cortices and in the basal ganglia, with subsequent increases in frontal and various association regions of the cerebral cortex occurring by 8 months of age. Little further change in rCGU was observed between 8 and 18 months, with adult values reached by 2 years.

Alternate Substrates to Glucose

The perinatal brain is capable of incorporating and metabolizing alternate substrates, most notably lactic acid and the ketone bodies, β-hydroxybutyrate and acetoacetate. In vitro studies of regional energy status and the availability of alternate substrates in rats have shown lactate concentrations to be elevated sixfold in newborn brain compared with the adult brain, and the β-hydroxybutyrate level to be double that of the adult, mature brain.[37]

With respect to the latter, both animal and human studies of the newborn have shown an enhanced capacity for the cerebral extraction of ketone bodies from blood compared with older infants and adults. The investigation of ketone body utilization in suckling rats suggests they may account for between 20% and 35% of cerebral energy metabolism in this age group.[7,8,38] Ketone body utilization peaks at postnatal day (PD) 14, and subsequently diminishes by PD21, at a time during which CGU is increasing and glucose becomes the major substrate for energy metabolism. These findings coincide with the capacity of the immature blood-brain barrier to transport ketone bodies at threefold greater rate compared with glucose.[39] Furthermore, those enzymes linked to ketone body metabolism in the brain display a rapid increase in activity after birth and a subsequent decline after weaning, in contrast to the pattern displayed by the key enzymes of glycolysis, whose activity increases with advancing age in an inverse relation to those of ketogenesis.[40]

Although ketone bodies appear to play a role in normal energy metabolism of the immature brain, whether they do under pathophysiologic circumstances of glucose deprivation seems unlikely. Data from human infants suggest that the capacity for hepatic ketone synthesis in the neonate is restricted. The findings demonstrate (1) low blood ketone levels, (2) a failure of ketone bodies to rise with fasting, and (3) a failure of ketone bodies to rise with hypoglycemia.[41,42] In contrast, lactic acid has been shown to be an important source of energy during hypoglycemia. Elegant studies in the newborn dog[43] during normoglycemia show that 95% of cerebral energy requirements are met by glucose with ketone bodies and lactate contributing

1% and 4%, respectively. With insulin-induced hypoglycemia and a concomitant reduction in CGU, lactate was able to support 58% of cerebral oxidative metabolism. Subsequent experiments showed that, under these conditions, there was no significant decline in brain high-energy phosphate levels.[44]

Recent findings from 35 newborns, at risk and hypoglycemic, show that the infants had glucose, ketone bodies, and lactate concentrations measured in their blood within the first 48 hours of birth. In this study, Harris et al. (2015) found that with glucose concentrations in the severe to moderate hypoglycemic range, β-hydroxybutyrate levels remained low (2.03 mean mmol/L), whereas lactate concentrations generally increased (3.06 mean mmol/L). The authors suggested that under circumstances of hypoglycemia, lactate may serve as a better fuel for neuroprotection than ketone bodies.[44a] Other investigators have also shown a preferential utilization of lactate over either glucose or ketone bodies in the newborn rat and dog and a sparing effect on glucose utilization during hypoglycemia.[45–47,49]

Glucose Transporters

The mechanism by which glucose is transported from blood into brain across cell membranes occurs by a Na^+-glucose cotransporter protein that is energy independent. These facilitative glucose transporter proteins are a family of structurally related proteins. Twelve glucose transporters (GLUTs) have been identified and labeled as GLUT1 through GLUT12.[50] Within the brain, GLUT1 and GLUT3 are predominant. GLUT1 is the most prevalent of the glucose transporters and is highly expressed in all blood-tissue barriers, including the blood-brain barrier. GLUT3 is the predominant isoform in neurons. GLUT5 has been detected in the microglia of both humans and rats.

The expression of glucose transporter proteins, not surprisingly, reflects the energy demands of the brain. Hence, analysis of cerebral cortical microvessels and membranes in the newborn rat demonstrates that all GLUT proteins are low during the first week of life. During the second and third postnatal weeks, GLUT proteins increase, particularly in the deep gray matter structures of the thalamus and hypothalamus, coincident with enhanced utilization of glucose as a fuel. Similarly, and in an almost linear fashion, GLUT proteins in the cortex and hippocampus increase from 20% to 100% of adult values between 7 and 30 PDs during a recognized period of rapid neuronal maturation and synaptogenesis.[51–53]

Definitions

Ambiguity surrounding a precise definition of "neonatal hypoglycemia" continues[54] and has been emphasized by a number of reviews in the recent past.[4,55–57] Koh et al., as far back as 1988,[58] surveyed 36 pediatric textbooks and 178 pediatric consultants searching for agreement on the definition of neonatal hypoglycemia. Perhaps not surprisingly, there was none, with definitions ranging from less than 1 mmol/L to less than 4 mmol/L. In 1937, Hartmann and Jaudon[12] published a series of 286 neonates and infants with "significant hypoglycemia" as determined by recurrent or persistent low "true" blood glucose values. Only those infants with clinical manifestations were considered. These authors defined hypoglycemia as follows: mild (2.2–2.78 mmol/L), moderate (1.11–2.22 mmol/L), or extreme (<1.11 mmol/L). Their approach incorporated the important concept that the definition of hypoglycemia must represent a continuum of values that deviate from the biologic norm. This latter concept is particularly relevant today as definitions of "treatable" hypoglycemia take into account gestational age, multisystem organ complications, and neurophysiologic and/or clinical symptomatology.

Difficulty in arriving at an absolute value for hypoglycemia in the newborn stems from the obvious factors that encompass a dynamic and vulnerable biologic process. Hypoglycemia simply refers to an *abnormally low blood glucose concentration*. In this context, the definition of "abnormal" becomes relevant, given that hypoglycemia—or euglycemia, for that matter—is an evolving, dynamic process, itself dependent on a large number of variables.

Absolute glucose concentrations below which the term hypoglycemia can be applied have been defined based on statistical measures (within two standard deviations of the mean). Hence, serial plasma glucose determinations in term healthy newborn infants revealed an initial drop to 55 to 60 mg/dL (3.05 mmol/L) within the first 2 hours of life, followed by a rise to 70 mg/dL (3.88 mmol/L) from 3 to 72 hours, and levels in excess of 80 mg/dL (4.44 mmol/L) beyond the third day.[20] Values below the fifth percentile were therefore considered by these authors as representing statistical hypoglycemia.

Lubchenco and Bard[27] studied the incidence of hypoglycemia as determined by gestational age and birth weight. Their work showed that preterm AGA infants played a mean glucose concentration of 48 mg/dL (2.6 mmol/L) compared with 54 mg/dL (3.0 mmol/L) in the term AGA infants. In the SGA infants born at term, there was a further shift to the left with mean glucose concentrations of 44 mg/dL (2.4 mmol/L).

In more recent studies of glucose concentrations in healthy term infants, Hoseth et al.[18] studied 223 term breast-fed newborns serially over the first 96 hours and found the lowest blood glucose values occurred within the first hours of life, with an overall range of 1.4 to 5.3 mmol/L (25.6–97 mg/dL; median 3.1 mmol/L, 57 mg/dL). Similar results were reported by a study of more than 200 term healthy newborns[21] in whom a mean glucose concentration of 2.8 mmol/L (51 mg/dL) was found. In both of these studies, 12% to 14% of the children had blood glucose concentrations less than 2.6 mmol/L (47 mg/dL), mostly during the first day of life.

A meta-analysis[59] analyzing 10 studies, inclusive of 723 healthy term AGA infants, suggested parameters that are less than the fifth percentile of norm for the definition of neonatal hypoglycemia. In this regard, thresholds for hypoglycemia would be on a sliding scale based on time after birth and include values less than 1.6, 2.2, and 2.67 mmol/L (<29, 40, and 49 mg/dL) at 1 to 2, 3 to 47, and 48 to 72 hours of age, respectively.

Based on the preceding findings, it is reasonable to state that normal glucose concentrations in term healthy infants have a wide range, with the lowest concentrations occurring during the first few hours of life. Within this range, the risk of neurologic sequelae is remote, and routine testing for blood glucose concentrations has been suggested to be unnecessary.[54]

Controversy and Question

These data do not, however, direct themselves to the more controversial and clinically relevant questions that remain somewhat unanswered. Hence, the definition of neonatal hypoglycemia remains nonspecific and is dependent on gestational age, appropriateness of fetal growth, the age of the newborn at the time of sampling, and whether or not the infant has fed. Given these parameters, current data suggest that hypoglycemia is not clinically evident, nor perhaps relevant, until values are less than 1.1 mmol/L (<20 mg/dL). We therefore need to ask the following question:

1. Are there other parameters or markers of hypoglycemia that suggest an association with resultant encephalopathy?

Symptomatic Versus Asymptomatic Hypoglycemia

Most common among the features of hypoglycemic encephalopathy is an alteration in the level of consciousness, described as lethargy or somnolence. Irritability, high-pitched cry, or exaggerated primitive reflexes may also be found. Newborns are often described as being jittery, and this may progress to seizures, apnea, hypotonia, and coma.[60]

In this regard, a number of investigators have shown that perhaps the more relevant way to define hypoglycemia is to do so based on whether or not the infant is symptomatic. Koivisto et al.[61] reported on 151 children, divided into three groups described as follows: the (1) symptomatic-convulsive group (n = 8), (2) symptomatic-nonconvulsive group (n = 77), and (3) asymptomatic group (n = 66). In this group of patients, feeding was not initiated for the first 24 hours of life. Symptoms were characterized by the presence of tremor, cyanosis, pallor, limpness, irritability, apathy, or tachypnea, which disappeared with glucose therapy. Hypoglycemia was defined as a glucose concentration less than 20 mg/dL (1.1 mmol/L). The findings indicated that 50% of the symptomatic convulsive group and 12% of the symptomatic nonconvulsive group had neurologic abnormalities on follow-up compared with only 6% of both the asymptomatic and control groups. In a study by Singh et al.,[62] 107 infants with severe hypoglycemia (<25 mg/dL) were evaluated over 15 months. Symptoms were present in 40%. Neurodevelopment in asymptomatic infants was normal.

Moore and Perlman[63] described three cases of profound hypoglycemia in term breast-fed newborns in whom seizures developed following discharge from hospital. All were symptomatic with pallor, jitteriness, poor feeding, but had nevertheless been sent home on early discharge. All of the patients showed glucose concentrations less than 1.1 mmol/L (<20 mg/dL). Late follow-up suggested that two of the three infants had normal findings, and one was significantly delayed.

Alkalay et al.[64] reviewed reports of hypoglycemia over the past four decades. Their criterion for inclusion, albeit retrospective, was the presence of neurologic sequelae, considered to be directly or primarily the result of hypoglycemia. The study was inclusive of both AGA and SGA infants as well as preterm infants. Their findings indicated that, of the study patients reported, more than 95% had plasma glucose concentrations less than 25 mg/dL (1.4 mmol/L). The incidence in this group with neurologic abnormality was 21%.

To correlate a critical threshold of blood glucose concentration with neurologic dysfunction, several studies have evaluated neurophysiologic parameters in association with hypoglycemia. Koh et al.[65] reported abnormalities in sensory evoked potentials in children when blood glucose concentrations fell below 2.6 mmol/L (<47 mg/dL). A glucose concentration of less than 18 mg/dL (<1.0 mmol/L) was associated with an isoelectric electroencephalogram (EEG), suggesting the potential for injury.[66] Unfortunately, only four of these children were younger than 1 month of age. Cowett et al.,[67] who studied term and preterm infants, found no such correlation, and Pryds et al.[68] also found no correlation between hypoglycemic glucose concentrations and brain auditory evoked response (BAER) and EEG patterns.

In a very recent study by Caksen et al.[69] the authors examined 110 infants with hypoglycemia using magnetic resonance imaging (MRI). There seemed to be no difference in glucose concentrations between the symptomatic versus asymptomatic patients, all of whom had mean values less than 1.0 mmol/L (<18 mg/dL). However, the symptomatic infants were more likely to have abnormal MRI findings compared with the asymptomatic infants.

Duration of Hypoglycemia

Alkalay et al. found that the minimal age at which hypoglycemia was detected was 10 hours, suggesting that a prolonged period of hypoglycemia was required before neurologic sequelae or symptomatology become evident.[64] Others have similarly suggested prolonged hypoglycemia as a prerequisite for damage. Lucas et al.[70] determined the neurologic outcome of 661 preterm infants. Moderate hypoglycemia, defined in their study as less than 2.6 mmol/L (<47 mg/dL), occurred in 433 infants, of whom 104 displayed recurrent events on 3 or more separate days. A strong correlation existed between the number of separate days in which hypoglycemia was recorded and reduced mental and motor development scores at 18 months corrected age. When hypoglycemia was present on 5 or more days, the incidence of cerebral palsy or developmental delay was increased by a factor of 3.5.

A more recent study conducted by Duvanel et al.[26] illustrated similar results. Eighty-five SGA preterm newborns were tested for hypoglycemia (defined as <2.6 mmol/L; <47 mg/dL). In their cohort, 73% met the criteria for hypoglycemia, and recurrent episodes were once again strongly correlated with persistent neurodevelopmental and physical growth deficits to 5 years of age.

A primate study determining the effect of prolonged insulin-induced hypoglycemia on outcome[71] also showed that the longer the duration of hypoglycemia, the greater the degree of abnormal behavioral outcome. However, even in those in whom hypoglycemia was produced for 10 hours, the effects were transient and reversible when training was done for the behavioral task. Blood glucose concentrations were less than 25 mg/dL. Unfortunately, no neuropathologic examination was reported for this group of animals.

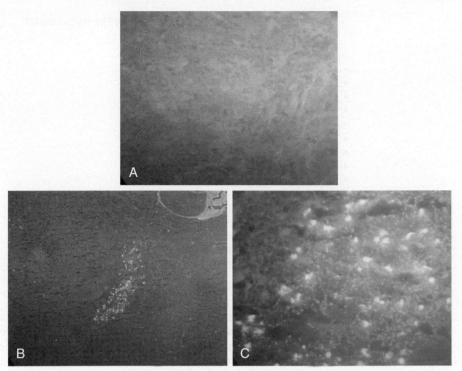

Fig. 9.1 Photographs indicating Fluoro-Jade (FJ) staining of neuronal cells in thalamic nuclei of coronal sections. A, Sham (5× magnification) shows no cells stained with FJ, whereas in experimental animals, staining is indicated by both 5× (B) and 40× (C) magnification of FJ-stained neurons within the thalamus in animals experiencing chronic hypoglycemia of less than 1.1 mmol/L for greater than 12 hours. FJ is a stain that labels degenerating neurons.

In our own laboratory, we have recently completed a study in newborn rat pups undergoing insulin-induced hypoglycemia to various degrees and for variable durations. Neuropathologic assessment was determined following a series of behavioral tests. In this experiment, the mortality rate was significantly increased among rat pups that achieved profound levels of hypoglycemia, below 1.0 mmol/L (<18 mg/dL). In survivors of prolonged hypoglycemia (>12 hours), behavioral assessments were no different than controls. However, brain pathology indicated a significant increase in cell death among those achieving severe hypoglycemia in specific nuclei of the thalamus (Fig. 9.1). Moreover, these pathologic alterations were accompanied by alterations in excitatory amino acid release and free radical production (unpublished data, 2008).

In a more mature model of recurrent moderate hypoglycemia, rat pups received 5 U/kg of insulin twice daily from PD10 to PD19. Although glucose levels were not recorded, those pups receiving insulin displayed heightened levels of anxiety during juvenile age equivalent and diminished social play behavior as adolescents. Though it is not a model of neonatal hypoglycemia, the study confirms the need for a prolonged period of hypoglycemia to obtain an abnormal phenotype.[72]

To provide basic guidelines by which to define hypoglycemia, Cornblath[73] issued a consensus statement regarding "operational thresholds" for blood glucose concentrations. These researchers defined operational threshold as that concentration of plasma or blood glucose at which clinicians should consider intervention. In that regard, they felt that term, healthy, asymptomatic full-term infants need not have routine monitoring of their glucose concentrations. On the other hand, any infant with clinical manifestations compatible with hypoglycemia should be tested, and intervention should be taken for those with values less than 45 mg/dL (2.5 mmol/L). For infants at risk of hypoglycemia owing to alterations in maternal metabolism, intrinsic neonatal problems, or endocrine or metabolic disturbances, glucose monitoring

---

Box 9.1   DIFFERENTIAL DIAGNOSIS OF SEVERE RECURRENT HYPOGLYCEMIA

Hyperinsulinism
- Beta-cell hyperplasia
- Nesidioblastosis
- Macrosomia
- Beckwith-Weidmann syndrome

Endocrine Abnormalities
- Panhypopituitarism
- Hypothyroidism
- Growth hormone deficiency
- Cortisol deficiency

Hereditary Metabolic Disorders
- Abnormalities of carbohydrate metabolism
- Amino acid disorders (maple syrup urine disease)
- Organic acid disorders
- Fatty acid oxidation defects

Glucose Transporter Defects

---

should begin as soon after birth as possible. For values less than 36 mg/dL (2.0 mmol/L), close surveillance should be maintained and intervention is recommended if concentrations remain low, regardless of the presence or absence of symptoms. In those infants in whom very low concentrations are detected (<20–25 mg/dL; 1.1–1.4 mmol/L), therapeutic intervention should be initiated immediately. Newborns being fed by continuous parenteral nutrition will have persistently high insulin levels. As a result, their ability to manifest significant ketogenesis and the means by which to use alternate substrates will be impaired. Under these circumstances, prudent caution suggests maintaining glucose concentrations in the higher therapeutic ranges (>45 mg/dL; 2.5 mmol/L).

More recent recommendations from the American Academy of Pediatrics (AAP)[56] and the Pediatric Endocrine Society (PES)[74] essentially substantiate Cornblath's early work, though controversy continues to persist (Box 9.1).[75]

While this consensus certainly addresses many of the concerns regarding the circumstances under which clinicians should be vigilant in their approach to the diagnosis and treatment of hypoglycemia, it does not answer several other important questions regarding the newborn in particular. Before attempting to answer these questions, further understanding of the epidemiology and pathophysiology of hypoglycemia would be in order.

Causes of Hypoglycemia

Although it is not the intent of this chapter to discuss the underlying causes of hypoglycemia, a list of etiologies is found in Box 9.1.

Incidence

The reported incidence of hypoglycemia depends on those variables also specific to the definition. Sexson et al.[23] found 8.1% of 232 infants had glucose values less than 30 mg/dL (1.6 mmol/L) in the first hours of life, with 20.6% having glucose concentrations less than 40 mg/dL (2.2 mmol/L). When a value less than 30 mg/dL was used as the definition, Lubchenco et al.[27] studied the incidence of hypoglycemia according to gestational age and weight and found the overall incidence to be 32% for SGA infants, and 10%, and 11.5% for AGA and LGA infants, respectively. With a definition of less than 20 mg/dL, the incidence obviously decreases. Of the 73% of SGA infants studied by Duvanel et al.[26] who had hypoglycemia, 30% would have had 6 or more episodes with glucose values between 1.6 and 2.6 mmol/L.

Pathophysiology of Hypoglycemia

Cerebral Blood Flow, Glucose Utilization, and Cerebral Energy Metabolism

As the major metabolic fuel for cerebral energy production is glucose, there is an inextricable link between the demands for energy production and the supply and extraction of substrate. In that regard, studies in newborn dogs[76] displayed an inverse linear relationship between blood glucose concentrations and cerebral blood flow (CBF). Therefore increases in CBF ranging from 150% to 450% of normal occurred as blood glucose concentrations decreased from 40 mg/dL to less than 5 mg/dL (2.2 to <0.3 mmol/L). Increases followed ontogeny and were more predominant in brainstem structures compared with other major regions of the brain. The same phenomenon is seen in human infants. Pryds et al.[68] found CBF increased by 200% above normal at levels of blood glucose below 30 mg/dL (1.6 mmol/L).

Vannucci's group of collaborators found similar results and, importantly, looked at the alterations in white matter glucose utilization during hypoglycemia.[77] In this study blood glucose concentrations were reduced to ~1.0 mmol/L. Hypoglycemia was associated with increases in regional CBF (rCBF) ranging from 170% (white matter) to 250% (thalamus). In both of the former studies, there was a direct relation between CBF and mean arterial pressure. Regional CGU, was unchanged in 11 of the 16 structures measured, but significantly, was reduced by 30% to 45% in the occipital white matter structures and cerebellum. Calculations of the extent to which glucose transport into the brain during hypoglycemia was enhanced by the increases in CBF suggested that glucose delivery contributed minimally (<10%) to the maintenance of CGU. Earlier studies had also shown that with hypoglycemia to levels as low as less than 1.0 mmol/L, the cerebral metabolic rate for oxygen ($CMRO_2$) decreased to 50% of normal. At this same level, cerebral metabolic rates for lactate increase 10-fold and became the dominant fuel for oxidative metabolism in the newborn dog brain.[43] Later experiments showed that using a similar experimental paradigm of hypoglycemia, high-energy phosphate reserves (phosphocreatine, adenosine triphosphate [ATP]) remained within normal concentrations.[44] From this group of studies, the authors concluded that CBF autoregulation is lost during hypoglycemia in the newborn, and that rather than glucose delivery, low energy demands serve to maintain glucose homeostasis and preclude tissue glucose deficiencies. They further hypothesized that alternate cerebral energy fuels, predominantly in the form of lactate, substitute for glucose at levels of blood glucose below 1 mmol/L.

Cerebral Biochemical Alterations During Hypoglycemia

Little work has been done on the biochemical perturbations that arise as a result of hypoglycemia in the immature brain. Much of what is known in this regard is derived from experiments done in the adult animal exposed to insulin-induced hypoglycemia. However, given the information discussed in the previous section, important comparisons between the adult and newborn brain can be made, and perhaps some tentative conclusions drawn.

As in the newborn, CBF increases during hypoglycemia. In the adult, this is where the similarities end. Hence in adult models of hypoglycemia, cerebral high-energy phosphate levels (ATP, phosphocreatine) plummet to levels less than 20% of normal as blood glucose concentrations fall below 1 mmol/L (<20 mg/dL). In concert with this depletion of high-energy reserves, neurophysiologic monitoring reveals an isoelectric EEG, a marked increase in intracellular Ca^{2+}, and a 10-fold and 4-fold rise in extracellular concentrations of the excitatory amino acids (EAAs) aspartate and glutamate, respectively.[78–80] Hence, at least in the adult, it now appears that the mechanism of neuronal death as a result of hypoglycemia is similar to that of hypoxia-ischemia (energy depletion → EEA → Ca^{2+} influx → free radical production → cell death).

As indicated earlier, the preservation of cerebral energy status in the newborn, even at very low concentrations of glucose, is accompanied by a preservation of neurophysiologic function as demonstrated by EEG. A possible underlying cause

Table 9.1 COMPARISON OF PATHOPHYSIOLOGIC MECHANISMS RESPONSIBLE FOR BRAIN DAMAGE IN ADULT VERSUS NEWBORN ANIMALS

Mechanism	Adult	Newborn
Cerebral blood flow	Increased	Increased
Cerebral uptake of glucose	Increased	Increased
Cerebral energy reserves	Depleted	Maintained
Utilization of alternate substrates	Neutral	Increased
Glucose utilization	Increased	Decreased

of cellular injury in the newborn may, however, be related to the release of EEAs. Silverstein et al.[81] induced hypoglycemia by insulin injection in 7-day-old immature rats. Blood glucose concentrations gradually diminished over time to 30 to 40 mg/dL in the first hour after injection, 20 mg/dL in the second hour, and to less than 5 mg/dL by 3 to 4 hours after injection. Their results indicated a direct correlation between decreasing glucose levels and increasing concentrations of extracellular glutamate. In hypoglycemic newborn human infants, Aral et al.[82] also reported on their finding of increased concentrations of glutamate and aspartate in the cerebrospinal fluid.

In more recent studies, neonatal rats of 7 days of age were made hypoglycemic, and antioxidant factors and cell death factors were measured in the cerebral cortices at 1 month of age. Anju et al. found that levels of superoxide dismutase and glutathione peroxidase, both powerful endogenous antioxidants, were significantly reduced in the hypoglycemic groups compared with controls. Apoptotic cell death, as measured by Bax, caspase-3 and caspase-8, were activated and increased in the cerebral cortices of these rat pups as well. Glucose concentrations in the rats were maintained at less than 40 mg/dL. The authors point to this experiment as indicating the role of oxidative stress in brain injury following hypoglycemia and the role of reduced glucose concentrations in inhibiting neuronal antioxidant capacity.[83]

Beyond the previous experimental data, there is very little information regarding the underlying mechanisms of hypoglycemic brain injury in the newborn. In comparing the newborn response to hypoglycemia with that of the adult (Table 9.1), several important differences become evident, particularly in relation to the controversy surrounding hypoglycemic brain injury. In this regard, then, the newborn appears to respond to hypoglycemia with physiologic alterations that appear to protect the brain from damage. Hence, CBF increases, glucose utilization is reduced, alternate substrates are able to substitute for demands of energy production, and as a result, cerebral energy reserves are preserved, at least in experimental animals. These metabolic adaptations beg the question as to whether or not hypoglycemia per se does cause brain damage, certainly an area of ongoing controversy.

Hypoglycemia and Brain Damage

Evidence of pathologic injury to the brain as a result of neonatal hypoglycemia has been particularly difficult to obtain. In this regard, in vitro cell culture studies, as well as animal models of pure hypoglycemia, have been helpful in documenting the effects of significantly low blood glucose concentrations on brain pathology.

In vitro nuclear magnetic resonance (NMR) studies on energy metabolism of neurons and astroglia under various pathologic conditions has shown that hypoglycemia per se did not significantly alter the high-energy reserves of either neurons or glia, even at levels as low as 0.1 mmol/L.[84] In our own laboratory, immature astrocytes in culture were exposed to a substrate-free medium (absence of glucose and amino acids). Under these circumstances, which do not allow for the utilization of any alternate substrate, the immature cells were able to survive for almost twice as long as the mature astrocytes. Although not strictly an indication of the effects of hypoglycemia, the study clearly points out the resistance of immature cells to substrate deprivation.[85]

Brierly et al.[86] investigated the effects of insulin-induced hypoglycemia in a group of adolescent primates. Physiologic parameters were controlled. Six of the 10 animals in which blood glucose was lowered to less than 20 mg/dL (1.1 mmol/L) for 2 hours or more displayed selective neuronal necrosis throughout the cerebral cortices, with particular vulnerability in the parieto-occipital region, as well as the hippocampus, caudate, and putamen. Similar findings were present in primates exposed to severe (<20 mg/dL) and prolonged hypoglycemia of more than 6 hours. In these animals neuropathologic alterations primarily occurred in the basal ganglia, cerebral cortex, and the hippocampus.[87]

In the adult rat, Auer and colleagues[88–93] have done extensive work defining the neuropathologic consequences of severe hypoglycemia. In a series of papers, this group defined the timing, evolution, and distribution of hypoglycemic brain damage in the rat. These investigators defined severe hypoglycemia as that level of blood glucose that caused electrocerebral silence.[94] Their previous studies had shown that glucose concentrations under these circumstances were between 0.12 and 1.36 mmol/L. Over the course of these investigations, they described several important features of hypoglycemic brain damage that distinguish it from ischemic injury. These include the following: (1) infarction of brain tissue does not occur with hypoglycemia, (2) a superficial to deep gradient in the density of neuronal necrosis is seen in the cerebral cortex, (3) the caudate-putamen is involved more heavily near the white matter and near the angle of the lateral ventricle, and (4) the hippocampus shows dense neuronal necrosis at the crest of the dentate gyrus (which is always spared in ischemia), and a gradient of increasing damage in the medial aspect of CA1.[89,90,95] Interestingly, white matter injury was not particularly addressed in these studies.

In the human neonate, there is clearly a paucity of neuropathologic papers that allow some insight into the distribution of injury in the newborn brain as a result of hypoglycemia. Anderson et al.[96] described six neonates who had been diagnosed with hypoglycemia and died within the first year of life for other non-CNS related causes. Blood glucose concentrations were less than 20 mg/dL in all cases. In four of the six neonates, the duration of hypoglycemia was longer than 36 hours. All infants were symptomatic. Histopathologically, the researchers observed widespread necrosis of neuronal and glial cells in the cerebral cortex, hippocampus, and basal ganglia. Within the cortex, the authors commented on a greater degree of involvement in the occipital region than the frontal region. They also noted no predilection for the boundary zones between major blood vessels that often distinguish ischemic lesions. Larroche et al.[97] emphasized the white matter–damaging potential of hypoglycemia and demonstrated prominent periventricular leukomalacia in their series of newborns dying of hypoglycemia.

Neuroimaging Abnormalities

The recognition of specific patterns of abnormality on CT and MRI scans of infants with diagnosed hypoglycemia has been a relatively recent finding in the literature. Spar et al.[98] described a newborn with well-documented hypoglycemia for at least 15 hours. The MRI scan, completed at 19 days of age, demonstrated a predominance of bilateral tissue loss in the parenchyma of the occipital lobes. Barkovich et al.[99] described his group of five patients with hypoglycemia in the newborn period and emphasized the findings of white matter damage in the parietal and occipital lobes. Globus pallidus injury was present in only one of the infants described. Kinnala et al.[100] published their findings of 18 full-term infants with blood glucose concentrations below 45 mg/dL (2.5 mmol/L). All were symptomatic. Only three of the infants described had hypoglycemia for longer than 24 hours; the longest duration was 33 hours. The mean blood glucose value was 25 mg/dL (1.4 mmol/L), with only two of the infants displaying glucose values below 5 mg/dL (0.3 mmol/L). Four of the infants showed hyperintensity lesions on T1-weighted images either in the occipital periventricular regions or the thalamus. Ninety-four percent of the infants were developmentally normal at follow-up. Murakami et al.[101] confirmed these latter results in his retrospective review of brain MRI in eight term infants, all of whom were symptomatic and had blood glucose concentrations below 20 mg/dL (1.1 mmol/L). Once again, abnormalities were consistently found in the parieto-occipital white matter in all but one of the children.

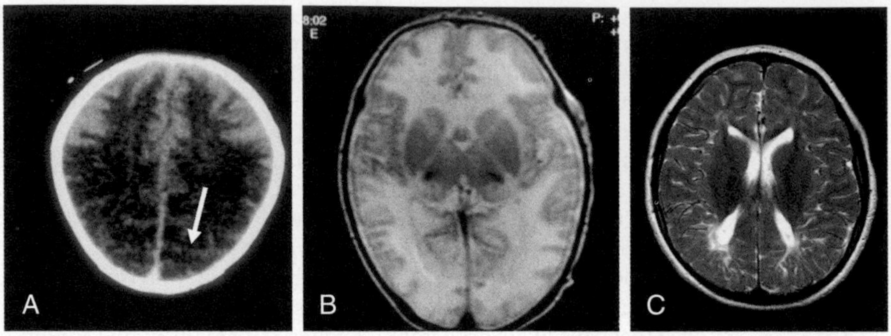

Fig. 9.2 Series of images from a term infant with normal Apgar scores and hypoglycemia at 20 hours of age. A, Computed tomographic scan on day 3 of life. Note the areas of attenuation bilaterally in the occipital regions. B, T2-weighted magnetic resonance imaging (MRI) scan on day 10 of life. Loss of cortex in the occipital region and hyperintense putamen is noted. C, T2-weighted MRI scan at 7 years of age shows chronic alterations with focal white matter and cortical injury in the occipital regions.

Within the past decade, a pattern of predominantly parieto-occipital white matter abnormalities, often in association with abnormal signal in the deep gray matter structures of the thalamus and/or basal ganglia, has been identified on follow-up of those neonates who had experienced symptomatic hypoglycemia. Although the number of studies and patients is few overall, the abnormalities appear to be relatively distinct for the syndrome of neonatal hypoglycemia. Alkalay et al.[102] reported a single case of term hypoglycemia and reviewed the literature of associated imaging findings. Blood glucose findings were always below 25 mg/dL (1.4 mmol/L); they were generally low for a prolonged period of time, and patients were symptomatic. When neuroimaging was done in this group, findings were abnormal, with more than 80% showing consistent abnormalities of the occipital lobes, similar to those displayed in Fig. 9.2.

A more recent study correlated brain MRI and neurodevelopmental outcome with symptomatic hypoglycemia. Burns et al.[103] examined 35 term infants with symptomatic hypoglycemia (mean glucose concentration <1.0 mmol/L) and without evidence of other complicating features, such as hypoxia-ischemia. White matter injury was present in 94% of the patients, although only 29% were noted to have a predominantly posterior localization. Cortical abnormalities were seen in 51% of patients; 40% of the abnormalities were deep gray matter thalamic and basal ganglia lesions. Of the total, 65% displayed neurodevelopmental abnormalities at 18 months of age, correlating in large part to the severity of the white matter lesions.

In this study, the majority of blood glucose values recorded (86%) were less than 1.5 mmol/L. Interestingly, however, two-thirds of the values were reported as being only transient in nature, resolving readily with treatment, while the other third were prolonged or recurrent.

Metabolically, these neuroimaging findings are consistent with studies by Mujsce et al.[77] that showed a reduction in CGU in the occipital white matter of newborn dogs during insulin-induced hypoglycemia. These findings occurred in contrast to the preservation of glucose utilization in other regions of the brain and an increase in brainstem structures. These data suggest an uncoupling of supply and demand requirements for glucose in this region of the newborn brain, and an outstripping of the available substrate supply for energy production, resulting in the enhanced sensitivity of the occipital regions.

Studies involving isolated hypoglycemia in the newborn remain relatively uncommon. Gataullina et al. studied 50 newborns and children with varying etiologies of metabolic hypoglycemia between 1 day and 5 years of age. Their cohort included predominantly patients with congenital hyperinsulinemia, fatty acid oxidation disorders, and glycogen storage disease. Interestingly, they found that rather than being associated with etiology, MRI findings showed topographic regionalization based on age. In this regard, patients who were between 1 day and 6 months of age showed lesions predominantly in the posterior white matter, as has been previously described. Patients between 6 and 22 months of age has lesions within the basal ganglia, and those older than 22 months showed parietotemporal cortex abnormalities. The authors suggested these changes may be dependent on maturational changes to the brain.[104]

Given the previous findings, several aspects of hypoglycemia and its effect on the newborn brain can be summarized:

1. The definition of hypoglycemia within statistical boundaries has been reasonably consistent as being abnormal if less than 2.5 mmol/L (<47 mg/dL) and severe if less than 1.1 mmol/L (<20 mg/dL).
2. The definition and risk of hypoglycemia are not static but depend on the gestational age of the infant at birth, weight of the infant, and timing of the evaluation of glucose as it relates to the age of the infant from birth, and whether or not feeding has been implemented.
3. A consistent association of hypoglycemia and neurologic injury has occurred only when the infant has, in addition to evidence of low blood concentrations of glucose, been symptomatic and generally continued to have hypoglycemia for a prolonged period.

Controversy and Question

While these parameters provide important information regarding the approach to hypoglycemia in the otherwise healthy infant, because glucose is a metabolically active substance in constant flux, confounding factors may influence whether or not hypoglycemia contributes to brain injury and at what level that might occur. Hence, disorders that the newborn faces alter the metabolic requirements of the brain, tipping the balance of supply and demand toward injury. Common examples in the newborn whereby the demand for glucose may outstrip its supply include hypoxia-ischemia and seizures, the latter being a complication of both hypoxia-ischemia and hypoglycemia itself. In these circumstances[105] we ask these questions:

1. Does hypoglycemia contribute to the brain damage caused by hypoxia-ischemia or seizures in the newborn infant?
2. Are additional risk factors associated with the onset of hypoglycemia or poor outcome?

Hypoglycemia and Hypoxia-Ischemia, Seizures

Hypoglycemia is deleterious when superimposed on hypoxia-ischemia. Vannucci and Vannucci[106] subjected newborn rat pups to anoxia in 100% nitrogen. The experimental group was rendered hypoglycemic to 0.75 mmol/L (14 mg/dL) by intraperitoneal insulin injection. Normoglycemic animals survived 10 times as long as those that were hypoglycemic. In newborn dogs made hypoglycemic in combination with asphyxia, brain ATP concentrations fell by 61% compared with those pups with hypoglycemia alone, in whom ATP was preserved.

In determining the combined effects of substrate utilization and hypoxia-ischemia in the neonate,[9] Yager et al.[107] subjected 7-day-old rat pups to hypoglycemia by either fasting them for 12 hours or by subcutaneous injection of insulin. Both control and experimental rat pups underwent hypoxia-ischemia by exposure to 8% oxygen combined with unilateral common carotid artery ligation. Although hypoglycemia was only mild in nature—5.4, 4.3, and 3.4 mmol/L (99, 79, and 62 mg/dL) for control, insulin, and fasted groups, respectively—brain damage was significantly greater in the insulin-treated animals than either of the other two groups. Fasted animals had the least damage, presumably owing to the enhanced ketogenesis and alternative substrate utilization displayed by this group.

Seizures are associated with an increase in energy demands, and hence a severalfold increase in glucose utilization. The increased demand produces a decrease in brain glucose stores, placing the brain in a vulnerable position. Hence it is not surprising that during hypoglycemia, supplies of glucose are further depleted and a deficit in energy reserves might be expected. Thus in the newborn puppy, significant depletion of cerebral high-energy phosphate stores, as measured by phosphorus 31 (^{31}P) NMR spectroscopy, occurred when seizures and hypoglycemia were combined, as compared with seizures alone.[108] In a model of neonatal hypoxia-ischemia and subsequent seizures,[109] Yager and his colleagues showed that those rat pups experiencing seizures and hypoxia-ischemia had significantly greater brain damage, particularly in the hippocampus, compared with those animals that were exposed only to hypoxia-ischemia. In a follow-up study, these investigators found that the former group of rat pups displayed a prolonged and irrecoverable period of brain energy depletion, accompanied also by diminished brain glucose concentrations during the postischemic seizures. The investigators concluded that this relative decrease in the concentration of brain glucose, compared with controls, during the postischemic seizures were responsible for the increase in brain damage seen in this model.[110] These data serve to highlight the importance of controlling seizures, particularly in the face of hypoglycemia.

In the human newborn, several studies have reviewed the effects of compounding hypoglycemia and perinatal asphyxia. Salhab et al.[111] retrospectively reviewed 185 term infants with perinatal asphyxia defined by a cord pH of less than 7.00. Fifteen percent[27] of the infants had an initial blood glucose concentration below 40 mg/dL (2.2 mmol/L). These authors found a significant contribution of hypoglycemia to abnormal outcome compared with those infants with blood glucose values above 40 mg/dL. The authors did not comment on the duration of hypoglycemia. Additional complicating features were also present.

Recent reviews on the subject of hypoglycemic brain injury in the newborn have consistently come to similar conclusions.[112] In one study, 4021 patients admitted to a neonatal intensive care unit between 1990 and 2006 were reviewed.[113] Sixty newborns were identified as meeting the study criteria for hypoglycemia, in whom there was an equal distribution of males and females. The patients were divided into two groups, one of which had abnormal developmental outcome (developmental delay, cerebral palsy, or epilepsy), and the other had normal outcome. Both groups had an equal incidence of small-for-gestational age births. The newborns who had abnormal outcomes were significantly more likely to have severe hypoglycemia of less than 15 mg/dL for a prolonged duration of 14 hours or longer compared with the infants with normal outcomes. In addition however, the newborns in the abnormal outcome group were also more likely to have additional perinatal risk factors, such as hypoxia and neonatal seizures, that were believed to contribute to the hypoglycemic brain injury syndrome.

In a study determining whether damage caused by hypoxic-ischemic encephalopathy (HIE) can be differentiated from that caused by hypoglycemia, in infants exposed to both, Wong et al. examined 179 term infants with MRI at 3 days of age.[113a] Blood glucose data were correlated with MRI and with clinical data of MRI. Hypoglycemia below 46 mg/dL was present in 34 of the cases. MRI findings had a positive predictive value of 82% and a negative predictive value of 78%. Selective posterior white matter injury and pulvinar edema were present and most predictive of clinical hypoglycemia.

An important study of the role of hypoglycemic and hyperglycemic newborns experiencing mild to moderate HIE who underwent cooling as treatment determined the effect of glucose alterations on outcome. A total of 234 infants were examined. Fifty-seven percent of the infants had an abnormal glucose value within 12 hours of birth. Unfavorable outcomes were significant and present in 81% of neonates with hypoglycemia and 67% of those with hyperglycemia compared with 48% of those who were normoglycemic. These findings remained after adjusting for adjusting for birth weight, Apgar score, pH, Sarnat stage, and hypothermia therapy. The findings clearly indicate a role for abnormal glucose metabolism in worsening HIE outcome.[114]

Case History

Not infrequently medicolegal questions arise surrounding the contribution of perinatal asphyxia to children who have developmental disability.[105] Hypoglycemia is often among the confounding factors.

A male infant was born at 42 weeks' gestation following a normal pregnancy. The delivery was forceps assisted. The infant's birth weight was 3.27 kg. Thick meconium was present, and the infant was suctioned for significant amounts. Apgar scores were 2 and 4 at 1 and 5 minutes, respectively. Approximately 3.5 hours after birth, the infant still displayed evidence of a neonatal encephalopathy and clinical seizures developed. The blood glucose value was determined to be 54 mg/dL (3.0 mmol/L). Seizures persisted intermittently that day. Blood glucose concentrations measured at 14 and 24 hours after delivery were 20 and 59 mg/dL (1.1 and 3.3 mmol/L), respectively. The EEG revealed multifocal areas of electrographic seizures. Computed tomography revealed bilateral occipital infarcts. This young man, now in his teens, has bilateral cortical blindness and mild developmental delay.

Clearly this infant illustrates a number of complexities. First, there is some evidence of perinatal asphyxia (interruption of placental blood flow), although a cord pH was not available, with respect to modestly depressed Apgar scores. Although he has cortical blindness, there is minimal developmental delay, suggesting the majority of injury was, in fact, in the occipital cortical regions. The question is to what extent, if any, did hypoglycemia contribute to the injury?

Although the patient was not severely hypoglycemic at birth, depressed glucose levels certainly persisted for at least 24 hours. The levels occurred concurrently with repetitive seizures, a circumstance of increased metabolic demand, on a background of a diffuse brain insult. Clinically this child did express a neonatal encephalopathy with both altered neurologic status and seizures. The outcome suggests that the injury, however, was relatively restricted to the occipital cortices. Hence, in the current scenario, hypoglycemia on the background of perinatal asphyxia not only contributed to the brain damage incurred but may have had the greatest effect, despite only one value that would have been categorized as severe hypoglycemia.

The findings are consistent with the available data suggesting that the otherwise normal neonatal brain is relatively tolerant of hypoglycemia. However, when superimposed on a brain that has been compromised by hypoxia-ischemia or seizures or both, hypoglycemia may exact damage, even when the levels of glucose are only borderline for hypoglycemia.[109]

Outcome

Given the complexities surrounding the definition and diagnosis of hypoglycemia in the newborn period, it is not surprising that there are difficulties in determining the neurologic morbidity surrounding this clinical entity. Several important papers regarding definition (see earlier text) and those looking at clinical prognosis allow us to make important observations regarding the thresholds to be assumed for the hypoglycemic neonate. Hence, Lucas et al.[48] detailed the neurologic outcome of a multicenter study of 661 preterm infants weighing less than 1850 g. Developmental outcome was determined at 18 months of age. The authors excluded variables independent of glucose concentrations and found that reduced mental and motor developmental scores were inversely related to the number of days that glucose concentrations were below 2.6 mmol/L (47 mg/dL), whereas with values above this concentration, no relationship was found. The relative risk of neurodevelopmental impairment in infants with hypoglycemia compared with those with no hypoglycemia was 3.5 times as great for those with blood glucose values below 2.6 mmol/L for more than 5 days.

A study by Stenninger et al.[115] reviewed the long-term neurologic morbidity in 13 children with neonatal hypoglycemia defined as blood glucose concentrations below 1.5 mmol/L (27 mg/dL) and compared them with 15 children without neonatal hypoglycemia. Neurodevelopmental assessments were done at approximately 7.75 years of age. These investigators found that children with neonatal hypoglycemia had significantly more difficulties in a screening test for minimal brain dysfunction and were more likely to be hyperactive, impulsive, and inattentive. These children also had lower developmental scores than did controls.

Brand et al.[116] evaluated 75 healthy term large-for-gestational age infants of nondiabetic mothers. The glucose value considered to be significant for hypoglycemia was less than 2.2 mmol/L (<40 mg/dL). Intravenous glucose treatment was started if the infant was symptomatic. They concluded that transient neonatal hypoglycemia was not harmful to psychomotor development when evaluated at 4 years of age. Alternatively, Kaiser et al. determined outcome in a group of newborns between 23 and 42 weeks' gestation with transient hypoglycemia. Of the 1943 normoglycemic and hypoglycemic infants found retrospectively, those with transient hypoglycemia values between less than 35 mg/dL and less than 45 mg/dL showed decreased proficiency in literacy and mathematics on fourth grade achievement tests compared with matched controls.[117]

A recent systematic review[118] of neurodevelopment following neonatal hypoglycemia in the first week of life evaluated 18 studies. Sixteen of the studies were felt to be of poor quality and 2 were of high quality, although they could not be pooled for data analysis. Unfortunately, the review concluded that "none of the studies provided a valid estimate of the effect of hypoglycemia on neurodevelopment"—a further indication that this topic requires significantly more research regarding the overall outcome of infants experiencing hypoglycemia at birth, in the various scenarios that may occur.[55]

Perhaps the most definitive of studies was published in 2015. Of 614 patients, 216 newborns had hypoglycemia, with blood glucose concentrations less than 47 mg/dL. Hypoglycemia, when treated to maintain a blood glucose concentration of at least 47 mg/dL, was not associated with an increased risk of the primary outcomes of neurosensory impairment or processing difficulty, defined as an executive function score more than 1.5 standard deviations from the mean.[119] Moreover, Tin et al. followed up on children with neonatal hypoglycemia who were first described in 1988. Fifteen years later they confirmed the earlier study. They examined infants born at less than 32 weeks' gestation between 1990 and 1991 with follow-up to 2 years of age. Of more than 500 infants, approximately 8% had blood glucose values of 2.5 mmol/L or lower measured within the first 10 days of life. No differences in physical or cognitive abilities were noted between this group and control children. Eighty-one percent of these children followed up 15 years later for psychometric testing also showed no difference from controls.[120]

Clearly, given the findings of studies illustrated in the preceding text and others, outcome following hypoglycemia, whether transient or of long duration, remains controversial. Nonetheless, this author would err on the side of caution, weighing the majority of evidence suggesting a negative effect of hypoglycemia, particularly of extended duration and glucose values less than 2.5 mmol/L (45 mg/dL) on outcome, and advocating for therapeutic intervention in newborns presenting with evidence of hypoglycemia meeting these levels, whether on a single measurement or multiple measurements.

Treatment

Despite the issues surrounding neonatal hypoglycemia, a review of the literature as outlined in this chapter clearly allows for the appropriate recognition of those infants at risk for significant hypoglycemia and the institution of a plan for monitoring and therapeutic intervention. Given the information available to us today, it appears that term infants born without complication and without symptomatology are highly unlikely to be at risk of neurodevelopmental abnormalities unless

1. Blood glucose concentrations are less than 1.1 mmol/L (<20 mg/dL)
2. The newborn is symptomatic and/or
3. Hypoglycemia is prolonged (hours)

In evaluating a newborn whose perinatal course has been complicated by small size for gestational age, perinatal asphyxia, seizures, sepsis, or other disorders that suggest an imbalance between substrate supply and demand for cerebral energy production, a broader definition of hypoglycemia should be used. Hence, under these circumstances infants with blood glucose concentrations below 45 mg/dL (<2.5 mmol/L), particularly on more than one occasion, should be aggressively treated and followed up. Newer techniques of continuous blood glucose monitoring of the newborn will provide a much greater and more accurate determination of glucose concentrations following birth and allow for early determination of those at risk.[121]

Clearly, there are infants who will require specific forms of therapy for their underlying metabolic and endocrinologic abnormalities. In the vast majority of infants, glucose alone will be the predominant therapeutic intervention. Although relatively large boluses of high concentration glucose have been advised in the past, it is probably best to avoid hyperglycemia and its attendant risks of rebound hypoglycemia. Lilien et al.[122] showed that a minibolus of 200 mg/kg (2 mL of 10% glucose over 1 minute) immediately followed by a continuous infusion of 8 mg/kg per minute results in the rapid correction of blood glucose concentrations and stable values of between 70 and 80 mg/dL (3.8–4.4 mmol/L). Continuous monitoring is, of course, required, and after glucose concentrations appear to have stabilized for 12 to 24 hours, the infusion can be decreased by 2 mg/kg per minute every 6 to 12 hours. In rare circumstances in which hypoglycemia does not respond to this regimen, to infusions of up to 12 mg/kg per minute, or recurs with tapering, hydrocortisone can be administered at a dose of 5 mg/kg every 12 hours.

Conclusions

Despite the fact that hypoglycemia remains a common disorder of the newborn, consensus has been difficult to reach regarding definition, diagnosis, outcome, and treatment. Several important points however, can be made, as follows:
1. The definition of hypoglycemia is not absolute and is highly dependent on the age, weight, timing of evaluation, whether the baby was fed, and on extenuating and complicating factors. Hence, it should be assessed on a per-patient basis.
2. Healthy term infants of appropriate weight, and who are fed early, are not at risk for hypoglycemic injury.
3. Significant hypoglycemia, with the potential to result in abnormal neurodevelopmental outcome, occurs in those newborns in whom (a) blood glucose concentrations are below 1.1 mmol/L (<20 mg/dL), (b) hypoglycemia is prolonged, and (c) neurologic symptoms are present.
4. A high level of sensitivity for hypoglycemia needs to be applied to all newborns who are compromised by small size for gestational age, perinatal asphyxia (interruption of placental blood flow), seizures, sepsis, or other pathologies that increase metabolic requirements. In these circumstances, a broader definition should be applied, and glucose concentrations should be maintained at levels of at least 40 mg/dL or higher.

With improved neuroradiologic techniques such as MRI and PET scanning becoming increasingly available, studies to determine the correlation between hypoglycemia and outcome will further help to clarify issues surrounding the effects of hypoglycemia on brain pathology and neurobehavioral outcome.

Long-term epidemiologic studies correlating the severity and duration of hypoglycemia with neurologic consequences are required and can be complemented by appropriate parallel investigations in animal models of neonatal hypoglycemia.

Currently, increasing attention to the rising incidence of gestational diabetes will ultimately help to provide the opportunity for prevention of neonatal hypoglycemia. Several guidelines are currently available for the close monitoring of maternal diabetes and the placement of appropriate protocols for blood glucose monitoring of the newborn following delivery.[123]

REFERENCES

1. Aynsley-Green A, Hawdon JM. Hypoglycemia in the neonate: current controversies. *Acta Paediatr Jpn, Overseas Ed.* 1997;39(suppl 1):S12–S16.
2. Kalhan S, Peter-Wohl S. Hypoglycemia: what is it for the neonate? *Am J Perinatol.* 2000;17(1):11–18.
3. Hawdon JM. Best practice guidelines: neonatal hypoglycaemia. *Early Hum Dev.* 2010;86(5):261.
4. Rozance PJ, Hay WW Jr. Describing hypoglycemia—definition or operational threshold? *Early Hum Dev.* 2010;86(5):275–280.
5. Hotu S, Carter B, Watson PD, Cutfield WS, Cundy T. Increasing prevalence of type 2 diabetes in adolescents. *J Pediatr Child Health.* 2004;40(4):201–204.
6. Jensen DM, Damm P, Moelsted-Pedersen L, et al. Outcomes in type 1 diabetic pregnancies: a nationwide, population-based study. *Diabetes Care.* 2004;27(12):2819–2823.
7. Nehlig A. Respective roles of glucose and ketone bodies as substrates for cerebral energy metabolism in the suckling rat. *Dev Neurosci.* 1996;18(5–6):426–433.
8. Nehlig A, Pereira de Vasconcelos A. Glucose and ketone body utilization by the brain of neonatal rats. *Prog Neurobiol.* 1993;40(2):163–221.
9. Vannucci RC, Yager JY. Glucose, lactic acid, and perinatal hypoxic-ischemic brain damage. *Pediatr Neurol.* 1992;8(1):3–12.
10. Burchell A, Gibb L, Waddell ID, Giles M, Hume R. The ontogeny of human hepatic microsomal glucose-6-phosphatase proteins. *Clin Chem.* 1990;36(9):1633–1637.
11. Bier DM, Leake RD, Haymond MW, et al. Measurement of "true" glucose production rates in infancy and childhood with 6,6-dideuteroglucose. *Diabetes.* 1977;26(11):1016–1023.
12. Hartmann A, Jaudon JC. Hypoglycemia. *J Pediatr.* 1937;(11):1–36.

13. Aynsley-Green A. Metabolic and endocrine interrelations in the human fetus and neonate. *Am J Clin Nutr*. 1985;41(suppl 2):399–417.
14. Aynsley-Green A, Soltesz G, Jenkins PA, Mackenzie IZ. The metabolic and endocrine milieu of the human fetus at 18–21 weeks of gestation. II. Blood glucose, lactate, pyruvate and ketone body concentrations. *Biol Neonate*. 1985;47(1):19–25.
15. Soltesz G, Harris D, Mackenzie IZ, Aynsley-Green A. The metabolic and endocrine milieu of the human fetus and mother at 18–21 weeks of gestation. I. Plasma amino acid concentrations. *Pediatric Res*. 1985;19(1):91–93.
16. Bozzetti P, Ferrari MM, Marconi AM, et al. The relationship of maternal and fetal glucose concentrations in the human from midgestation until term. *Metab Clin Exp*. 1988;37(4):358–363.
17. Heck LJ, Erenberg A. Serum glucose levels in term neonates during the first 48 hours of life. *J Pediatr*. 1987;110(1):119–122.
18. Hoseth E, Joergensen A, Ebbesen F, Moeller M. Blood glucose levels in a population of healthy, breast fed, term infants of appropriate size for gestational age. *Arch Dis Child Fetal Neonatal Ed*. 2000;83(2):F117–F119.
19. Tanzer F, Yazar N, Yazar H, Icagasioglu D. Blood glucose levels and hypoglycaemia in full term neonates during the first 48 hours of life. *J Trop Pediatr*. 1997;43(1):58–60.
20. Srinivasan G, Pildes RS, Cattamanchi G, Voora S, Lilien LD. Plasma glucose values in normal neonates: a new look. *J Pediatr*. 1986;109(1):114–117.
21. Diwakar KK, Sasidhar MV. Plasma glucose levels in term infants who are appropriate size for gestation and exclusively breast fed. *Arch Dis Child Fetal Neonatal Ed*. 2002;87(1):F46–F48.
22. Ward Platt M, Deshpande S. Metabolic adaptation at birth. *Semin Fetal Neonatal Med*. 2005;10(4):341–350.
23. Sexson WR. Incidence of neonatal hypoglycemia: a matter of definition. *J Pediatr*. 1984;105(1):149–150.
24. Hawdon JM, Ward Platt MP, Aynsley-Green A. Patterns of metabolic adaptation for preterm and term infants in the first neonatal week. *Arch Dis Child*. 1992;67(4 Spec No):357–365.
25. Jackson L, Burchell A, McGeechan A, Hume R. An inadequate glycaemic response to glucagon is linked to insulin resistance in preterm infants? *Arch Dis Child Fetal Neonatal Ed*. 2003;88(1):F62–F66.
26. Duvanel CB, Fawer CL, Cotting J, Hohlfeld P, Matthieu JM. Long-term effects of neonatal hypoglycemia on brain growth and psychomotor development in small-for-gestational-age preterm infants. *J Pediatr*. 1999;134(4):492–498.
27. Lubchenco LO, Bard H. Incidence of hypoglycemia in newborn infants classified by birth weight and gestational age. *Pediatrics*. 1971;47(5):831–838.
28. Hawdon JM, Weddell A, Aynsley-Green A, Ward Platt MP. Hormonal and metabolic response to hypoglycaemia in small for gestational age infants. *Arch Dis Child*. 1993;68(3 Spec No):269–273.
29. Bazaes RA, Salazar TE, Pittaluga E, et al. Glucose and lipid metabolism in small for gestational age infants at 48 hours of age. *Pediatrics*. 2003;111(4 Pt 1):804–809.
30. Duckrow RB, LaManna JS, Rosenthal M. Disparate recovery of resting and stimulated oxidative metabolism following transient ischemia. *Stroke; J Cerebral Cir*. 1981;12(5):677–686.
31. Chugani HT, Phelps ME, Mazziotta JC. Positron emission tomography study of human brain functional development. *Ann Neurol*. 1987;22(4):487–497.
32. Chugani HT, Phelps ME. Maturational changes in cerebral function in infants determined by 18FDG positron emission tomography. *Science*. 1986;231(4740):840–843.
33. Chugani HT, Hovda DA, Villablanca JR, Phelps ME, Xu WF. Metabolic maturation of the brain: a study of local cerebral glucose utilization in the developing cat. *J Cereb Blood Flow Metab*. 1991;11(1):35–47.
34. Chance B, Leigh JS Jr, Nioka S, Sinwell T, Younkin D, Smith DS. An approach to the problem of metabolic heterogeneity in brain: ischemia and reflow after ischemia. *Ann NY Acad Sci*. 1987;508:309–320.
35. Kinnala A, Nuutila P, Ruotsalainen U, et al. Cerebral metabolic rate for glucose after neonatal hypoglycaemia. *Early Hum Dev*. 1997;49(1):63–72.
36. Kinnala A, Suhonen-Polvi H, Aarimaa T, et al. Cerebral metabolic rate for glucose during the first six months of life: an FDG positron emission tomography study. *Arch Dis Child Fetal Neonatal Ed*. 1996;74(3):F153–F157.
37. Lust WD, Pundik S, Zechel J, Zhou Y, Buczek M, Selman WR. Changing metabolic and energy profiles in fetal, neonatal, and adult rat brain. *Metab Brain Dis*. 2003;18(3):195–206.
38. Cremer JE. Substrate utilization and brain development. *J Cereb Blood Flow Metab*. 1982;2(4):394–407.
39. DeVivo DC, Leckie MP, Agrawal HC. The differential incorporation of beta-hydroxybutyrate and glucose into brain glutamate in the newborn rat. *Brain Res*. 1973;55(2):485–490.
40. Booth RF, Patel TB, Clark JB. The development of enzymes of energy metabolism in the brain of a precocial (guinea pig) and non-precocial (rat) species. *J Neurochem*. 1980;34(1):17–25.
41. Anday EK, Stanley CA, Baker L, Delivoria-Papadopoulos M. Plasma ketones in newborn infants: absence of suckling ketosis. *J Pediatr*. 1981;98(4):628–630.
42. Stanley CA, Anday EK, Baker L, Delivoria-Papadopolous M. Metabolic fuel and hormone responses to fasting in newborn infants. *Pediatrics*. 1979;64(5):613–619.
43. Hernandez MJ, Vannucci RC, Salcedo A, Brennan RW. Cerebral blood flow and metabolism during hypoglycemia in newborn dogs. *J Neurochem*. 1980;35(3):622–628.

44. Vannucci RC, Nardis EE, Vannucci SJ, Campbell PA. Cerebral carbohydrate and energy metabolism during hypoglycemia in newborn dogs. *Am J Physiol*. 1981;240(3):R192–R199.
44a. Harris DL, Weston PJ, Harding JE. Lactate, rather than ketones, may provide alternative cerebral fuel in hypoglycemic newborns. *Arch Dis Child Fetal Neonatal Ed*. 2015;100:F161–F164.
45. Young RS, Petroff OA, Chen B, Aquila WJ Jr, Gore JC. Preferential utilization of lactate in neonatal dog brain: in vivo and in vitro proton NMR study. *Biol Neonate*. 1991;59(1):46–53.
46. Vicario C, Medina JM. Metabolism of lactate in the rat brain during the early neonatal period. *J Neurochem*. 1992;59(1):32–40.
47. Miller AL, Kiney CA, Staton DM. Effects of lactate on glucose metabolism of developing rat brain. *Brain Res*. 1984;316(1):33–40.
48. Maran A, Cranston I, Lomas J, Macdonald I, Amiel SA. Protection by lactate of cerebral function during hypoglycaemia. *Lancet*. 1994;343(8888):16–20.
49. Dombrowski GJ Jr, Swiatek KR, Chao KL. Lactate, 3-hydroxybutyrate, and glucose as substrates for the early postnatal rat brain. *Neurochem Res*. 1989;14(7):667–675.
50. Simpson IA, Carruthers A, Vannucci SJ. Supply and demand in cerebral energy metabolism: the role of nutrient transporters. *J Cereb Blood Flow Metab*. 2007;27(11):1766–1791.
51. Powers WJ, Rosenbaum JL, Dence CS, Markham J, Videen TO. Cerebral glucose transport and metabolism in preterm human infants. *J Cereb Blood Flow Metab*. 1998;18(6):632–638.
52. Vannucci SJ, Maher F, Simpson IA. Glucose transporter proteins in brain: delivery of glucose to neurons and glia. *Glia*. 1997;21(1):2–21.
53. Vannucci SJ. Developmental expression of GLUT1 and GLUT3 glucose transporters in rat brain. *J Neurochem*. 1994;62(1):240–246.
54. Nicholl R. What is the normal range of blood glucose concentrations in healthy term newborns? *Arch Dis Child*. 2003;88(3):238–239.
55. Hay WW Jr, Raju TN, Higgins RD, Kalhan SC, Devaskar SU. Knowledge gaps and research needs for understanding and treating neonatal hypoglycemia: workshop report from Eunice Kennedy Shriver National Institute of Child Health and Human Development. *J Pediatr*. 2009;155(5):612–617.
56. Committee on Fetus and Newborn, Adamkin DH. Postnatal glucose homeostasis in late-preterm and term infants. *Pediatrics*. 2011;127(3):575–579.
57. Adamkin DH. Neonatal hypoglycemia. *Semin Fetal Neonatal Med*. 2017;22(1):36–41.
58. Koh TH, Eyre JA, Aynsley-Green A. Neonatal hypoglycaemia—the controversy regarding definition. *Arch Dis Child*. 1988;63(11):1386–1388.
59. Alkalay AL, Sarnat HB, Flores-Sarnat L, Elashoff JD, Farber SJ, Simmons CF. Population meta-analysis of low plasma glucose thresholds in full-term normal newborns. *Am J Perinatol*. 2006;23(2):115–119.
60. Volpe JJ. *Neurology of the Newborn*. 4th ed. Philadelphia: WB Saunders; 2001.
61. Koivisto M, Blanco-Sequeiros M, Krause U. Neonatal symptomatic and asymptomatic hypoglycaemia: a follow-up study of 151 children. *Dev Med Child Neurol*. 1972;14(5):603–614.
62. Singh M, Singhal PK, Paul VK, et al. Neurodevelopmental outcome of asymptomatic & symptomatic babies with neonatal hypoglycaemia. *Indian J Med Res*. 1991;94:6–10.
63. Moore AM, Perlman M. Symptomatic hypoglycemia in otherwise healthy, breastfed term newborns. *Pediatrics*. 1999;103(4 Pt 1):837–839.
64. Alkalay AL, Flores-Sarnat L, Sarnat HB, Farber SJ, Simmons CF. Plasma glucose concentrations in profound neonatal hypoglycemia. *Clin Pediatr*. 2006;45(6):550–558.
65. Koh TH, Aynsley-Green A, Tarbit M, Eyre JA. Neural dysfunction during hypoglycaemia. *Arch Dis Child*. 1988;63(11):1353–1358.
66. Oliveira AJ, Nunes ML, Haertel LM, Reis FM, da Costa JC. Duration of rhythmic EEG patterns in neonates: new evidence for clinical and prognostic significance of brief rhythmic discharges. *Clin Neurophysiol*. 2000;111(9):1646–1653.
67. Cowett RM, Howard GM, Johnson J, Vohr B. Brain stem auditory-evoked response in relation to neonatal glucose metabolism. *Biol Neonate*. 1997;71(1):31–36.
68. Pryds O, Greisen G, Friis-Hansen B. Compensatory increase of CBF in preterm infants during hypoglycaemia. *Acta Paediatr Scand*. 1988;77(5):632–637.
69. Caksen H, Guven AS, Yilmaz C, et al. Clinical outcome and magnetic resonance imaging findings in infants with hypoglycemia. *J Child Neurol*. 2011;26(1):25–30.
70. Lucas A, Morley R, Cole TJ. Adverse neurodevelopmental outcome of moderate neonatal hypoglycaemia. *BMJ*. 1988;297(6659):1304–1308.
71. Schrier A, Wilhelm PB, Church RM, et al. Neonatal hypoglycemia in the rhesus monkey: effect on development and behavior. *Infant Behav Dev*. 1990;13(2):189–207.
72. Moore H, Craft TK, Grimaldi LM, Babic B, Brunelli SA, Vannucci SJ. Moderate recurrent hypoglycemia during early development leads to persistent changes in affective behavior in the rat. *Brain Behav Immun*. 2010;24(5):839–849.
73. Cornblath M, Hawdon JM, Williams AF, et al. Controversies regarding definition of neonatal hypoglycemia: suggested operational thresholds. *Pediatrics*. 2000;105(5):1141–1145.
74. Thornton PS, Stanley CA, De Leon DD, et al. Recommendations from the Pediatric Endocrine Society for Evaluation and Management of Persistent Hypoglycemia in Neonates, Infants, and Children. *J Pediatr*. 2015;167(2):238–245.
75. Rasmussen AH, Wehberg S, Fenger-Groen J, Christesen HT. Retrospective evaluation of a national guideline to prevent neonatal hypoglycemia. *Pediatr Neonatol*. 2017;58(5):398–405.
76. Anwar M, Vannucci RC. Autoradiographic determination of regional cerebral blood flow during hypoglycemia in newborn dogs. *Pediatric Res*. 1988;24(1):41–45.

77. Mujsce DJ, Christensen MA, Vannucci RC. Regional cerebral blood flow and glucose utilization during hypoglycemia in newborn dogs. *Am J Physiol*. 1989;256(6 Pt 2):H1659–H1666.

78. Butcher SP, Sandberg M, Hagberg H, Hamberger A. Cellular origins of endogenous amino acids released into the extracellular fluid of the rat striatum during severe insulin-induced hypoglycemia. *J Neurochem*. 1987;48(3):722–728.

79. Sandberg M, Butcher SP, Hagberg H. Extracellular overflow of neuroactive amino acids during severe insulin-induced hypoglycemia: in vivo dialysis of the rat hippocampus. *J Neurochem*. 1986;47(1):178–184.

80. Uematsu D, Greenberg JH, Reivich M, Karp A. Cytosolic free calcium and NAD/NADH redox state in the cat cortex during in vivo activation of NMDA receptors. *Brain Res*. 1989;482(1):129–135.

81. Silverstein FS, Simpson J, Gordon KE. Hypoglycemia alters striatal amino acid efflux in perinatal rats: an in vivo microdialysis study. *Ann Neurol*. 1990;28(4):516–521.

82. Aral YZ, Gucuyener K, Atalay Y, et al. Role of excitatory aminoacids in neonatal hypoglycemia. *Acta Paediatr Jpn*. 1998;40(4):303–306.

83. Anju TR, Akhilraj PR, Paulose CS. Oxidative stress and cell death in the cerebral cortex as a long-term consequence of neonatal hypoglycemia. *Can J Physiol Pharmacol*. 2016;94(9):1015–1022.

84. Alves PM, Fonseca LL, Peixoto CC, Almeida AC, Carrondo MJ, Santos H. NMR studies on energy metabolism of immobilized primary neurons and astrocytes during hypoxia, ischemia and hypoglycemia. *NMR Biomed*. 2000;13(8):438–448.

85. Hertz L, Yager JY, Juurlink BH. Astrocyte survival in the absence of exogenous substrate: comparison of immature and mature cells. *Int J Dev Neurosci*. 1995;13(6):523–527.

86. Brierly JB, Brown AW, Meldrum BS. *The Neuropathology of Insulin Induced Hypoglycemia in Primate*. In: Brierly JB, Meldrum BS, eds. Philadelphia: JB Lippincott; 1971.

87. Myers RE, Kahn KJ. Insulin induced hypoglycemia in the non-human primate. *II: Long Term Neuropathological Consequences*. In: Brierly JB, Meldrum BS, eds. Philadelphia: JB Lippincott; 1971:195–206.

88. Auer R, Kalimo H, Olsson Y, Wieloch T. The dentate gyrus in hypoglycemia: pathology implicating excitotoxin-mediated neuronal necrosis. *Acta Neuropathol (Berl)*. 1985;67(3–4):279–288.

89. Auer RN, Kalimo H, Olsson Y, Siesjo BK. The temporal evolution of hypoglycemic brain damage. I. Light- and electron-microscopic findings in the rat cerebral cortex. *Acta Neuropathol (Berl)*. 1985;67(1–2):13–24.

90. Auer RN, Kalimo H, Olsson Y, Siesjo BK. The temporal evolution of hypoglycemic brain damage. II. Light- and electron-microscopic findings in the hippocampal gyrus and subiculum of the rat. *Acta Neuropathol (Berl)*. 1985;67(1–2):25–36.

91. Auer RN, Siesjo BK. Biological differences between ischemia, hypoglycemia, and epilepsy. *Ann Neurol*. 1988;24(6):699–707.

92. Auer RN, Siesjo BK. Hypoglycaemia: brain neurochemistry and neuropathology. *Baillieres Clin Endocrinol Metab*. 1993;7(3):611–625.

93. Auer RN, Wieloch T, Olsson Y, Siesjo BK. The distribution of hypoglycemic brain damage. *Acta Neuropathol (Berl)*. 1984;64(3):177–191.

94. Auer RN, Olsson Y, Siesjo BK. Hypoglycemic brain injury in the rat. Correlation of density of brain damage with the EEG isoelectric time: a quantitative study. *Diabetes*. 1984;33(11):1090–1098.

95. Kalimo H, Auer RN, Siesjo BK. The temporal evolution of hypoglycemic brain damage. III. Light and electron microscopic findings in the rat caudoputamen. *Acta Neuropathol (Berl)*. 1985;67(1–2):37–50.

96. Anderson JM, Milner RD, Strich SJ. Effects of neonatal hypoglycaemia on the nervous system: a pathological study. *J Neurol Neurosurg Psychiatry*. 1967;30(4):295–310.

97. Larroche JC. *Developmental Pathology of the Neonate*. In: Larroche JC, ed. New York: Excerpta Medica; 1977.

98. Spar JA, Lewine JD, Orrison WW Jr. Neonatal hypoglycemia: CT and MR findings. *AJNR Am J Neuroradiol*. 1994;15(8):1477–1478.

99. Barkovich AJ, Ali FA, Rowley HA, Bass N. Imaging patterns of neonatal hypoglycemia. *AJNR Am J Neuroradiol*. 1998;19(3):523–528.

100. Kinnala A, Rikalainen H, Lapinleimu H, Parkkola R, Kormano M, Kero P. Cerebral magnetic resonance imaging and ultrasonography findings after neonatal hypoglycemia. *Pediatrics*. 1999;103(4 Pt 1):724–729.

101. Murakami Y, Yamashita Y, Matsuishi T, Utsunomiya H, Okudera T, Hashimoto T. Cranial MRI of neurologically impaired children suffering from neonatal hypoglycaemia. *Pediatr Radiol*. 1999;29(1):23–27.

102. Alkalay AL, Flores-Sarnat L, Sarnat HB, Moser FG, Simmons CF. Brain imaging findings in neonatal hypoglycemia: case report and review of 23 cases. *Clin Pediatr*. 2005;44(9):783–790.

103. Burns CM, Rutherford MA, Boardman JP, Cowan FM. Patterns of cerebral injury and neurodevelopmental outcomes after symptomatic neonatal hypoglycemia. *Pediatrics*. 2008;122(1):65–74.

104. Gataullina S, De Lonlay P, Dellatolas G, et al. Topography of brain damage in metabolic hypoglycaemia is determined by age at which hypoglycaemia occurred. *Dev Med Child Neurol*. 2013;55(2):162–166.

105. Williams AF. Neonatal hypoglycaemia: clinical and legal aspects. *Semin Fetal Neonatal Med*. 2005;10(4):363–368.

106. Vannucci RC, Vannucci SJ. Cerebral carbohydrate metabolism during hypoglycemia and anoxia in newborn rats. *Ann Neurol*. 1978;4(1):73–79.

107. Yager JY, Heitjan DF, Towfighi J, Vannucci RC. Effect of insulin-induced and fasting hypoglycemia on perinatal hypoxic-ischemic brain damage. *Pediatr Res*. 1992;31(2):138–142.

108. Young RS, Cowan BE, Petroff OA, Novotny E, Dunham SL, Briggs RW. In vivo ^{31}P and in vitro ^{1}H nuclear magnetic resonance study of hypoglycemia during neonatal seizure. *Ann Neurol.* 1987;22(5):622–628.
109. Wirrell EC, Armstrong EA, Osman LD, Yager JY. Prolonged seizures exacerbate perinatal hypoxic-ischemic brain damage. *Pediatr Res.* 2001;50(4):445–454.
110. Yager JY, Armstrong EA, Miyashita H, Wirrell EC. Prolonged neonatal seizures exacerbate hypoxic-ischemic brain damage: correlation with cerebral energy metabolism and excitatory amino acid release. *Dev Neurosci.* 2002;24(5):367–381.
111. Salhab WA, Wyckoff MH, Laptook AR, Perlman JM. Initial hypoglycemia and neonatal brain injury in term infants with severe fetal acidemia. *Pediatrics.* 2004;114(2):361–366.
112. Rozance PJ, Hay WW. Hypoglycemia in newborn infants: features associated with adverse outcomes. *Biol Neonate.* 2006;90(2):74–86.
113. Montassir H, Maegaki Y, Ogura K, et al. Associated factors in neonatal hypoglycemic brain injury. *Brain Dev.* 2009;31(9):649–656.
113a. Wong DST, Poskitt KJ, Chau V, et al. Brain injury patterns in hypoglycemia in neonatal encephalopathy. *AJNR.* July 2013;1456–1461.
114. Basu SK, Kaiser JR, Guffey D, et al. Hypoglycaemia and hyperglycaemia are associated with unfavourable outcome in infants with hypoxic ischaemic encephalopathy: a post hoc analysis of the CoolCap Study. *Arch Dis Child Fetal Neonatal Ed.* 2016;101(2):F149–F155.
115. Stenninger E, Flink R, Eriksson B, Sahlen C. Long-term neurological dysfunction and neonatal hypoglycaemia after diabetic pregnancy. *Arch Dis Child Fetal Neonatal Ed.* 1998;79(3):F174–F179.
116. Brand PL, Molenaar NL, Kaaijk C, Wierenga WS. Neurodevelopmental outcome of hypoglycaemia in healthy, large for gestational age, term newborns. *Arch Dis Child.* 2005;90(1):78–81.
117. Kaiser JR, Bai S, Gibson N, et al. Association between transient newborn hypoglycemia and fourth-grade achievement test proficiency: a population-based study. *JAMA Pediatr.* 2015;169(10):913–921.
118. Boluyt N, van Kempen A, Offringa M. Neurodevelopment after neonatal hypoglycemia: a systematic review and design of an optimal future study. *Pediatrics.* 2006;117(6):2231–2243.
119. McKinlay CJ, Alsweiler JM, Ansell JM, et al. Neonatal glycemia and neurodevelopmental outcomes at 2 years. *N Engl J Med.* 2015;373(16):1507–1518.
120. Tin W, Brunskill G, Kelly T, Fritz S. 15-year follow-up of recurrent "hypoglycemia" in preterm infants. *Pediatrics.* 2012;130(6):e1497–e1503.
121. Beardsall K. Measurement of glucose levels in the newborn. *Early Hum Dev.* 2010;86(5):263–267.
122. Lilien LD, Pildes RS, Srinivasan G, Voora S, Yeh TF. Treatment of neonatal hypoglycemia with minibolus and intraveous glucose infusion. *J Pediatr.* 1980;97(2):295–298.
123. Williams A, Modder J. Management of pregnancy complicated by diabetes—maternal glycaemic control during pregnancy and neonatal management. *Early Hum Dev.* 2010;86(5):269–273.

9

CHAPTER 10

Hyperbilirubinemia and the Risk for Brain Injury

Jean-Baptiste Le Pichon, Sean M. Riordan, and Steven M. Shapiro

- Following AAP guidelines prevents most cases of kernicterus.
- Extreme hyperbilirubinemia requires emergent treatment with double volume exchange transfusion.
- Early auditory assessment is important because both ANSD and SNHL respond better to early treatments including cochlear implantation.
- Acute MRI findings are T1 hyperintensity of bilateral globus pallidus (GP), which then resolves to be later replaced by T2 hyperintensity.
- A novel term Kernicterus Spectrum Disorders (KSDs) is used to clinically define and categorize kernicterus subtypes and severity.

CASE HISTORY

BB is a white male infant, born at term gestation weighing 2980 g to a 25-year-old G1P0 mother, blood type B^+, via spontaneous vaginal delivery. Apgar scores were 8 and 9 at 1 and 5 minutes, respectively. The infant was blood type A^+, had a large cephalohematoma, and appeared jaundiced at 24 hours of life. He passed an automated auditory brainstem response (ABR) screening and was discharged at 58 hours with a transcutaneous bilirubin level of 13.2 mg/dL and a total serum bilirubin level of 14 mg/dL. One day later at follow-up, the pediatrician said he looked fine. He returned at 6 days of age with a history of lethargy but had regained his birth weight. The pediatrician estimated visually that the bilirubin level was about 5 mg/dL. On day 7 the infant was more lethargic and had feeding difficulty. On day 8 he was noted to have a high-pitched cry, downward deviation of the eyes, and episodic and then continual extension of arms, legs, neck, and trunk. He was evaluated in an emergency room. Cerebral spinal fluid (CSF) analysis was normal except for yellow color of the fluid. Total bilirubin level at 211 hours (8.8 days) of age was 45.6 mg/dL. He was placed under phototherapy lights with a blanket underneath, was intubated because of low oxygen (O_2) saturation, and received a double-volume exchange transfusion at 214 hours of age. Preexchange and postexchange total bilirubin values were 35.8 and 20.9 mg/dL, respectively. BB was intubated and sedated. Five days later, emerging from sedation, he was hypotonic with a setting sun sign and with episodic O_2 desaturation. He was treated with phenobarbital for presumed seizures. However, an electroencephalogram (EEG) was reported as normal except for some sharp waves over the left temporal region. He was discharged after a 10-day hospitalization. He has subsequently demonstrated feeding issues, incoordination of suck and swallow, hypertonia and dystonia, and delayed motor development. ABRs at 2.5 weeks and 2 months of age were absent, a finding consistent with auditory neuropathy/dyssynchrony, despite normal distortion product otoacoustic emissions (OAEs). Magnetic resonance imaging (MRI) done at 11 days of age showed increased signal intensity in the globus pallidus bilaterally on both T1- and T2-weighted images and

CASE HISTORY—cont'd

a resolving cephalohematoma. Because of reflux and failure to thrive, a gastrostomy tube was placed with Nissen fundoplication. Treatment with diazepam was instituted to treat increased tone. Phenobarbital dosage was tapered and then discontinued. Intermittent clonic activity was noted, but video EEGs repeatedly failed to demonstrate an electrographic correlate. At 1.5 years of age, BB had not developed speech or language, had not responded to sound amplification, and could not sit or crawl.

This case highlights the risk of visual assessment of jaundice. The serum bilirubin level at discharge, 14 mg/dL, was at the 95th percentile of the hour-specific nomogram developed by Bhutani and colleagues.[1] The bilirubin at the 95th percentile, the significant cephalohematoma, and an ABO blood group abnormality were predictive of a high subsequent bilirubin level. The infant had symptoms of acute bilirubin encephalopathy (ABE) that were not recognized until it was too late to prevent extreme hyperbilirubinemia, and as a result the child developed all the clinical signs, symptoms, and laboratory findings of kernicterus.

Definition and Epidemiology

The classic clinical syndrome caused by brain injury as the result of hyperbilirubinemia is called *kernicterus*. Kernicterus was originally a pathologic term referring to the yellow staining (*icterus*) of the deep nuclei of the brain (*kern,* relating to the basal ganglia). The term *chronic bilirubin encephalopathy* has been used interchangeably with kernicterus. *Acute bilirubin encephalopathy* (ABE) refers to the acute injury associated with bilirubin neurotoxicity in the neonatal period. Historically the terms *acute bilirubin encephalopathy* and *chronic bilirubin encephalopathy* or *kernicterus* have been used to describe the clinical symptoms associated with the neuropathology. With the growth of modern medicine clinical studies such as magnetic resonance imaging (MRI) and auditory brainstem responses (ABRs), also known as brainstem auditory evoked potentials (BAEPs) or responses (BAERs), have shown objective evidence of bilirubin encephalopathy as evidenced by characteristic neuropathologic lesions (MRI) and abnormal neurologic function (ABRs).

Classic kernicterus is a well-described clinical syndrome that involves (1) a dystonic or athetoid movement disorder, (2) an auditory processing disturbance now called auditory neuropathy spectrum disorder (ANSD) with or without hearing loss, (3) oculomotor impairment, especially impairment of upward gaze, (4) dysplasia of the enamel of deciduous (baby) teeth, and, perhaps less well-known, (5) hypotonia and ataxia owing to cerebellar involvement. It is important to emphasize that more subtle forms of brain injury caused by an excess of hyperbilirubinemia have also been described. These have been referred to by different terms, including subtle kernicterus, chronic bilirubin encephalopathy of the subtle type, and bilirubin-induced neurologic dysfunction (BIND). We now advocate use of the term *kernicterus spectrum disorders* (KSDs) to encompass the entire spectrum of bilirubin-induced neurologic disorders, ranging from subtle neurodevelopmental disorders in children with less than all of the clinical features of classic kernicterus, up to and including the most severe forms of classic kernicterus.[2]

Classic kernicterus is a rare disorder. However, the severity of the lifelong disability, especially deafness, abnormal tone, and the loss of motor control, can be profound. Studies in Canada find an incidence of 1 case per 44,000,[3] whereas in Denmark the incidence of kernicterus is estimated to be 1 case per 110,000 live births.[4–7] The incidence of extreme hyperbilirubinemia, defined as at or above the criteria for performing exchange transfusion (median 28.8 mg/dL, range 22.5–40.3 mg/dL), was 25 cases per 100,000.[5,8] A population-based survey in northern California found that 150 per 100,000 infants had total serum bilirubin (TSB) levels of 25 mg/dL or higher and 10 per 100,000 had levels of 30 mg/dL or higher.[9,10] In the United States, based on the Canadian estimate of 1 per 44,000 live births, at least 90 cases of severe kernicterus per year are predicted. The incidence in underdeveloped low- and

10

middle-income countries is much higher. A study in Nigeria revealed an incidence of 2.7%, equivalent to 1 in 37 live births.[11] A review by Bhutani and Johnson[12] estimated the risk of kernicterus in infants with TSB levels above 25 mg/dL to be about 1 in 17.6 cases in Canada and 1 in 16.2 cases in Denmark, and for TSB levels above 30 mg/dL, the risk of kernicterus was estimated to be as high as 1 in 7 cases.

The incidence of extreme hyperbilirubinemia and kernicterus depends on the care infants receive in the first few weeks of life, the vigilance of screening, and the ability to treat excessive hyperbilirubinemia should it occur. Incidence and prevalence studies are complicated by the lack of specific objective definitions of kernicterus or KSDs and the inconsistency of reporting kernicterus or hyperbilirubinemia in most countries. Further, the incidence and prevalence of subtle neurodevelopmental disorders, such as auditory processing disorders and visual motor disabilities resulting from hyperbilirubinemia, remain unknown, largely owing to a lack of recognition of the syndrome.

Precisely how to determine the risk of brain injury in a hyperbilirubinemic newborn is important not only for choosing the level of care but also for optimally allocating health care resources. The precise determination of risk of brain injury will allow not only better guidelines for treatment to prevent brain damage but also the reduction or elimination of unnecessary treatments. This chapter discusses new concepts of pathogenesis, approaches or strategies for diagnosis and treatment, gaps in knowledge, and recommendations for treatment.

History of KSD Prevalence

Through the decades from the 1950s to the 1980s, clinical practice evolved to essentially eliminate classic kernicterus; however, a reemergence of kernicterus occurred in the 1990s and continues to the present and is associated with changes in medical practice and health care delivery. Clearly, universal screening of infants combined with close follow-up, monitoring, and aggressive phototherapy treatment at relatively low bilirubin levels could eliminate most of the new cases of kernicterus, but the prevention of a devastating but very rare disorder must be balanced against the costs and possible risks of overtreating very large numbers of infants. Currently a postdischarge bilirubin level is now standard practice within 2 days of discharge or earlier, depending on the predischarge level to identify patients with spikes in bilirubin after discharge. Determining the bilirubin level at which toxicity is increased is a difficult issue for physicians in everyday practice. They must balance the gains of an early visit versus the concerns that increased surveillance will result in a greater use of resources (phototherapy), more parental anxiety, and reduced breastfeeding.

Pathogenesis of Bilirubin Neurotoxicity

Bilirubin neurotoxicity is highly selective, targeting specific neurons in the central nervous system (CNS). The clinical expression and neuropathology of kernicterus are likewise highly selective. The movement disorders, dystonia and athetosis, are likely the result of lesions in the basal ganglia (globus pallidus and subthalamic nucleus) and cerebellum. Lesions to brainstem nuclei result in auditory, vestibular, and oculomotor function impairment and poor truncal tone. Any explanation of pathogenesis must account for the selective neurotoxicity of bilirubin.[13]

Total bilirubin in the blood, called total plasma or TSB, is composed of unconjugated bilirubin (UCB) plus conjugated bilirubin, also known as indirect and direct bilirubin, respectively. Neurotoxic UCB is largely bound to blood proteins, especially albumin, and except in unusual circumstances (e.g., disruption of the blood-brain barrier [BBB]) albumin-bound UCB does not move out of blood into brain. However, unbound or "free" bilirubin (Bf) is capable of crossing the BBB and moving into the central nervous system (CNS). Bf formation is favored when bilirubin binding sites become saturated and with low pH.

It is useful to compartmentalize the concept of bilirubin neurotoxicity into (1) processes that cause the cells to be exposed to excess bilirubin (production and elimination), (2) those that interfere with the cell's ability to handle the excess bilirubin, and (3) the molecular mechanisms responsible for the cell's response to the stress caused by bilirubin neurotoxicity.

Overall bilirubin exposure is a combination of bilirubin production, binding, and excretion. Bilirubin is actively excreted from the cells in the CNS. The ability of cells to handle excess bilirubin may vary. Risk factors can affect one or more of the compartments defined previously. For example, acidosis decreases binding and increases unbound Bf, thus exposing the cell to more bilirubin. However, pH might also affect cellular enzymes, energy production, and transport. Other risk factors, such as prematurity, inflammation, and isoimmunization, may act in one or more specific compartments.

In the following discussion, we examine individually the contributions from each of the compartments defined earlier, starting with production and elimination and concluding with cellular and molecular mechanisms underlying bilirubin neurotoxicity. An essential concept for clinicians caring for children with hyperbilirubinemia is the importance of thinking in terms of Bf exposure rather than total bilirubin. The BBB excludes large molecules, including albumin and albumin-bound bilirubin from the CNS, and transports substances into and out of the CNS.[14] The endothelial cells of the BBB restrict diffusion of many toxic compounds to adjacent neurons and astrocytes but do not restrict the free diffusion of free (Bf), unbound, unconjugated bilirubin (UCB), which is permeable with single-pass uptake estimated to be as high as 28% in rats.[15] Therefore it is the free fraction of bilirubin that matters as it relates to bilirubin neurotoxicity.

Comprehensive reviews have been published about the molecular mechanism of bilirubin neurotoxicity.[14,16,17] Recent findings have shed new light on the molecular basis of jaundice,[18] possible molecular mechanisms underlying the neurologic selectivity of bilirubin neurotoxicity,[19,20] the role of unconjugated bilirubin in health and disease,[21] and the possibility of genetic factors leading to susceptibility or resistance to bilirubin neurotoxicity.[22]

Active Transport of Bilirubin

Specific transporters for bilirubin, such as multidrug resistance protein 1 (MRP1),[14] a member of the multidrug resistance–associated protein subfamily of adenosine triphosphate (ATP)-binding cassette transporters, may protect the CNS from exposure to excessive levels of bilirubin. Accumulating evidence indicates that bilirubin is removed from cells via MRP1.[14,16,23,24] MRP1 transports bilirubin with an affinity that is 10 times greater than that of other substrates[24] and may represent a mechanism by which bilirubin is transported out of the CNS and excreted into the circulation. It is hypothesized that when this transport system is overwhelmed, toxic levels of bilirubin can accumulate in the cell.

Mechanisms of Bilirubin Damage

It appears that bilirubin damages cells by both apoptotic and necrotic mechanisms and affects mitochondrial energy metabolism. Studies in cultured cells[14,25–27] are starting to clarify the roles of apoptosis, mitochondria, and other molecular mechanisms contributing to bilirubin neurotoxicity. Purified bilirubin can induce apoptosis in cultured rat brain neurons[26,27] by triggering the release of cytochrome c from mitochondria with caspase-3 activation and cleavage of poly(adenosine diphosphate [ADP]-ribose) polymerase, confirming the role of one of the pathways that underlies induction of apoptosis.[28] Studies have shown that bilirubin facilitates transmitter release in cochlear nucleus neurons via presynaptic protein kinase A activation, which might provide insight into the cellular mechanism underlying bilirubin-induced hearing dysfunction.[29] Apoptotic changes are also reported in the cerebellum[28,30] and brainstem of jaundiced Gunn rats (an animal model of hyperbilirubinemia)[30] and in the basal ganglia of kernicteric human infants, accounting for prominent signs of bilirubin neurotoxicity in each. Furthermore, Falcao and colleagues[31] have raised the possibility that neuroinflammation may be a significant contributor to bilirubin neurotoxicity.

Bilirubin and Calcium Homeostasis

Braun and Schulman[32] have proposed that bilirubin interferes with intracellular calcium homeostasis and have demonstrated decreased activity of calcium and calmodulin-dependent protein kinase II (CaMKII) in the Gunn rat model of kernicterus. Bilirubin inhibits CaMKII in vitro,[33] and its developmental expression is impaired in jaundiced (jj) Gunn rats.[34] Further, there is a selective decrease in expression of calcium-binding proteins (CBPs) in specific brainstem areas susceptible to bilirubin neurotoxicity in the CNS of kernicteric Gunn rats.[35,36] CaMKII regulates neurotransmitter release, calcium-regulated ion conductance, and neuroskeletal dynamics[37] and can trigger programmed cell death (apoptosis). It has also been proposed that bilirubin and increased calcium cause damage through an excitotoxic, N-methyl-D-aspartate (NMDA)-dependent mechanism,[38–40] although there is also evidence against this hypothesis.[41] My colleagues and I[42] have found that MK-801 (dizocilpine), an NMDA channel blocker, does not protect against bilirubin neurotoxicity in vitro in hippocampal neurons, nor does it protect against auditory dysfunction in vivo in the Gunn rat model of ABE.

Mechanisms of Auditory Dysfunction

Another study used the Gunn rat to investigate bilirubin-induced auditory deficits.[43] In vivo ABRs revealed severe auditory deficits within 18 hours of exposure to high bilirubin levels. Extracellular multielectrode array recordings following hyperbilirubinemia in an in vitro preparation of the auditory brainstem demonstrated transmission failure indicative of damage at a presynaptic site in the medial nucleus of the trapezoid body. Similarly, multiphoton imaging demonstrated that giant synapses in this nucleus were destroyed. These neurons express high levels of nitric oxide synthase (NOS); nitric oxide has been implicated in mechanisms of bilirubin toxicity elsewhere in the brain,[44] and antagonism of neuronal NOS by 7-nitroindazole was found to protect hearing during bilirubin exposure.[43]

Neuroprotective Action of Bilirubin

Somewhat paradoxically, bilirubin and heme oxygenase 2, the enzyme that catalyzes its formation, have been shown to have neuroprotective antioxidant properties. Neurons are susceptible to apoptotic death from oxidative stress. Work from the Snyder laboratory has begun to define the role of bilirubin and its precursor, biliverdin, in normal cells.[45–49] Depleting cultured HeLA cells and cortical neurons of biliverdin reductase by ribonucleic acid (RNA) interference leads to increased oxidative activity and renders cells more susceptible to caspase-dependent death from hyperoxia and hydrogen peroxide toxicity.[49] The antioxidant activity of these compounds is comparable to that of glutathione, long assumed to be the principal cellular antioxidant.[49] Hippocampal cultures from heme oxygenase 2 (but not 1) knockout mice are more susceptible to hydrogen peroxide toxicity,[45] and heme oxygenase 2 knockout mice are more susceptible to focal cerebral ischemia and excitotoxic injury.[46] Despite its extremely low concentration in the cell, bilirubin is recycled to greatly increase its effect.[49] Bararano and colleagues[49] have proposed that the potent physiologic antioxidant action of bilirubin is amplified when the detoxification of reactive oxygen species oxidizes bilirubin back to biliverdin, which is then reduced again by biliverdin reductase to form bilirubin. As this redox-amplification cycle is repeated, the antioxidant effect of bilirubin is multiplied. Although this redox-amplification cycle has been proposed to constitute the principal physiologic function of bilirubin, it should be noted that a protective action of modest levels of bilirubin does not alter the well-established dangers of kernicterus associated with major elevations of serum bilirubin.[48]

Reinforcing the concept that bilirubin has a protective/beneficial effect, numerous studies in adults have shown the beneficial effects of slight elevations of UCB throughout the life span—for example, the lower incidence of heart disease and stroke in individuals with Gilbert syndrome and a mild unconjugated hyperbilirubinemia. The evidence for molecular and clinical effects of bilirubin in health and disease has recently been reviewed and summarized by Gazzin and colleagues.[21]

Molecular Response to Hyperbilirubinemia

As just discussed, bilirubin is on the one hand a powerful antioxidant that has protective properties and modulates cell growth; however, in excess, it has deleterious properties that cause cell death and apoptosis, in part owing to oxidative stress. Cells exposed to bilirubin increase expression of a multifunctional neuroprotective protein DJ-1, an adaptive response that maintains cellular oxidative stress homeostasis.[50] Dogan and coworkers[51] have demonstrated a relationship between serum total

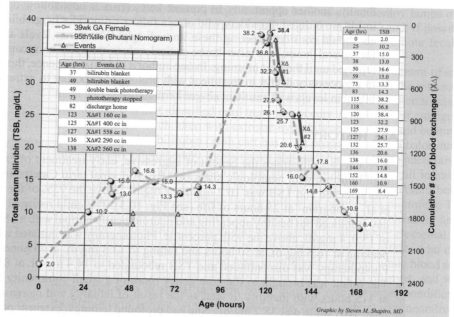

Fig. 10.4 Total serum bilirubin (*TSB*) levels with age in hours after birth in a 39-week gestational age girl. The measures TSB levels are connected with a dotted blue line. The first TSB of 2.0 mg/dL is a hypothetical estimate. Phototherapy is represented by a blue line, higher when the phototherapy was increased from double to triple lights. The two double-volume exchange transfusions are represented in red, with the secondary y-axis (on the right) representing the amount of blood exchanged.

Recommendation for the Diagnosis of KSD and Treatment of Its Clinical Manifestations

Once the child is stable, consideration should be given to obtaining an MRI scan of the head without contrast. Currently we recommend an MRI scan of the head and an ABR test. The MRI scan should be obtained with special attention to the globus pallidus (i.e., T1-weighted, T2-weighted, fluid-attenuated inversion recovery [FLAIR] sequences through the basal ganglia), the addition of thin sections with contiguous cuts and coronal sections through the basal ganglia may be helpful but are generally not necessary. The ABR test should be obtained with special attention to IWIs and CMs to determine the presence or absence of ANSD. It is not often appreciated that OAEs, also known as distortion product otoacoustic emissions (DPOAEs), do not detect the auditory abnormality owing to hyperbilirubinemia. Children completely deaf with severe ANSD have normal OAEs as neonates and in infancy. Therefore one must obtain an ABR (BAEP) test for diagnostic information. Because the number of children with abnormalities that then improve is unknown, early testing is important, with serial testing if the results are abnormal. A good neurologic examination with special attention to muscle tone and eye movements is also important. Serial neurologic evaluations during the first few months of life can be helpful in determining if brain injury has occurred. Early identification and treatment with physical therapy, occupational therapy, and speech therapy can be helpful. Some children with classic kernicterus have failure to thrive because of swallowing difficulties, gastroesophageal reflux, and excessive metabolic demands from their movement disorders. These children often benefit from placement of nasogastric or gastrostomy tubes, although they continue to be fed orally. If severe ANSD is present or the child is deaf or severely hearing impaired, cochlear implantation has proved beneficial. We agree with the current recommendations that this procedure be done as soon as possible. The parents of a large majority of patients with kernicterus who have undergone cochlear implantation have reported benefit. In severe cases, medications to treat dystonia and hypertonia are important.

Dystonia is a major source of impairments for children with kernicterus. We have often observed children with apparently intact intellect, virtually prisoners of in a body plagued with dystonia and athetosis. Anticholinergic medications have a long history of use in the treatment of dystonia. The rationale for the use of anticholinergics is based on the rich cholinergic input to the basal ganglia, notably on tonically activated muscarinic receptors.[99] Trihexyphenidyl, a cholinergic muscarinic antagonist, has been best studied. Although trihexyphenidyl has been useful in other dystonias, initial reports do not show that benefit in children with kernicterus.[100]

Baclofen, a gamma-aminobutyric acid ionotropic receptor family B ($GABA_B$) receptor antagonist, has been extensively used in the treatment of dystonia in both the oral form and intrathecally via a baclofen pump.[101] One major issue for children with kernicterus is that baclofen can worsen truncal hypotonia, a potentially significant problem for some children with kernicterus who need every little bit of truncal tone to hold their posture. Benzodiazepines, $GABA_A$ antagonists, have a limited role in the treatment of dystonia in kernicterus because of the side effect profile of this class of medications, including sialorrhea and sedation. Finally, botulinum toxin injections can provide significant relief to children with focal dystonias.[102]

In 2003 the U.S. Food and Drug Administration granted a humanitarian device exemption for use of the Medtronic deep brain stimulation device (Medtronic, Minneapolis, MN) in children with dystonia who are 7 years old or older. The data in children with primary dystonia have been promising; however, similar results are less encouraging for children with secondary dystonias.[103] We have implanted electrodes in the globus pallidus pars interna (GPi) bilaterally in four children with severe motor-predominant dystonic kernicterus. With intensive programming they have shown modest clinical improvements both immediately and several months after implantation. There have been encouraging reports in adults with choreoathetoid dystonia who had implants in the subthalamic nucleus.[104] We believe that implanting other basal ganglia regions in addition to GPi may improve the benefits provided by this therapeutic approach. Trials are currently underway at our center to probe this approach.

Expanding the Idea of Kernicterus as a Spectrum of Disorders

A more accurate definition of kernicterus is needed. The definition of classic kernicterus is well established in the literature, but new clinical cases have led to the concept of a spectrum of kernicterus. To emphasize this point we have suggested using the term KSDs. Indeed, kernicterus is not a single clinical entity; some children have an auditory-predominant form of kernicterus, whereas others have a motor-predominant form. In our Kernicterus Clinic, admittedly composed of a skewed population of children with KSDs, we have observed a small number of cases of auditory-predominant kernicterus in infants of 30 to 32 weeks' gestation who have TSB levels in the range of 20 to 25 mg/dL.[105,106] This is very consistent with the observation that neuronal sensitivities to bilirubin toxicity vary with gestational age (see earlier discussion), resulting in a different phenotype when the hyperbilirubinemic event occurs in a premature infant versus a term or near-term infant.

The genetic influences and susceptibilities for developing kernicterus are not completely known—for example, it is well established that males are more susceptible to bilirubin neurotoxicity than females, yet the etiology for this sexual difference remains unexplained. Identification of precisely when and how bilirubin becomes neurotoxic, both on a cellular (molecular) basis and to the whole organism, will improve understanding how and when to treat hyperbilirubinemic newborns. Better basic science can thus be expected to lead to a better treatment paradigm for jaundiced newborns.

Bilirubin Neurotoxicity in the Very Premature Infant

A significant gap in knowledge is determining when bilirubin neurotoxicity occurs in the premature infant. Guidelines that exist for administration of phototherapy and exchange transfusion are not evidence based, and there are currently no established guidelines for the extremely premature infants (<35 weeks' gestation).[107] Morris et al. have shown that aggressive phototherapy significantly reduced the rate of neurodevelopment impairments in infants with extremely low birth weight (<1000 g), albeit with a nonstatistically significant increase in mortality among infants weighing 501 to 750 g at birth.[108] Whether bilirubin encephalopathy contributes to neurodevelopmental disabilities or learning disorders in this population is unknown. We suspect that, if present, bilirubin is likely to cause some problems similar to those seen with classic kernicterus, including auditory processing disorders. As evidenced by data presented earlier in this chapter, the damage or developmental consequences of excessive bilirubin on the very immature CNS is likely to have significant differences from its effects on a more mature system. Furthermore, the role of bilirubin in common neurodevelopmental disorders, such as auditory processing disorders, cognitive disorders, sensory motor disorders, autism, and attention-deficit/hyperactivity disorder (ADHD), has yet to be established.

Kernicterus and KSDs in preterm infants present difficult but important challenges for the future. Because almost all prematurely born infants have hyperbilirubinemia, it is problematic to determine whether hyperbilirubinemia is the cause of subsequent neurodevelopmental disabilities. Nonetheless, the relative rarity of ANSD in the general population and in the population of children with hearing loss (0.23%) contrasts greatly with its accounting for 24% of at-risk infants from a regional perinatal center NICU.[109]

Difficulties in Assessing Kernicterus in Preterm Infants

Kernicterus in preterm infants may occur without the typical neurologic signs of ABE[84] or with neurologic signs different from those in term infants.[71] A retrospective study from Japan of eight preterm infants (<34 weeks' gestation, several of whom were born at less than 26 weeks' gestation) with a diagnosis of athetoid cerebral palsy made by consensus between pediatric neurologists and physical therapists[84] concluded that these infants had features similar to those in term infants with kernicterus. Yet none showed classic ABE during the neonatal period. Abnormal muscle tone and dystonic posture were recognized within 6 months corrected age in all. In infancy, MRI scans were performed on seven of the eight subjects, and all seven subjects showed abnormalities in the globus pallidus bilaterally, but after 1 year corrected age the abnormalities had resolved. ABRs, measured after discharge, were abnormal bilaterally in all seven infants. The researchers noted that a lack of acute neurologic symptoms in the preterm infants was common in infants in whom kernicterus later developed and concluded that the absence of characteristic neurologic symptoms does not exclude the possibility of kernicterus in preterm infants.

The issue of MRI abnormalities that disappear with time presents difficulties for diagnosis and recognition that clinical sequelae are due to bilirubin neurotoxicity. MRI and single-photon emission computed tomography (SPECT) from three of the patients from the study just described found high-intensity areas in the globus pallidus in the neonatal period, but on later MRI, only one had abnormalities, which were subtle.[110] However, SPECT performed at the time of the later MRI showed decreased perfusion in all three patients. It follows that SPECT imaging may be a useful measure of pathologic injury in the evaluation of KSDs.

Wennberg and colleagues[111] pointed out that 150,000 to 200,000 premature infants undergo phototherapy each year in the United States to avoid TSB levels thought to require exchange transfusion. Two measurable plasma variables that might explain the variation and the response to TSB are the unbound, unconjugated bilirubin concentration (free bilirubin) and the plasma concentration of photoisomers, although the question of whether photic isomers are toxic has not been convincingly resolved. These issues and questions are likely more important in the prevention of kernicterus and KSDs in prematurely born infants.

Gkoltsiou and associates[112] studied serial brain MRI and HUS findings in 11 infants with unconjugated bilirubin levels higher than 400 μmol/L (23.4 mg/dL) and/or neurologic signs suggestive of kernicterus. This study confirmed that in this cohort severe cerebral palsy occurred with relatively low TSB levels in preterm infants but only in those with high TSB levels in full-term infants. They concluded that HUS and MRI at preterm and term age were not reliable in excluding significant damage to the globus pallidus.

Amin and coworkers[113] found an association of apnea with ABE in premature infants born at 28 to 32 weeks gestational age who transient bilirubin encephalopathy. They identified 34 of 100 infants with bilirubin encephalopathy, as defined by abnormal ABR progression in temporal relation to hyperbilirubinemia. These infants had significantly more apneic and bradycardic events, required more treatment with continuous positive airway pressure and methylxanthines, and had higher bilirubin values than those with normal ABR progression. They concluded that premature infants with transient bilirubin encephalopathy, as defined by abnormal ABR progression in relation to hyperbilirubinemia, have more concurrent apneic events and require more prolonged respiratory support and medications.

One must conclude that bilirubin neurotoxicity in the premature infant is a pathologically different process than in the full-term infant. This has important consequences regarding the treatment of hyperbilirubinemia in the preterm infant and, while there are suggestions as to how to approach this population,[107] this issue is still in need of more research to make recommendations based on objective evidence.

Genetics of KSDs and Susceptibility to Bilirubin Neurotoxicity

We have emphasized throughout this chapter the need to understand the role of systematic measurements of bilirubin using TSB and, hopefully in the future, Bf to assess the level of risk of developing excessive hyperbilirubinemia and ultimately KSDs. However, individuals with relatively low levels of bilirubin (also known as low bilirubin kernicterus), defined as the occurrence of kernicterus at TSB levels below commonly recommended exchange transfusion thresholds,[71,114] can still sustain significant neurologic damage.[71,112,114–118] Watchko and Maisels[114] discuss factors that contribute to low bilirubin kernicterus in premature infants, including hypoalbuminemia, limited and/or impaired albumin–bilirubin binding, and comorbid CNS injuries. Similarly, there is evidence that patients with high to very high levels or levels above AAP recommendation for double-volume exchange transfusion can sometimes have very mild or no noticeable symptoms of damage. Newman et al.[119] obtained outcome data on 132 infants from a population of 106,000 infants in a large managed care organization with TSB values between 25 and 45 mg/dL who were treated with phototherapy or exchange transfusion and found no kernicterus after at least 2 years of follow-up. Wu et al.,[120] who studied a population of more than 500,000 infants in the same managed care organization, found kernicterus occurred only in infants with two or more risk factors for neurotoxicity (prematurity, G6PD deficiency, hypoalbuminemia, hypoxia-ischemia, and sepsis) and TSB levels greater than 5 mg/dL above the exchange transfusion threshold. Although it is clear that differences in outcome with similar TSB levels can be explained by differences in etiology, albumin binding, Bf, pH, inflammation, sepsis, and duration of exposure or other complicating factors, we believe that it is also likely that the biochemical and cellular pathways responsible for clearing and responding to excessive CNS bilirubin can be impacted by genetic differences.[22]

There are known genetic risk factors for developing excessive neonatal hyperbilirubinemia, but there are currently no studies available that have identified a major genetic factor in determining the inherent sensitivity of an individual to bilirubin neurotoxicity. Genetic studies are currently limited to conditions that increase bilirubin production or decrease binding or elimination (e.g., mutations that cause increased red blood cell fragility, such as those leading to a deficiency in G6PD) or RBC membranes abnormalities (e.g., hereditary spherocytosis or eliptocytosis). We recently reported an extremely rapid rise of TSB to 39 mg/dL at 32 hours of life[121] in a child with congenital thrombotic thrombocytopenic purpura, or Upshaw-Schulman syndrome, caused by a deficiency of ADAMTS13 protein, or von Willebrand factor–cleaving protease. Genetic defects that cause decreased elimination through decreased enzyme activity of key enzymes, such as uridine diphosphate (UDP)-glucuronosyltransferase 1A1 (*UGT1A1*) (Crigler-Najjar syndrome) and its regulation (Gilbert syndrome), are known genetic risk factors for hyperbilirubinemia and kernicterus.[122] These risk factors have been well described in the clinical setting, but there is no current evidence of a strong genetic link to an increased sensitivity to bilirubin neurotoxicity.

There have been recent examples of in vitro studies in human cell lines, as well as mouse and rat primary neuronal and glial cells, exposed to toxic levels bilirubin and then screened for changes in gene expression and protein levels.[123–127] Using the genes and pathways identified within these in vitro studies, combined with the well-known group of genes linked to elevated bilirubin levels and an in silico identification of differentially expressed genes in susceptible versus protected regions of the brain, we have developed a novel list of genes representing the most likely contributors to sensitivity to bilirubin neurotoxicity.[22] To use these lists of genes we have developed a modified version of the pathway genetic load (PGL) score.[128] This method represents a focused genetic analysis strategy to investigate whether there exists a significant number of deleterious mutations in a small set of genes thought to be key to a specific outcome. This analysis is based on the hypothesis that increases in sensitivity to bilirubin neurotoxicity result from the combination of multiple deleterious mutations present in key response genes. Although one or two of these mutations will not create a significant impact, the presence of multiple damaging mutations will combine to place a significant "load" on the pathway of interest and lead to an increased risk of damage in the presence of high levels of bilirubin.[22] If this hypothesis can be confirmed, then genetic testing could presumably be used to more accurately assess the risk of bilirubin neurotoxicity and future KSDs in jaundiced neonates.

Gaps in Knowledge

Although there has been significant progress in the understanding of how bilirubin causes brain damage, significant gaps in knowledge remain. An important gap in basic science knowledge relates to specific cellular and regional selectivity of the CNS to bilirubin toxicity. The current methods of assessing risk for kernicterus and KSD—that is, TSB measurement—do not measure the amount of bilirubin in brain tissue. Thus some infants with relatively low TSB values may have KSD, and undoubtedly many with relatively high TSB levels may be treated unnecessarily to prevent kernicterus in a few infants. Research is needed to investigate the sensitivity and reliability of new methods to better detect ABE, including clinical examination of newborn infants, additional biochemical measures of bilirubin toxicity such as Bf, and neurophysiology such as ABRs.

Conclusion

Great strides have been made in the management of neonatal jaundice, hyperbilirubinemia, and kernicterus in the past 25 years. The AAP practice parameter on the management of jaundice, published in 2004[55] and updated in 2009,[87] marked a shift in clinical practice that resulted in a large decrease in the number of children developing KSD. Yet as described in this chapter, much still remains to be done. The guidelines, as would be expected of any guidelines, are not perfect and will undoubtedly undergo several more revisions. Perhaps more significantly, we still have significant knowledge gaps in the effects of hyperbilirubinemia in preterm infants. And finally, we are just starting to uncover the genomics of bilirubin susceptibility. In this chapter, we hope to have highlighted these important areas of research and discoveries in the field related to hyperbilirubinemia that remain to be investigated in the years to come.

REFERENCES

1. Bhutani VK, Johnson L, Sivieri EM. Predictive ability of a predischarge hour-specific serum bilirubin for subsequent significant hyperbilirubinemia in healthy term and near-term newborns. *Pediatrics*. 1999;103(1):6–14.
2. Le Pichon JB, et al. The neurological sequelae of neonatal hyperbilirubinemia: definitions, diagnosis and treatment of the Kernicterus Spectrum Disorders (KSDs). *Curr Pediatr Rev*. 2017. [Epub ahead of print.]
3. Sgro M, et al. Incidence of chronic bilirubin encephalopathy in Canada, 2007–2008. *Pediatrics*. 2012;130(4):e886–890.
4. Bjerre JV, Petersen JR, Ebbesen F. Surveillance of extreme hyperbilirubinaemia in Denmark. A method to identify the newborn infants. *Acta Paediatr*. 2008;97(8):1030–1034.
5. Ebbesen F. Recurrence of kernicterus in term and near-term infants in Denmark. *Acta Paediatr*. 2000;89(10):1213–1217.
6. Ebbesen F, et al. Extreme hyperbilirubinaemia in term and near-term infants in Denmark. *Acta Paediatr*. 2005;94(1):59–64.
7. Manning D, et al. Prospective surveillance study of severe hyperbilirubinaemia in the newborn in the UK and Ireland. *Arch Dis Child Fetal Neonatal Ed*. 2007;92(5):F342–F346.
8. Bjerre JV, Ebbesen F. Incidence of kernicterus in newborn infants in Denmark. *Ugeskr Laeger*. 2006;168(7):686–691.
9. Newman TB, et al. Frequency of neonatal bilirubin testing and hyperbilirubinemia in a large health maintenance organization. *Pediatrics*. 1999;104(5 Pt 2):1198–1203.
10. Newman TB, Liljestrand P, Escobar GJ. Infants with bilirubin levels of 30 mg/dL or more in a large managed care organization. *Pediatrics*. 2003;111(6 Pt 1):1303–1311.
11. Ogunlesi TA, et al. The incidence and outcome of bilirubin encephalopathy in Nigeria: a bi-centre study. *Niger J Med*. 2007;16(4):354–359.
12. Bhutani VK, Johnson L. Kernicterus in the 21st century: frequently asked questions. *J Perinatol*. 2009;29(suppl 1):S20–S24.
13. Shapiro SM, Powers K. Kernicterus subtypes and their association with signs of neonatal encephalopathy. *Ann Neurol*. 2010;68(suppl 14):S117–S118.
14. Ostrow JD, et al. Molecular basis of bilirubin-induced neurotoxicity. *Trends Mol Med*. 2004;10(2):65–70.
15. Ives NK, Gardiner RM. Blood-brain barrier permeability to bilirubin in the rat studied using intracarotid bolus injection and in situ brain perfusion techniques. *Pediatr Res*. 1990;27(5):436–441.
16. Ostrow JD, et al. New concepts in bilirubin encephalopathy. *Eur J Clin Invest*. 2003;33(11):988–997.
17. Watchko JF. Kernicterus and the molecular mechanisms of bilirubin-induced CNS injury in newborns. *Neuromolecular Med*. 2006;8(4):513–529.
18. Gazzin S, et al. The molecular basis of jaundice: an old symptom revisited. *Liver Int*. 2017;37(8):1094–1102.
19. Watchko JF, Tiribelli C. Bilirubin-induced neurologic damage–mechanisms and management approaches. *N Engl J Med*. 2013;369(21):2021–2030.
20. Gazzin S, et al. Bilirubin accumulation and Cyp mRNA expression in selected brain regions of jaundiced Gunn rat pups. *Pediatr Res*. 2012;71(6):653–660.
21. Gazzin S, et al. A novel perspective on the biology of bilirubin in health and disease. *Trends Mol Med*. 2016;22(9):758–768.
22. Riordan SM, et al. A hypothesis for using pathway genetic load analysis for understanding complex outcomes in bilirubin encephalopathy. *Front Neurosci*. 2016;10:376.
23. Gennuso F, et al. Bilirubin protects astrocytes from its own toxicity by inducing up-regulation and translocation of multidrug resistance-associated protein 1 (Mrp1). *Proc Natl Acad Sci U S A*. 2004;101(8):2470–2475.
24. Rigato I, et al. The human multidrug-resistance-associated protein MRP1 mediates ATP-dependent transport of unconjugated bilirubin. *Biochem J*. 2004;383(Pt 2):335–341.
25. Rodrigues CM, et al. Bilirubin and amyloid-beta peptide induce cytochrome c release through mitochondrial membrane permeabilization. *Mol Med*. 2000;6(11):936–946.
26. Silva RF, Rodrigues CM, Brites D. Bilirubin-induced apoptosis in cultured rat neural cells is aggravated by chenodeoxycholic acid but prevented by ursodeoxycholic acid. *J Hepatol*. 2001;34(3):402–408.
27. Rodrigues CM, Sola S, Brites D. Bilirubin induces apoptosis via the mitochondrial pathway in developing rat brain neurons. *Hepatology*. 2002;35(5):1186–1195.
28. Hanko E, et al. Bilirubin induces apoptosis and necrosis in human NT2-N neurons. *Pediatr Res*. 2005;57(2):179–184.
29. Li CY, et al. Protein kinase A and C signaling induces bilirubin potentiation of GABA/glycinergic synaptic transmission in rat ventral cochlear nucleus neurons. *Brain Res*. 2010;1348:30–41.
30. Conlee JW, Shapiro SM. Morphological changes in the cochlear nucleus and nucleus of the trapezoid body in Gunn rat pups. *Hear Res*. 1991;57(1):23–30.
31. Falcao AS, et al. Bilirubin-induced immunostimulant effects and toxicity vary with neural cell type and maturation state. *Acta Neuropathol*. 2006;112(1):95–105.
32. Braun AP, Schulman H. The multifunctional calcium/calmodulin-dependent protein kinase: from form to function. *Annu Rev Physiol*. 1995;57:417–445.
33. Churn SB. Multifunctional calcium and calmodulin-dependent kinase II in neuronal function and disease. *Adv Neuroimmunol*. 1995;5(3):241–259.

34. Conlee JW, Shapiro SM, Churn SB. Expression of the alpha and beta subunits of Ca^{2+}/calmodulin kinase II in the cerebellum of jaundiced Gunn rats during development: a quantitative light microscopic analysis. *Acta Neuropathol.* 2000;99(4):393–401.
35. Shaia WT, et al. Immunohistochemical localization of calcium-binding proteins in the brainstem vestibular nuclei of the jaundiced Gunn rat. *Hear Res.* 2002;173(1–2):82–90.
36. Spencer RF, et al. Changes in calcium-binding protein expression in the auditory brainstem nuclei of the jaundiced Gunn rat. *Hear Res.* 2002;171(1–2):129–141.
37. Greengard P. Neuronal phosphoproteins. Mediators of signal transduction. *Mol Neurobiol.* 1987;1(1–2):81–119.
38. Hoffman DJ, et al. The in vivo effect of bilirubin on the *N*-methyl-D-aspartate receptor/ion channel complex in the brains of newborn piglets. *Pediatr Res.* 1996;40(6):804–808.
39. McDonald JW, et al. Role of glutamate receptor-mediated excitotoxicity in bilirubin-induced brain injury in the Gunn rat model. *Exp Neurol.* 1998;150(1):21–29.
40. Grojean S, et al. Bilirubin induces apoptosis via activation of NMDA receptors in developing rat brain neurons. *Exp Neurol.* 2000;166(2):334–341.
41. Warr O, Mort D, Attwell D. Bilirubin does not modulate ionotropic glutamate receptors or glutamate transporters. *Brain Res.* 2000;879(1–2):13–16.
42. Shapiro SM, et al. NMDA channel antagonist MK-801 does not protect against bilirubin neurotoxicity. *Neonatology.* 2007;92(4):248–257.
43. Haustein MD, et al. Acute hyperbilirubinaemia induces presynaptic neurodegeneration at a central glutamatergic synapse. *J Physiol.* 2010;588(Pt 23):4683–4693.
44. Brito MA, et al. *N*-Methyl-aspartate receptor and neuronal nitric oxide synthase activation mediate bilirubin-induced neurotoxicity. *Mol Med.* 2010;16(9–10):372–380.
45. Dore S, et al. Bilirubin, formed by activation of heme oxygenase-2, protects neurons against oxidative stress injury. *Proc Natl Acad Sci U S A.* 1999;96(5):2445–2450.
46. Dore S, et al. Heme oxygenase-2 is neuroprotective in cerebral ischemia. *Mol Med.* 1999;5(10):656–663.
47. Greenberg DA. The jaundice of the cell. *Proc Natl Acad Sci U S A.* 2002;99(25):15837–15839.
48. Sedlak TW, Snyder SH. Bilirubin benefits: cellular protection by a biliverdin reductase antioxidant cycle. *Pediatrics.* 2004;113(6):1776–1782.
49. Baranano DE, et al. Biliverdin reductase: a major physiologic cytoprotectant. *Proc Natl Acad Sci U S A.* 2002;99(25):16093–16098.
50. Deganuto M, et al. A proteomic approach to the bilirubin-induced toxicity in neuronal cells reveals a protective function of DJ-1 protein. *Proteomics.* 2010;10(8):1645–1657.
51. Dogan M, et al. Evaluation of oxidant and antioxidant status in infants with hyperbilirubinemia and kernicterus. *Hum Exp Toxicol.* 2011;30(11):1751–1760.
52. Conlee JW, Shapiro SM. Development of cerebellar hypoplasia in jaundiced Gunn rats: a quantitative light microscopic analysis. *Acta Neuropathol.* 1997;93(5):450–460.
53. Falcao AS, et al. Bilirubin-induced inflammatory response, glutamate release, and cell death in rat cortical astrocytes are enhanced in younger cells. *Neurobiol Dis.* 2005;20(2):199–206.
54. Falcao AS, et al. Role of multidrug resistance-associated protein 1 expression in the in vitro susceptibility of rat nerve cell to unconjugated bilirubin. *Neuroscience.* 2007;144(3):878–888.
55. American Academy of Pediatrics Subcommittee on. H. Management of hyperbilirubinemia in the newborn infant 35 or more weeks of gestation. *Pediatrics.* 2004;114(1):297–316.
56. Brooks JC, et al. Evidence suggests there was not a "resurgence" of kernicterus in the 1990s. *Pediatrics.* 2011;127(4):672–679.
57. Johnson L, Brown AK. A pilot registry for acute and chronic kernicterus in term and near-term infants. *Pediatrics.* 1999;104(3):736.
58. Ahlfors CE, Wennberg RP. Bilirubin-albumin binding and neonatal jaundice. *Semin Perinatol.* 2004;28(5):334–339.
59. Wennberg RP, et al. Toward understanding kernicterus: a challenge to improve the management of jaundiced newborns. *Pediatrics.* 2006;117(2):474–485.
60. Ahlfors CE. Bilirubin-albumin binding and free bilirubin. *J Perinatol.* 2001;21(suppl 1):S40–S42. discussion S59–S62.
61. Wennberg RP, et al. Abnormal auditory brainstem response in a newborn infant with hyperbilirubinemia: improvement with exchange transfusion. *J Pediatr.* 1982;100(4):624–626.
62. Amin SB, et al. Bilirubin and serial auditory brainstem responses in premature infants. *Pediatrics.* 2001;107(4):664–670.
63. Funato M, et al. Vigintiphobia, unbound bilirubin, and auditory brainstem responses. *Pediatrics.* 1994;93(1):50–53.
64. Nwaesei CG, et al. Changes in auditory brainstem responses in hyperbilirubinemic infants before and after exchange transfusion. *Pediatrics.* 1984;74(5):800–803.
65. Wennberg R. Bilirubin transport and toxicity. *Mead Johnson Symp Perinat Dev Med.* 1982;19:25–31.
66. Sugama S, Soeda A, Eto Y. Magnetic resonance imaging in three children with kernicterus. *Pediatr Neurol.* 2001;25(4):328–331.
67. Martich-Kriss V, Kollias SS, Ball WS Jr. MR findings in kernicterus. *AJNR Am J Neuroradiol.* 1995;16(suppl 4):819–821.
68. Yilmaz Y, et al. Magnetic resonance imaging findings in patients with severe neonatal indirect hyperbilirubinemia. *J Child Neurol.* 2001;16(6):452–455.
69. Penn AA, et al. Kernicterus in a full term infant. *Pediatrics.* 1994;93(6 Pt 1):1003–1006.

70. Johnston MV, Hoon AH Jr. Possible mechanisms in infants for selective basal ganglia damage from asphyxia, kernicterus, or mitochondrial encephalopathies. *J Child Neurol*. 2000;15(9):588–591.

71. Govaert P, et al. Changes in globus pallidus with (pre)term kernicterus. *Pediatrics*. 2003;112(6 Pt 1):1256–1263.

72. Harris MC, et al. Developmental follow-up of breastfed term and near-term infants with marked hyperbilirubinemia. *Pediatrics*. 2001;107(5):1075–1080.

73. Saluja S, et al. Auditory neuropathy spectrum disorder in late preterm and term infants with severe jaundice. *Int J Pediatr Otorhinolaryngol*. 2010;74(11):1292–1297.

74. Wisnowski JL, et al. Magnetic resonance imaging abnormalities in advanced acute bilirubin encephalopathy highlight dentato-thalamo-cortical pathways. *J Pediatr*. 2016;174:260–263.

75. Watchko JF. Bilirubin-induced neurotoxicity in the preterm neonate. *Clin Perinatol*. 2016;43(2):297–311.

76. Wisnowski JL, et al. Magnetic resonance imaging of bilirubin encephalopathy: current limitations and future promise. *Semin Perinatol*. 2014;38(7):422–428.

77. Johnson L, Brown A, Bhutani V. BIND-A clinical score for bilirubin induced neurologic dysfunction in newborns. *Pediatrics*. 1999;104(3):746–747.

78. Volpe JJ. Bilirubin and brain injury. In: Volpe JJ, ed. *Neurology of the Newborn*. Philadelphia: WB Saunders; 2001:490–514.

79. Radmacher PG, et al. A modified Bilirubin-induced neurologic dysfunction (BIND-M) algorithm is useful in evaluating severity of jaundice in a resource-limited setting. *BMC Pediatr*. 2015;15:28.

80. Amin SB. Bilirubin binding capacity in the preterm neonate. *Clin Perinatol*. 2016;43(2):241–257.

81. Amin SB, Bhutani VK, Watchko JF. Apnea in acute bilirubin encephalopathy. *Semin Perinatol*. 2014;38(7):407–411.

82. Amin SB. Clinical assessment of bilirubin-induced neurotoxicity in premature infants. *Semin Perinatol*. 2004;28(5):340–347.

83. Fahn S, Jankovic J. *Principles and Practice of Movement Disorders*. Philadelphia: Churchill Livingstone/Elsevier; 2007. x, 652 pp, 8pp of plates.

84. Okumura A, et al. Kernicterus in preterm infants. *Pediatrics*. 2009;123(6):e1052–e1058.

85. Shapiro SM. Chronic bilirubin encephalopathy: diagnosis and outcome. *Semin Fetal Neonatal Med*. 2010;15(3):157–163.

86. Shapiro SM. Kernicterus. In: Stevenson DK, Maisels MJ, Watchko J, eds. *Care of the Jaundiced Neonate*. New York: McGraw-Hill; 2012:229–242.

87. Maisels MJ, et al. Hyperbilirubinemia in the newborn infant > or =35 weeks' gestation: an update with clarifications. *Pediatrics*. 2009;124(4):1193–1198.

88. Bhutani VK, Johnson L. A proposal to prevent severe neonatal hyperbilirubinemia and kernicterus. *J Perinatol*. 2009;29(suppl 1):S61–67.

89. Hansen TW. Acute management of extreme neonatal jaundice—the potential benefits of intensified phototherapy and interruption of enterohepatic bilirubin circulation. *Acta Paediatr*. 1997;86(8):843–846.

90. Smitherman H, Stark AR, Bhutani VK. Early recognition of neonatal hyperbilirubinemia and its emergent management. *Semin Fetal Neonatal Med*. 2006;11(3):214–224.

91. Gourley GR, et al. Neonatal jaundice and diet. *Arch Pediatr Adolesc Med*. 1999;153(2):184–188.

92. Johnson L, et al. Clinical report from the pilot USA Kernicterus Registry (1992 to 2004). *J Perinatol*. 2009;29(suppl 1):S25–S45.

93. Hansen TW. The role of phototherapy in the crash-cart approach to extreme neonatal jaundice. *Semin Perinatol*. 2011;35(3):171–174.

94. Gourley GR, Arend RA. Beta-glucuronidase and hyperbilirubinaemia in breast-fed and formula-fed babies. *Lancet*. 1986;1(8482):644–646.

95. Gottstein R, Cooke RW. Systematic review of intravenous immunoglobulin in haemolytic disease of the newborn. *Arch Dis Child Fetal Neonatal Ed*. 2003;88(1):F6–F10.

96. Johnson L, Boggs TR. Bilirubin-dependent brain damage: incidence and indications for treatment. In: Odell GB, Schaffer R, Sionpoulous AP, eds. *Phototherapy in the Newborn: An Overview*. Washington, DC: National Academy of Sciences; 1974:122–149.

97. de Vries LS, Lary S, Dubowitz LM. Relationship of serum bilirubin levels to ototoxicity and deafness in high-risk low-birth-weight infants. *Pediatrics*. 1985;76(3):351–354.

98. Kaplan M, et al. Gilbert syndrome and glucose-6-phosphate dehydrogenase deficiency: a dose-dependent genetic interaction crucial to neonatal hyperbilirubinemia. *Proc Natl Acad Sci U S A*. 1997;94(22):12128–12132.

99. Picciotto MR, Higley MJ, Mineur YS. Acetylcholine as a neuromodulator: cholinergic signaling shapes nervous system function and behavior. *Neuron*. 2012;76(1):116–129.

100. Sanger TD, et al. Prospective open-label clinical trial of trihexyphenidyl in children with secondary dystonia due to cerebral palsy. *J Child Neurol*. 2007;22(5):530–537.

101. Jankovic J. Medical treatment of dystonia. *Mov Disord*. 2013;28(7):1001–1012.

102. Ramirez-Castaneda J, Jankovic J. Long-term efficacy, safety, and side effect profile of botulinum toxin in dystonia: a 20-year follow-up. *Toxicon*. 2014;90:344–348.

103. Katsakiori PF, et al. Deep brain stimulation for secondary dystonia: results in 8 patients. *Acta Neurochir (Wien)*. 2009;151(5):473–478, discussion 478.

104. Vidailhet M, et al. Bilateral pallidal deep brain stimulation for the treatment of patients with dystonia-choreoathetosis cerebral palsy: a prospective pilot study. *Lancet Neurol*. 2009;8(8):709–717.

10

105. Shapiro SM. Definition of the clinical spectrum of kernicterus and bilirubin-induced neurologic dysfunction (BIND). *J Perinatol*. 2005;25(1):54–59.
106. Shapiro SM, Bhutani VK, Johnson L. Hyperbilirubinemia and kernicterus. *Clin Perinatol*. 2006;33(2):387–410.
107. Maisels MJ, et al. An approach to the management of hyperbilirubinemia in the preterm infant less than 35 weeks of gestation. *J Perinatol*. 2012;32(9):660–664.
108. Morris BH, et al. Aggressive vs. conservative phototherapy for infants with extremely low birth weight. *N Engl J Med*. 2008;359(18):1885–1896.
109. Berg AL, et al. Newborn hearing screening in the NICU: profile of failed auditory brainstem response/passed otoacoustic emission. *Pediatrics*. 2005;116(4):933–938.
110. Okumura A, et al. Single photon emission computed tomography and serial MRI in preterm infants with kernicterus. *Brain Dev*. 2006;28(6):348–352.
111. Wennberg RP, Ahlfors CE, Aravkin AY. Intervention guidelines for neonatal hyperbilirubinemia: an evidence based quagmire. *Curr Pharm Des*. 2009;15(25):2939–2945.
112. Gkoltsiou K, et al. Serial brain MRI and ultrasound findings: relation to gestational age, bilirubin level, neonatal neurologic status and neurodevelopmental outcome in infants at risk of kernicterus. *Early Hum Dev*. 2008;84(12):829–838.
113. Amin SB, Charafeddine L, Guillet R. Transient bilirubin encephalopathy and apnea of prematurity in 28 to 32 weeks gestational age infants. *J Perinatol*. 2005;25(6):386–390.
114. Watchko JF, Maisels MJ. The enigma of low bilirubin kernicterus in premature infants: why does it still occur, and is it preventable? *Semin Perinatol*. 2014;38(7):397–406.
115. Odutolu Y, Emmerson AJ. Low bilirubin kernicterus with sepsis and hypoalbuminaemia. *BMJ Case Rep*. 2013;2013.
116. Moll M, et al. Are recommended phototherapy thresholds safe enough for extremely low birth weight (ELBW) infants? A report on 2 ELBW infants with kernicterus despite only moderate hyper-bilirubinemia. *Neonatology*. 2011;99(2):90–94.
117. Kamei A, et al. Proton magnetic resonance spectroscopic images in preterm infants with bilirubin encephalopathy. *J Pediatr*. 2012;160(2):342–344.
118. Ahdab-Barmada M, Moossy J. The neuropathology of kernicterus in the premature neonate: diagnostic problems. *J Neuropathol Exp Neurol*. 1984;43(1):45–56.
119. Newman TB, et al. Outcomes among newborns with total serum bilirubin levels of 25 mg per deciliter or more. *N Engl J Med*. 2006;354(18):1889–1900.
120. Wu YW, et al. Risk for cerebral palsy in infants with total serum bilirubin levels at or above the exchange transfusion threshold: a population-based study. *JAMA Pediatr*. 2015;169(3):239–246.
121. Thornton KM, et al. An unusual case of rapidly progressive hyperbilirubinemia. *Case Rep Pediatr*. 2013;2013:284029.
122. Watchko JF. Genetics and pediatric unconjugated hyperbilirubinemia. *J Pediatr*. 2013;162(6):1092–1094.
123. Calligaris R, et al. A transcriptome analysis identifies molecular effectors of unconjugated bilirubin in human neuroblastoma SH-SY5Y cells. *BMC Genomics*. 2009;10:543.
124. Barateiro A, et al. ER stress, mitochondrial dysfunction and calpain/JNK activation are involved in oligodendrocyte precursor cell death by unconjugated bilirubin. *Neuromolecular Med*. 2012;14(4):285–302.
125. Vaz AR, et al. Pro-inflammatory cytokines intensify the activation of NO/NOS, JNK1/2 and caspase cascades in immature neurons exposed to elevated levels of unconjugated bilirubin. *Exp Neurol*. 2011;229(2):381–390.
126. Fernandes A, et al. MAPKs are key players in mediating cytokine release and cell death induced by unconjugated bilirubin in cultured rat cortical astrocytes. *Eur J Neurosci*. 2007;25(4):1058–1068.
127. Silva SL, et al. Features of bilirubin-induced reactive microglia: from phagocytosis to inflammation. *Neurobiol Dis*. 2010;40(3):663–675.
128. Huebinger RM, Garner HR, Barber RC. Pathway genetic load allows simultaneous evaluation of multiple genetic associations. *Burns*. 2010;36(6):787–792.

CHAPTER 11

Neonatal Meningitis: Current Treatment Options

David Kaufman, Santina Zanelli, and Pablo J. Sánchez

- As many as 40% of infants with meningitis who have a gestational age of ≥34 weeks do not have a positive blood culture at the time of their diagnosis.
- Urine culture is an important part of a sepsis evaluation since urinary tract infection is relatively common in neonates who are greater than 72 hours of age.
- For late-onset sepsis, a penicillinase-resistant, semisynthetic penicillin such as oxacillin or nafcillin in combination with an aminoglycoside is the preferred choice.
- The treatment of gram-negative meningitis initially includes the addition of a third or fourth generation cephalosporin such as cefotaxime or cefepime[77,78] or a carbapenem antibiotic such as meropenem.
- For meningitis due to gram-negative bacilli, the duration of antimicrobial therapy is a minimum of 21 days.
- For meningitis due to group B streptococcus, a minimum of 10 days of antimicrobial therapy is recommended.
- Among infants with gram-negative enteric meningitis approximately 20% to 30% of affected infants die, and neurologic sequelae are found in 35% to 50% of survivors.

Bacterial meningitis occurs in approximately 0.4 neonates per 1000 live births. It is defined as inflammation of the meninges that is manifested by an elevated number of white blood cells in the cerebrospinal fluid (CSF). It often is associated with elevated protein content and a low glucose concentration in CSF. Meningitis generally results as a consequence of hematogenous dissemination of bacteria via the choroid plexus and into the central nervous system (CNS) during a sepsis episode. Invasion of the meninges occurs in about 10% to 20% of infants with bacteremia. Rarely, meningitis develops secondary to extension from infected skin through the soft tissues and skull as may occur with an infected cephalohematoma or direct spread from skin surfaces, as in infants with myelomeningoceles or other congenital malformations of the neural tube. In addition, ventriculoperitoneal shunts or ventricular reservoirs may be the primary site of infection. A potential but infrequent complication of meningitis is brain abscess that results from hematogenous spread of bacteria into tissue that has incurred anoxic injury or severe vasculitis with hemorrhage or infarction.

Virtually all organisms that cause neonatal infection or sepsis can result in central nervous disease with severe consequences for the developing brain.[1-5] A list of these pathogens is provided in Box 11.1. It is imperative that a correct and timely diagnosis with a specific organism be made because treatment decisions vary by causative agent.[6]

Box 11.1   CAUSATIVE AGENTS OF NEONATAL MENINGITIS[a]

1. Bacteria   Aerobic:

        Gram-positive: group B streptococcus, group A streptococcus, *Enterococcus* spp., *Streptococcus bovis*, viridans streptococci, *Staphylococcus aureus*, coagulase-negative staphylococci, *Listeria monocytogenes*, *Streptococcus pneumoniae*, others[b]
        Gram-negative: *Escherichia coli*, *Klebsiella* spp., *Enterobacter* spp., *Serratia* spp., *Proteus* spp., *Citrobacter* spp., *Salmonella* spp., *Pseudomonas aeruginosa*, *Haemophilus influenzae*, *Neisseria gonorrhoeae*, *Neisseria meningitidis*, others[c]

        Anaerobic:
        Gram-positive: *Clostridium* spp., *Peptostreptococcus* spp.
        Gram-negative: *Bacteroides fragilis*
        Genital mycoplasmas: *Ureaplasma* spp., *Mycoplasma hominis*
        Spirochetes: *Treponema pallidum*, *Borrelia burgdorferi*
        Mycobacteria: *Mycobacteria tuberculosis*

2. Viruses   Herpes simplex virus, cytomegalovirus, enteroviruses, human immunodeficiency virus, varicella-zoster virus, rubella virus, human parvovirus B19, lymphocytic choriomeningitis virus, Zika virus

3. Fungi   *Candida* spp., *Malassezia* spp., *Aspergillus* spp., *Trichosporon beigelis*, Cryptococcus, *Coccidioides immitis*

4. Protozoa   *Toxoplasma gondii*

[a]For a more complete listing, see Palazzi DL, Klein JO, Baker CJ. Bacterial sepsis and meningitis. In: Remington JS, Klein JO, Wilson CB, Baker CJ, eds. *Infectious Diseases of the Fetus and Newborn Infant.* 6th ed. Philadelphia: WB Saunders; 2006:247–295.
[b]For others, see Giacoia GP. Uncommon pathogens in newborn infants. *J Perinatol.* 1994;14:134–144.

    The case of a preterm infant is presented and discussed to illustrate and highlight the multifaceted nature of this disease. The objective of this chapter is to review the current management of neonatal bacterial meningitis, in the hope of ameliorating the destructive nature of many of these organisms and ultimately improving the outcome of these high-risk infants.

CASE HISTORY

A preterm infant weighing 1004 g was born at 28 weeks' gestation to a 24-year-old mother by cesarean section. The pregnancy was complicated by premature rupture of membranes 2 weeks before delivery, and the mother developed intrapartum fever and was diagnosed with chorioamnionitis. She received antenatal steroids and antimicrobial therapy consisting of ampicillin and gentamicin. At delivery, the infant was floppy with poor respiratory effort, and he required intubation and admission to the neonatal intensive care unit (NICU). Apgar scores were 3 at 1 minute and 7 at 5 minutes. The infant's vital signs were normal, and antimicrobial therapy with ampicillin and gentamicin was initiated after a blood culture was obtained. Hyaline membrane disease was diagnosed and the infant received exogenous surfactant therapy.

Question 1: What Risk Factors Predispose This Infant to Have Early-Onset Bacterial Meningitis?

Because meningitis is a complication of bacteremia; the risk factors are similar to those that contribute to neonatal sepsis—namely prematurity, prolonged rupture of fetal membranes (≥18 hours), maternal urinary tract infection, and maternal intrapartum fever or chorioamnionitis.[7] Immune dysfunction as well as lack of transplacentally acquired maternal immunoglobulin G (IgG) antibodies in premature infants also may increase risk of sepsis and CNS infection. Recently, lower neonatal 25-hydroxyvitamin D levels have been associated with early-onset sepsis.[8]

Likewise, clinical signs suggestive of bacterial meningitis are similar to those of neonatal sepsis. In the full-term infant, fever, lethargy, hypotonia, irritability, apnea, poor feeding, high-pitched cry, emesis, seizures, and bulging fontanelle are prominent clinical signs, whereas in preterm infants, respiratory decompensation consisting of an increased number of apneic episodes predominates. Neonates with meningitis are never "asymptomatic."[9]

The widespread and routine use of intrapartum antimicrobial chemoprophylaxis since 1996 has significantly reduced the rate of early-onset group B streptococcal (GBS) infection by more than 70%.[11,12] Fortunately there has not been a reciprocal increase in early-onset bacterial infections caused by gram-negative organisms among all newborns in the United States.[13,14] However, among very low-birth-weight (VLBW) infants with birth weight of 1500 g of less, a shift toward more gram-negative infections has occurred.[15,16] Among the NICUs of the National Institute of Child Health and Human Development (NICHD) Neonatal Research Network centers, intrapartum antimicrobial chemoprophylaxis resulted in a significant decrease in early-onset GBS infection while the rate of infections caused by *Escherichia coli* increased significantly from 3 to 7 cases per 1000 live births.[15,17] More recently, another NICHD Neonatal Research Network study documented rates of culture-confirmed early-onset sepsis among almost 400,000 live births at Network centers.[16] The overall rate of early-onset sepsis, defined as a positive blood or cerebrospinal fluid bacterial culture at less than 72 hours of age, was 0.98 infections per 1000 live births with rates inversely related to birth weight (BW; 401–1500 g BW, 10.96/1000; 1501–2500 g BW, 1.38/1000; >2500 g BW, 0.57/1000). Among cases of early-onset meningitis, 44% were due to *E. coli* while only 19% were due to GBS. The majority of *E. coli* isolates were resistant to ampicillin, an antibiotic that is often used for intrapartum GBS chemoprophylaxis. Even more concerning was the finding that 3% of *E. coli* isolates were resistant to the third-generation cephalosporin agents.

Question 2: Do Infants With Meningitis Have Positive Blood Cultures?

As many as 40% of infants with meningitis who have a gestational age of 34 weeks or more do not have a positive blood culture at the time of their diagnosis.[18] Similarly, among VLBW infants, almost one-half of cases of meningitis occur with sterile blood cultures.[19,20] Therefore it is imperative that a lumbar puncture be performed if sepsis or meningitis is suspected.[21,22] Evaluation of CSF indices and Gram stain not only will establish a diagnosis but also will help guide initial therapy. Normal CSF indices are provided in Table 11.1.[23–30]

Meningitis in preterm infants admitted to the NICU with respiratory distress syndrome is very uncommon.[31–34] Therefore performance of a lumbar puncture in these infants in whom sepsis is not suspected is not mandatory. Similar data are available for full-term infants.[9,35] However, if the blood culture yields a pathogenic organism, then evaluation of CSF should be done.[22] A lumbar puncture is contraindicated when there is cardiorespiratory instability. Delay in performing a lumbar puncture only delays a potential diagnosis of meningitis and can lead to prolonged and possibly inappropriate antibiotic use.[19,36]

CONTINUATION OF CASE HISTORY

The infant was extubated and continuous positive airway pressure therapy was started on the first day of age. Trophic feedings were initiated on the second day of age, and a percutaneous intravenous central venous catheter was placed for parenteral nutrition. She achieved full enteral feedings on the 20th day. Over the subsequent 2 days, she developed lethargy, hyperglycemia, and increased episodes of apnea that resulted in reinitiation of mechanical ventilation. Two blood cultures were obtained, and antimicrobial therapy with nafcillin and gentamicin was initiated.

Table 11.1 CEREBROSPINAL FLUID INDICES IN NEONATES

Birth Weight (g)	Age (Days)	No. of Patients	Red Blood Cells (/mm³) Mean ± SD (Range)	White Blood Cells (/mm³) Mean ± SD (Range)	Polymorphonuclear Leukocytes (%) Mean ± SD (Range)	Glucose (mg/dL) Mean ± SD (Range)	Protein (mg/dL) Mean ± SD (Range)
Preterm Neonate[a]							
≤1000	0–7	6	335 ± 709 (0–1780)	3 ± 3 (1–8)	11 ± 20 (0–50)	70 ± 17 (41–89)	162 ± 37 (115–222)
	8–28	17	1465 ± 4062 (0–19,050)	4 ± 4 (0–14)	8 ± 17 (0–66)	68 ± 48 (41–89)	159 ± 77 (95–370)
	29–84	15	808 ± 1843 (0–6850)	4 ± 3 (0–11)	2 ± 9 (0–36)	49 ± 22 (41–89)	137 ± 61 (76–260)
1001–1500	0–7	8	407 ± 853 (0–2450)	4 ± 4 (1–10)	4 ± 10 (0–28)	74 ± 19 (41–89)	136 ± 35 (85–176)
	8–28	14	1101 ± 2643 (0–9750)	7 ± 11 (0–44)	10 ± 19 (0–60)	59 ± 23 (41–89)	137 ± 46 (54–227)
	29–84	11	661 ± 1198 (0–3800)	8 ± 8 (0–23)	11 ± 19 (0–48)	47 ± 13 (41–89)	122 ± 47 (45–187)
Full-Term Neonate[b]							
	0–30	108	≤1000/mm³	7.3 ± 13.9 (0–130) median 4	0.8 ± 6.2 (0–65) median 0	51.2 ± 12.9 (62% of serum glucose)	64.2 ± 24.2

[a]From Rodriguez AF, Kaplan SL, Mason EO Jr. Cerebrospinal fluid values in the very low birth weight infant. *J Pediatr.* 1990;116:971–874.
[b]From Ahmed A, Hickey SM, Ehrett S, et al. Cerebrospinal fluid values in the term neonate. *Pediatr Infect Dis J.* 1996;15:298–303.

Question 3: What Is the Optimal Evaluation for Possible Late-Onset Sepsis in Preterm Infants in the NICU?

Infants suspected of having late-onset sepsis in the NICU should have a complete evaluation that consists of a complete blood cell (CBC) count, a urinanalysis, and culture. In critically ill hospitalized neonates, it is very difficult to distinguish infection from noninfectious clinical deteriorations; however, there should be a low threshold for performing a lumbar puncture. Unfortunately, there is no laboratory or clinical finding that has a sensitivity of 100% for the diagnosis of neonatal sepsis.[37,38] Such laboratory tools as CBC count; C-reactive protein; interleukin (IL)-6, IL-8, IL-10; and procalcitonin have suboptimal sensitivity and specificity to replace the blood culture as the gold standard, but these tests may be useful to support a diagnosis of infection when their results are abnormal and accompanied by clinical signs of infection.[39–41] Polymerase chain reaction for detection of bacterial and fungal DNA ultimately may lead to an earlier diagnosis.[42]

It is important to obtain a CBC count with platelets for reasons other than diagnosis. Neonatal sepsis may result in neutropenia, which is associated with a high mortality rate. The finding of an absolute neutrophil count of 500/mm^3 or less may prompt the administration of intravenous immunoglobulin (IvIg 750 mg/kg); the use of IvIg has been associated with improvement in the peripheral neutrophil count presumably from improved neutrophil egress from the bone marrow in infants with sepsis.[43,44] Routine use of IvIg infusions for suspected sepsis is not recommended, however, as studies have not demonstrated benefit in early or late morbidity or mortality.[45] Recombinant granulocyte or granulocyte-macrophage colony-stimulating factors can be considered if IvIg is unsuccessful in improving the neutrophil count.[46,47] Another reason for performance of a CBC count is evaluation of the platelet count because disseminated intravascular coagulation may result in severe thrombocytopenia. In addition, thrombocytopenia may be an early marker of disseminated candidiasis.[48]

Debate continues as to whether multiple blood cultures should be performed. Certainly with bacterial organisms that are frequent blood culture contaminants, such as coagulase-negative staphylococci (CoNS), the diagnosis of sepsis is best confirmed by the finding of two or more positive cultures from multiple sites or body fluids that are normally sterile.[49,50] Two peripheral vein blood cultures are recommended in an infant with a suspected late-onset infection. However, given the difficulty of obtaining blood cultures, this often means obtaining a blood culture from a central catheter and another from a peripheral blood vessel. The value of obtaining a blood culture from a central venous catheter has been debated, because a positive central line culture may represent colonization rather than true infection. The isolation of CoNS from only one blood culture when only one is obtained is problematic and of uncertain significance. Because many of these positive cultures represent contamination with skin microflora, the practice of obtaining only one blood culture often leads to prolonged and unnecessary antibiotic therapy. In addition, performance of two blood cultures may increase the likelihood of isolating a causative agent. This practice leads to more prudent antibiotic use—a major goal in the NICU where antimicrobial resistance is an emerging but preventable problem.[4,51]

Urine culture is an important part of the evaluation because urinary tract infection is relatively common in neonates older than 72 hours of age.[52,53] Urine should be obtained by suprapubic bladder aspiration whenever possible, and the finding of any growth is significant. Alternatively, a catheterized urine specimen may be obtained, recognizing that urethral or perineal bacterial or fungal contamination in these small infants may complicate the assessment of results. In general, the presence of at least 50,000 colonies per milliliter of a single organism is considered a true urinary tract infection, whereas lower colony counts are more indicative of contamination.[54] In addition, microscopic analysis for evidence of pyuria is useful to support its diagnosis. Bag specimens should never be obtained for the evaluation of possible urinary tract infection.

11

A chest radiograph should be obtained if respiratory decompensation is present. A lumbar puncture should generally be performed in infants evaluated for possible late-onset sepsis for reasons stated in answer to Question 2. Risk factors for meningitis in preterm infants include low gestational age and prior bloodstream infection.[19] In VLBW infants, the average age of late-onset meningitis is 26 days (median 19 days; range 4–102 days).[19] Therapeutic decisions with regard to antibiotic choices can be made only if one knows whether the CNS is involved.

Question 4: What Is the Empirical Antimicrobial Choice for Possible Late-Onset Sepsis in the NICU?

In general, antimicrobial therapy for neonatal sepsis is dependent on the agents commonly seen in that particular nursery and their susceptibility pattern. For early-onset sepsis, ampicillin combined with an aminoglycoside, usually gentamicin, has been the empiric therapy of choice since group B *Streptococcus*, other streptococcal species, *Listeria monocytogenes*, and gram-negative bacilli predominate.[16]

For late-onset sepsis, a penicillinase-resistant, semisynthetic penicillin such as oxacillin or nafcillin in combination with an aminoglycoside is the preferred choice.[50,55,56] For CNS infections, nafcillin is preferred because of improved penetration. Because approximately 50% of all bloodstream infections are due to CoNS, some experts recommend vancomycin instead of a semisynthetic penicillin because CoNS are almost uniformly resistant to these agents. This practice has led to widespread use of vancomycin in NICUs with its attendant risk for emergence of vancomycin-resistant organisms.

The use of a penicillinase-resistant penicillin antibiotic such as nafcillin to treat a possible staphylococcal infection in this infant is based on the goal of reducing vancomycin use in NICUs. Clinical experience and intervention trials suggest that such a practice is safe.[55,57–61] Bloodstream infections caused by CoNS are rarely fulminant or fatal, and they are not associated with an increased case-fatality rate over that seen among uninfected VLBW infants.[62] The clinical outcome of CoNS bacteremia is similar whether the initial antibiotic therapy is vancomycin or another agent that does not reliably treat CoNS infections.[58–60] In addition, only one of five evaluations for sepsis yields a causative organism.[62] The observation that more than 80% of blood cultures that yield CoNS are positive by 24 hours of incubation makes it possible for the clinician to change antibiotic therapy in a timely fashion if needed.[63] An additional concern of vancomycin therapy has been the association of prior vancomycin use with subsequent development of gram-negative bacteremia among hospitalized pediatric patients.[64] The emergence of community-associated methicillin-resistant *Staphylococcus aureus* (CA-MRSA) in NICUs may limit the use of such a policy in NICUs where the prevalence of CA-MRSA is high.[61,65–67] However, by routine screening for MRSA and appropriate isolation precautions for colonized infants, MRSA can be controlled if not eradicated in NICUs.[68]

Aminoglycosides have been the time-honored choice for empiric treatment of infections caused by gram-negative bacilli.[69] Once-daily or extended dosing of gentamicin is used frequently in both full-term and preterm infants based on sound pharmacodynamic and pharmacokinetic considerations.[70] Such a dosing schedule may maximize the bactericidal activity of the aminoglycoside while minimizing its potential toxicity. A retrospective review by Jackson et al.[71] reported the occurrence of hypocalcemia in 3.5% of term and near-term newborns who received gentamicin once daily for 4 days or longer after a change in dosing regimen from every 12 hours to every 24 hours. Although it is known that aminoglycosides enhance urinary calcium excretion, it is not known whether this is potentiated by higher doses of gentamicin.

Aminoglycosides have the distinct advantage of exerting less selective pressure for development of resistance in closed units like the NICU, thus minimizing the risk of emergence of resistant bacteria.[72] This is in contrast to the rapid emergence of cephalosporin resistance when these agents are provided routinely for possible late-onset sepsis.[73,74] When used for empirical therapy of early-onset infection, cefotaxime has been associated with increased neonatal mortality.[75] However, because CSF penetration of aminoglycosides is poor, their use in meningitis is problematic. If a lumbar puncture is not performed as part of the initial evaluation for possible sepsis, and only an aminoglycoside is used, then effective therapy for gram-negative meningitis may not be provided. Delay in the determination of whether a neonate has meningitis will delay optimal therapy for this condition.

CONTINUATION OF CASE HISTORY

Within 24 hours of collection, the blood cultures yielded gram-negative rods. Cefotaxime was added to the antibiotic regimen. *E. coli* was subsequently identified from the blood cultures. A lumbar puncture was then performed that demonstrated 4160 white blood cells/mm^3 (90% polymorphonuclear cells, 10% mononuclear cells); 8320 red blood cells/mm^3; protein of 433 mg/dL; and glucose of 84 mg/dL (serum glucose of 180 mg/dL). Culture of CSF yielded *E. coli*.

Question 5: What Is the Treatment of Meningitis in Neonates, Particularly That Caused by Gram-Negative Bacilli?

Table 11.2 provides the recommended antimicrobial treatment for neonatal meningitis based on causative organism.[76] The treatment of gram-negative meningitis initially includes the addition of a third- or fourth-generation cephalosporin such as cefotaxime or cefepime,[77,78] or a carbapenem antibiotic such as meropenem.[69,79,80] Meningitis caused by gram-negative enteric bacilli is challenging because eradication of the organism from CSF is often delayed. Moreover, many of these pathogens are now resistant to ampicillin, and aminoglycoside concentrations are typically low in CSF. Cefotaxime has superior in vitro and CSF bactericidal activity and is the agent of choice. Recently there has been a shortage of cefotaxime in the United States; ceftazidime or cefepime are suitable alternative agents.[81] The cephalosporin agent is combined with an aminoglycoside at least until sterilization of CSF has been achieved. There is no experience or studies using once-daily dosing of aminoglycosides for neonatal meningitis, although from a pharmacodynamic standpoint, such a dosing schedule may be preferred as it should achieve higher CSF concentrations.[69] Continued treatment of gram-negative bacillary meningitis is based on in vitro susceptibility tests. Ampicillin may be used in the infrequent cases when the organism is susceptible.

Of concern is the production by gram-negative bacteria of both chromosomally determined β-lactamases and plasmid-determined extended-spectrum β-lactamases (ESBLs), both of which can result in resistance to the third-generation cephalosporin antibiotics, even during therapy.[82–84] Chromosomally determined β-lactamases are seen in *Enterobacter* spp., *Serratia* spp., *Pseudomonas aeruginosa*, *Citrobacter* spp., and indole-positive *Proteus*, whereas ESBLs are present in the Enterobacteriaceae, especially *Klebsiella pneumoniae* and *E. coli*. Treatment of infections caused by gram-negative bacteria that produce ESBLs with a third-generation cephalosporin such as cefotaxime has been associated with significantly higher mortality in adults.[82] It is therefore recommended that treatment of such infections should be with a carbapenem antibiotic (meropenem or imipenem), possibly in combination with an aminoglycoside.[83] Recently carabapenem resistance has emerged among gram-negative bacilli.[85,86] Studies on the impact of these organisms in NICUs and the appropriate antimicrobial therapy of neonatal infections with these organisms are needed.[87]

The treatment of GBS meningitis is ampicillin or penicillin G. No GBS resistance to penicillin G in the United States has been documented despite its extensive use in mothers and neonates. However, a report from Japan noted the emergence of penicillin resistance among some isolates of group B streptococci.[88] Despite the in vitro resistance of GBS to aminoglycosides, the addition of gentamicin to a

Table 11.2 RECOMMENDED THERAPY FOR NEONATAL MENINGITIS[61]

Meningitis	Therapy[a]	Comment
Initial therapy, CSF abnormal but organism unknown	Ampicillin IV *and* gentamicin IV, IM *and* cefotaxime IV	Cefotaxime is added if meningitis suspected or cannot be excluded. Alternatives to ampicillin in nursery-acquired infections: vancomycin or nafcillin. Alternatives to cefotaxime: ceftazidime, cefepime
Bacteroides fragilis spp. *Fragilis*[b]	Metronidazole IV	Alternative: meropenem
Coliform bacteria[c]	Cefotaxime IV, IM, *and* gentamicin	Discontinue gentamicin when clinical and microbiologic response documented. Alternative: ampicillin if organism susceptible; meropenem or cefepime for multiresistant organisms. Lumbar intrathecal or intraventricular gentamicin usually not beneficial
Chryseobacterium (*Flavobacterium*) *meningosepticum*	Vancomycin IV *and* rifampin IV, PO	Alternatives: clindamycin, ciprofloxacin
Group A streptococcus[d]	Penicillin G *or* ampicillin IV	
Group B streptococcus[b]	Ampicillin *or* penicillin G IV *and* gentamicin IV, IM	Discontinue gentamicin when clinical and microbiologic response documented
Enterococcal spp.[d]	Ampicillin IV, IM, *and* gentamicin IV, IM; for ampicillin-resistant organisms: vancomycin *and* gentamicin	Gentamicin only if synergy documented
Other streptococcal species[d]	Penicillin *or* ampicillin IV, IM	
Gonococcal[e]	Ceftriaxone IV, IM *or* cefotaxime IV, IM	Duration of therapy uncertain (5–10 days?)
Haemophilus influenzae[d]	Cefotaxime IV, IM	Ampicillin if β-lactamase negative
Listeria monocytogenes[d]	Ampicillin IV, IM, *and* gentamicin IV, IM	Gentamicin is synergistic in vitro with ampicillin but can be discontinued when sterilization achieved
Staphylococcus epidermidis (or any coagulase-negative staphylococci)[e]	Vancomycin IV	Add rifampin if cultures persistently positive. Alternative: linezolid
Staphylococcus aureus[c]	MSSA: nafcillin IV; MRSA: vancomycin IV	Gentamicin may provide synergy; rifampin if cultures persistently positive
Pseudomonas aeruginosa[c]	Ceftazidime IV, IM *and* aminoglycoside IV, IM	Meropenem *or* cefepime are suitable alternatives
Candida spp.[f]	Amphotericin B deoxycholate (AmB-D) X 3–6 weeks	Alternatives: AmB-lipid complex, AmB-liposomal, fluconazole for susceptible strains (*Candida krusei* usually resistant). Addition of fluconazole to amphotericin if cultures persistently positive
Ureaplasma spp.[d]	Doxycycline IV *or* azithromycin IV	Alternatives: ciprofloxacin
Mycoplasma hominis[d]	Clindamycin *or* doxycycline IV	Alternatives: ciprofloxacin

[a]Minimum duration of therapy as indicated below:
[b]4 days.
[c]21 days; for gram-negative meningitis, at least 14 days after CSF is sterilized, whichever is longer.
[d]10 days.
[e]7–10 days.
[f]4 weeks (or 30 mg/kg total dose of amphotericin deoxycholate).
IM, Intramuscularly; *IV*, intravenously; *MSSA*: methicillin-susceptible *S. aureus*; *MRSA*: methicillin-resistant *S. aureus*; *O*, orally.
Adapted from Bradley JS, Nelson JD. 2015 *Nelson's Pediatric Antimicrobial Therapy*. 21st ed. Elk Grove Village, IL: American Academy of Pediatrics; 2015.

penicillin agent provides synergy. In general, gentamicin can be discontinued once CSF sterilization is documented by a repeat lumbar puncture performed 24 to 48 hours after initiation of therapy. With more severe cases of meningitis, some experts continue gentamicin for about 1 week; the benefit of such an approach is unproven.

Similar considerations are applicable in the preterm infant in whom meningitis develops while in the NICU. Potential pathogens include *S. aureus*, CoNS, enterococci, and multiply resistant pathogens such as methicillin-resistant *S. aureus* and gentamicin- or cephalosporin-resistant gram-negative enteric bacilli. Empirical therapy may include a combination of ampicillin, nafcillin, or vancomycin and an aminoglycoside, cefotaxime, or even meropenem, depending on the predominant pathogens seen in that NICU. Ceftazidime or meropenem with or without an aminoglycoside should be used for *P. aeruginosa* meningitis. *Chryseobacterium* (formerly *Flavobacterium*) *meningosepticum*, a multiply resistant gram-negative bacilli, is a rare cause of meningitis that requires treatment with vancomycin and rifampin, or even ciprofloxacin.

Meningitis caused by anaerobic bacteria is infrequent and is usually caused by *Bacteroides fragilis* and *Clostridium* spp., mostly *C. perfringens*.[89] The mortality rate is high. Penicillin, ampicillin, cephalosporins, and vancomycin are active against many gram-positive anaerobes. They have little if any activity against most anaerobic gram-negative bacilli; metronidazole is the agent of choice for meningitis secondary to these organisms. Carbapenem antibiotics such as meropenem and imipenem have excellent anaerobic activity against both gram-positive and negative organisms and can also be used.

The treatment of neonatal infections caused by *Ureaplasma urealyticum* and *Mycoplasma hominis* is complicated by the susceptibility patterns of these organisms as they usually are resistant to most antibiotics commonly used in neonates.[90] For infections caused by *U. urealyticum*, doxycycline is recommended, with azithromycin as an alternative. For *M. hominis*, clindamycin or doxycycline is preferred, with ciprofloxacin as an alternative. Although the exact duration of therapy is not known, a 10- to 14-day course seems reasonable when there is associated clinical improvement and microbiologic eradication during that period.

Neonatal fungal infection of the CNS is usually caused by *Candida* species.[91] Amphotericin deoxycholate remains the treatment of choice,[92] and it has been used successfully as monotherapy.[93] Amphotericin B lipid formulations may be used if renal toxicity occurs while the infant is receiving the deoxycholate preparation. Fluconazole has excellent CNS penetration and is frequently added to amphotericin therapy in cases of persistent fungemia or poor clinical response.[94,95] There is limited experience in neonates with the use of newer azoles such as voriconazole that are active against more resistant fungi such as *Candida krusei* and *Candida glabrata*.[96–98] Echinocandins such as caspofungin and micafungin at currently recommended dosages do not penetrate well into the CNS.[99–101]

CONTINUATION OF CASE HISTORY

A lumbar puncture was repeated 24 hours after diagnosis of meningitis and the CSF showed 6900 white blood cells/mm³ (90% polymorphonuclear cells, 10% mononuclear cells); 2400 red blood cells/mm³; protein of 550 mg/dL; and glucose of 21 mg/dL. Culture of CSF again yielded *E. coli* that was resistant to ampicillin but susceptible to cefotaxime, ceftazidime, and gentamicin with minimum inhibitory concentrations of 2 µg/mL.

Question 6: Should Other Therapies Be Considered?

Meningitis secondary to gram-negative bacilli is associated with persistently positive CSF cultures despite appropriate therapy. The median duration of positive CSF cultures is 3 days, and the duration of positivity has correlated with long-term prognosis. In addition, the duration of positive CSF culture will have an impact on the total length of therapy. For these reasons, it is recommended that a repeat lumbar puncture be performed to determine both occurrence and timing of CSF sterilization. The timing of the repeat lumbar puncture will be determined in part by the clinical findings and initial spinal fluid analysis.

Ventriculitis occurs in at least 70% of cases; however, ventricular fluid is poorly accessible to systemically administered antibiotics.[101a] Therefore both lumbar intrathecal and intraventricular gentamicin have been used for treatment of gram-negative meningitis.[102,103] Among infants who received parenteral drug alone or parenteral plus intrathecal therapy (1 mg/day for at least 3 days), no differences in either the case-fatality rate or neurologic residua were observed by the Neonatal Meningitis Cooperative Study Group.[102] These investigators subsequently studied the use of intraventricular gentamicin (2.5 mg); there was higher mortality among infants who received intraventricular gentamicin (43%) in combination with ampicillin and gentamicin than in those who received systemic antibiotics alone (13%).[103] Subsequent evaluation of ventricular fluid from infants who received intraventricular gentamicin showed significantly greater concentrations of tumor necrosis factor and IL-1β in their CSFs, indicating that greater inflammatory injury may result from this form of therapy.[104] In general, intraventricular therapy is not recommended, although it remains an option in those infants who already have a ventricular drain in place and persistently positive CSF cultures.

CONTINUATION OF CASE HISTORY

A cranial ultrasound performed on days 2 and 7 after presentation did not demonstrate abscess formation or new intracranial hemorrhage, but it did show mild ventricular dilatation, and echogenic debris and septations were visualized within the ventricular system (Fig. 11.1). The infant continued to receive cefotaxime and was nearing 21 days of therapy.

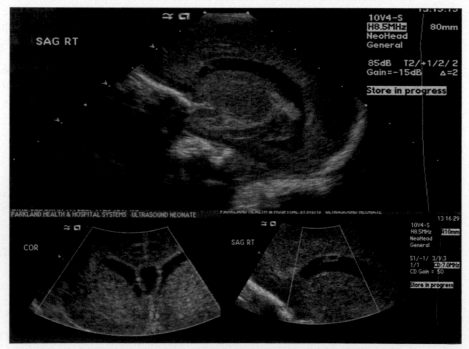

Fig. 11.1   Cranial ultrasound performed on a 2-week-old extremely low-birth-weight infant with meningitis caused by *Escherichia coli*. There are echogenic debris and septation consistent with purulent material within the dilated lateral ventricle.

Question 7: What Is the Duration of Treatment for Meningitis in Neonates?

Unfortunately, there are no randomized studies of duration of antibiotic therapy for neonatal meningitis. In general, duration of therapy is dependent on the causative organism, site(s) of infection, clinical severity, and course. This is usually 7 days for uncomplicated bacteremia, 7 to 10 days for sepsis and pneumonia, and 14 to 21 days for meningitis, depending on the causative agent. Normalization of the C-reactive protein or other inflammatory markers such as IL-8 or IL-10 has been used to discontinue antibiotic therapy in infants with sepsis.[105,106] Although this approach seems reasonable, more studies involving high-risk neonates with serious infections such as meningitis are needed before such a strategy can be recommended routinely.

For meningitis caused by gram-negative bacilli, the duration of antimicrobial therapy is a minimum of 21 days or 2 weeks after the first sterile CSF culture, whichever is longest. Earlier discontinuation of antimicrobial therapy may result in bacterial relapse. Performance of another lumbar puncture after 21 days of treatment in infants with gram-negative enteric meningitis and before discontinuation of antibiotic therapy may be useful to determine the adequacy of therapy. Markedly abnormal CSF findings, such as glucose concentration less than 25 mg/dL, protein content higher than 300 mg/dL, or more than 50% polymorphonuclear cells, without other explanation warrant continued antimicrobial therapy to prevent relapse.

For meningitis caused by group B streptococcus, a minimum of 10 days of antimicrobial therapy is recommended. The decision of whether to perform an "end of therapy" lumbar puncture in these neonates can be based on clinical course. If the infant has experienced complications such as seizures, significant hypotension, or prolonged positive CSF cultures, or if the neuroimaging is abnormal, then it probably is prudent to do it.

The optimal duration of therapy for meningitis caused by other microorganisms is not known. Meningitis secondary to *S. aureus* should be treated with at least 3 weeks of antibiotic therapy. In general, cerebral abscess requires more prolonged therapy of 4 to 6 weeks, depending on whether it is surgically drained or there is persistence of abnormalities on neuroimaging.

Question 8: When Should Neuroimaging Be Considered, and What Type of Examination Is Recommended?

The timing and the reason for performing neuroimaging studies are important considerations in the decision of which type of study should be performed. Cranial ultrasonography is safe, convenient, and readily available; it can be done at the bedside and does not require sedation. It provides rapid and reliable information on ventricular size and whether there is development of hydrocephalus.[107] It is therefore useful to perform an ultrasound early in the course when the infant is too critical to transport to radiology. Cranial ultrasonography also will provide information on periventricular white matter injury; initially, ischemia may be manifested by increased periventricular echogenicity, which may progress to cystic periventricular leukomalacia in later studies (Fig. 11.2).[108,109] Ultrasonography, however, does not allow for optimal evaluation of parenchymal abnormalities such as infarct or abscess nor of presence of subdural empyema, all known complications of neonatal meningitis.

Computed tomography will provide information on whether the course of meningitis has been complicated by a cerebral abscess, hydrocephalus, or subdural collections. In general, however, computed tomography scans should be avoided except when neuroimaging is required on an emergent basis as its use has been associated with subsequent neurodevelopmental impairment and increased risk for cancer.[110,111]

Magnetic resonance imaging (MRI) is the best currently available modality for evaluation of the neonatal brain. It provides excellent information on the status of the white matter, cortex, subdural and epidural spaces, and even the posterior fossa in cases of tuberculous meningitis (Fig. 11.3). In addition, it has been used in preterm infants

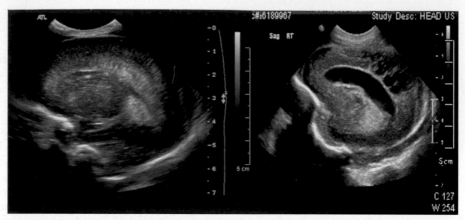

Fig. 11.2   Cranial ultrasound performed on an extremely low-birth-weight infant with meningitis that demonstrates echogenic periventricular white matter *(left)* with subsequent progression to cystic periventricular leukomalacia *(right)*.

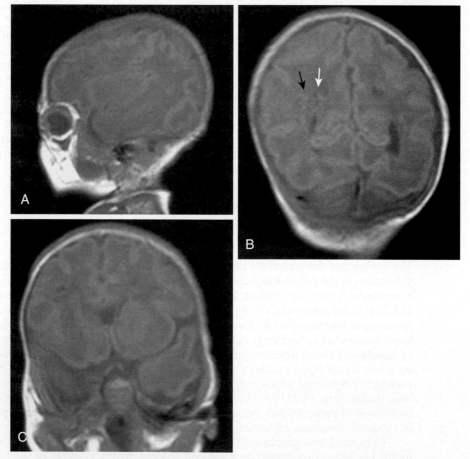

Fig. 11.3   Magnetic resonance imaging of the brain of an infant who 4 weeks earlier had *Pseudomonas aeruginosa* sepsis and meningitis. A, On the T2-weighted images, small foci of high signal are seen in the periventricular white matter in the frontoparietal and occipital regions. These represent areas of cystic encephalomalacia, consistent with periventricular leukomalacia. B, Small foci of hemosiderin deposition *(black arrow)* is seen in the posterior right temporo-occipital region along with cystic encephalomalacia changes *(white arrows)*. C, Coronal image of periventricular white matter.

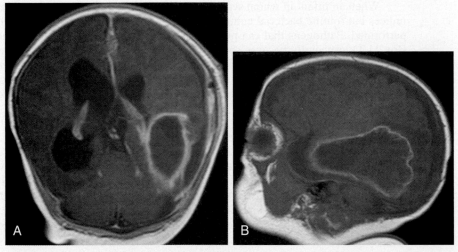

Fig. 11.4 Magnetic resonance image of brain of 3-week-old full-term infant with meningitis and cerebral abscess caused by *Serratia marcescens*. Following gadolinium administration, a large ring-enhancing lesion is seen that extends from the posterior aspect of the temporal lobe into the adjacent parietal and occipital white matter.

to predict neurodevelopmental outcome.[112] For these reasons, infants with suspected cerebral injury either because of abnormalities on ultrasonography, seizures, persistent CSF abnormalities, or meningitis caused by organisms such as *Citrobacter koseri* (formerly *Citrobacter diversus*) or fungi that are associated with abscess formation should have brain MRI performed. Cerebral abscess formation complicates the course of about 70% of cases of *C. koseri* meningitis, whereas it occurs in fewer than 10% of meningitis cases caused by other gram-negative enteric bacilli (Fig. 11.4).[113,114] Microabscesses also are not infrequent with neonatal fungal meningitis. For these reasons, many experts recommend that at least one brain MRI be performed for every case of neonatal meningitis.[115] In addition, all infants with meningitis require hearing evaluation.

Question 9: Should Other Adjunctive Therapies Be Provided to an Infant With Meningitis?

Dexamethasone has been shown in some studies to decrease neurologic morbidity in older infants and children with meningitis.[116–118] No studies are available in neonates, and its use is not recommended. In a rabbit model of *E. coli* meningitis, the addition of dexamethasone to standard antibiotic therapy was associated with an increase in hippocampal neuronal apoptosis.[119]

The prolonged use of broad-spectrum antimicrobial agents, especially third-generation cephalosporins and carbapenems, has been associated with development of systemic candidiasis in preterm infants with birth weight less than 1000 g.[120] Prophylactic fluconazole has been shown to decrease the incidence of candidiasis in these infants,[121–123] and its use should be considered in preterm infants with meningitis who require prolonged broad-spectrum antimicrobial therapy.[124] No data from randomized controlled clinical trials are available in infants with a birth weight greater than 1500 g.

Question 10: What If the Infant's CSF Is Abnormal but Routine Bacterial Cultures of CSF and Blood Are Sterile?

The most frequent reason for a sterile CSF culture despite CSF changes indicative of meningitis is previous antimicrobial therapy. However, intraventricular hemorrhage can result in inflammatory changes such as pleocytosis with predominance of polymorphonuclear cells, elevated protein concentration, and hypoglycorrhachia in the absence of an infectious process, making the performance of a lumbar puncture before initiation of antimicrobial therapy important.

11

When an infant in whom sepsis and meningitis is suspected has abnormal CSF indices but routine bacterial cultures are sterile, a repeat lumbar puncture should be performed. Pathogens that can produce aseptic meningitis should be excluded (see Box 11.1), especially because specific therapy is available for some of them. CSF should be tested for the presence of anaerobic bacteria, *M. hominis*, *Ureaplasma* spp., fungi,[125] and viruses such as herpes simplex, cytomegalovirus,[126] enteroviruses, and parechoviruses by culture or polymerase chain reaction[42] as appropriate.

CONTINUATION OF CASE HISTORY

The infant's CSF evaluation was markedly improved after 21 days of cefotaxime, and MRI examination revealed only mild ventriculomegaly. At discharge to home at 3 months of age, he passed an automated auditory brainstem response test. At 22 months corrected gestational age, he had mild impairment in both mental and psychomotor development indexes by Bayley Scales of Infant Development.

Question 11: What Is the Outcome of Meningitis in Neonates?

Despite improvements in neonatal care and antibiotic therapy, significant morbidity and mortality persist.[127] Among preterm infants with birth weights 1000 g, infants with meningitis are more likely to have low (<70) mental and psychomotor indices, cerebral palsy, vision impairment, and head circumference below the 10th percentile than uninfected infants of similar birth weight and gestation.[128]

Among infants with gram-negative enteric meningitis, the case-fatality rate and morbidity remain high. Approximately 20 T to 30% of affected infants die, and neurologic sequelae are found in 35% to 50% of survivors.[102,103,129] These include hydrocephalus (30%), seizure disorder (30%), developmental delay (30%), cerebral palsy (25%), and hearing loss (15%). Ten percent have severe sequelae defined as failure to develop beyond the age at which the disease occurred or requirement of custodial care. It is hoped that prediction of late morbidity will be aided by the use of brain MRI performed toward the end of therapy.

Among infants with GBS meningitis, the mortality rate is about 25%, and among survivors, another 25% to 30% of children have major neurologic sequelae such as spastic quadriplegia, profound intellectual disability, hemiparesis, deafness, or cortical blindness; 15% to 20% have mild to moderate sequelae, and 50% to 60% are normal compared with sibling controls.[130,131] The occurrence of seizures during the acute illness has been associated with a poor prognosis; these children are more likely to die or sustain major sequelae. On the other hand, children not identified early as having major sequelae performed intellectually, socially, and academically in a manner similar to other family members.

Conclusion

Meningitis is a serious infection for which early therapy is mandatory to improve both short- and long-term outcomes. This is possible only by the timely recognition of its occurrence, thus making performance of a lumbar puncture for CSF analysis and culture the key to rapid institution of effective antimicrobial therapy. Ultimately, however, its prevention will be achieved when neonatal sepsis is controlled, an elusive but not impossible goal in neonatal medicine.[132]

REFERENCES

1. Kaufman D, Fairchild KD. Clinical microbiology of bacterial and fungal sepsis in very-low-birth-weight infants. *Clin Microbiol Rev*. 2004;17(3):638–680.
2. Palazzi DL, Klein JO, Baker CJ. Bacterial sepsis and meningitis. In: Remington JS, Klein JO, Wilson CB, Baker CJ, eds. *Infectious Diseases of the Fetus and Newborn Infant*. 6th ed. Philadelphia: WB Saunders; 2006:247–295.

11

3. Giacoia GP. Uncommon pathogens in newborn infants. *J Perinatol.* 1994;14(2):134–144.
4. Cantey JB, Milstone AM. Bloodstream infections: epidemiology and resistance. *Clin Perinatol.* 2015;42(1):1–16, vii.
5. Cantey JB, Farris AC, McCormick SM. Bacteremia in early infancy: etiology and management. *Curr Infect Dis Rep.* 2016;18(1):1.
6. Cantey JB. Optimizing the use of antibacterial agents in the neonatal period. *Pediatr Drugs.* 2016;18(2):109–122.
7. Schrag S, Gorwitz R, Fultz-Butts K, et al. Prevention of perinatal group B streptococcal disease. Revised guidelines from CDC. *MMWR Recomm Rep.* 2002;51(RR-11):1–22.
8. Cetinkaya M, Cekmez F, Buyukkale G, et al. Lower vitamin D levels are associated with increased risk of early-onset neonatal sepsis in term infants. *J Perinatol.* 2015;35(1):39–45.
9. Johnson CE, Whitwell JK, Pethe K, et al. Term newborns who are at risk for sepsis: are lumbar punctures necessary? *Pediatrics.* 1997;99(4):E10.
10. Smith PB, Cotten CM, Garges HP, et al. A comparison of neonatal gram-negative rod and gram-positive cocci meningitis. *J Perinatol.* 2006;26(2):111–114.
11. Schrag SJ, Zywicki S, Farley MM, et al. Group B streptococcal disease in the era of intrapartum antibiotic prophylaxis. *N Engl J Med.* 2000;342(1):15–20.
12. Verani JR, McGee L, Schrag SJ. Prevention of perinatal group B streptococcal disease–revised guidelines from CDC, 2010. *MMWR Recomm Rep.* 2010;59(RR-10):1–36.
13. Schrag SJ, Hadler JL, Arnold KE, et al. Risk factors for invasive, early-onset *Escherichia coli* infections in the era of widespread intrapartum antibiotic use. *Pediatrics.* 2006;118(2):570–576.
14. Baltimore RS, Huie SM, Meek JI, et al. Early-onset neonatal sepsis in the era of group B streptococcal prevention. *Pediatrics.* 2001;108(5):1094–1098.
15. Stoll BJ, Hansen N, Fanaroff AA, et al. Changes in pathogens causing early-onset sepsis in very-low-birth-weight infants. *N Engl J Med.* 2002;347(4):240–247.
16. Stoll BJ, Hansen NI, Sanchez PJ, et al. Early onset neonatal sepsis: the burden of group B streptococcal and *E. coli* disease continues. *Pediatrics.* 2011;127(5):817–826.
17. Stoll BJ, Hansen NI, Higgins RD, et al. Very low birth weight preterm infants with early onset neonatal sepsis: the predominance of gram-negative infections continues in the National Institute of Child Health and Human Development Neonatal Research Network, 2002–2003. *Pediatr Infect Dis J.* 2005;24(7):635–639.
18. Garges HP, Moody MA, Cotten CM, et al. Neonatal meningitis: what is the correlation among cerebrospinal fluid cultures, blood cultures, and cerebrospinal fluid parameters? *Pediatrics.* 2006;117(4):1094–1100.
19. Stoll BJ, Hansen N, Fanaroff AA, et al. To tap or not to tap: high likelihood of meningitis without sepsis among very low birth weight infants. *Pediatrics.* 2004;113(5):1181–1186.
20. Cohen-Wolkowiez M, Smith PB, Mangum B, et al. Neonatal Candida meningitis: significance of cerebrospinal fluid parameters and blood cultures. *J Perinatol.* 2007;27(2):97–100.
21. Wiswell TE, Baumgart S, Gannon CM, et al. No lumbar puncture in the evaluation for early neonatal sepsis: will meningitis be missed? *Pediatrics.* 1995;95(6):803–806.
22. Malbon K, Mohan R, Nicholl R. Should a neonate with possible late onset infection always have a lumbar puncture? *Arch Dis Child.* 2006;91(1):75–76.
23. Ahmed A, Hickey SM, Ehrett S, et al. Cerebrospinal fluid values in the term neonate. *Pediatr Infect Dis J.* 1996;15(4):298–303.
24. Bonadio WA. The cerebrospinal fluid: physiologic aspects and alterations associated with bacterial meningitis. *Pediatr Infect Dis J.* 1992;11(6):423–431.
25. Pappu LD, Purohit DM, Levkoff AH, et al. CSF cytology in the neonate. *Am J Dis Child.* 1982;136(4):297–298.
26. Portnoy JM, Olson LC. Normal cerebrospinal fluid values in children: another look. *Pediatrics.* 1985;75(3):484–487.
27. Rodriguez AF, Kaplan SL, Mason EO Jr. Cerebrospinal fluid values in the very low birth weight infant. *J Pediatr.* 1990;116(6):971–974.
28. Sarff LD, Platt LH, McCracken GH Jr. Cerebrospinal fluid evaluation in neonates: comparison of high-risk infants with and without meningitis. *J Pediatr.* 1976;88(3):473–477.
29. Naidoo BT. The cerebrospinal fluid in the healthy newborn infant. *S Afr Med J.* 1968;42(35):933–935.
30. O'Shea TM, Klinepeter KL, Meis PJ, Dillard RG. Intrauterine infection and the risk of cerebral palsy in very low-birthweight infants. *Paediatr Perinat Epidemiol.* 1998;12(1):72–83.
31. Eldadah M, Frenkel LD, Hiatt IM, et al. Evaluation of routine lumbar punctures in newborn infants with respiratory distress syndrome. *Pediatr Infect Dis J.* 1987;6(3):243–246.
32. Hendricks-Munoz KD, Shapiro DL. The role of the lumbar puncture in the admission sepsis evaluation of the premature infant. *J Perinatol.* 1990;10(1):60–64.
33. MacMahon P, Jewes L, de Louvois J. Routine lumbar punctures in the newborn–are they justified? *Eur J Pediatr.* 1990;149(11):797–799.
34. Weiss MG, Ionides SP, Anderson CL. Meningitis in premature infants with respiratory distress: role of admission lumbar puncture. *J Pediatr.* 1991;119(6):973–975.
35. Isaacs D, Dobson S. When to do a lumbar puncture in a neonate. *Arch Dis Child.* 1989;64(10):1513–1514.
36. Bergin SP, Thaden JT, Ericson JE, et al. Neonatal *Escherichia coli* bloodstream infections: clinical outcomes and impact of initial antibiotic therapy. *Pediatr Infect Dis J.* 2015;34(9):933–936.
37. Laborada G, Rego M, Jain A, et al. Diagnostic value of cytokines and C-reactive protein in the first 24 hours of neonatal sepsis. *Am J Perinatol.* 2003;20(8):491–501.

38. Verboon-Maciolek MA, Thijsen SF, Hemels MA, et al. Inflammatory mediators for the diagnosis and treatment of sepsis in early infancy. *Pediatr Res.* 2006;59(3):457–461.
39. Manroe BL, Weinberg AG, Rosenfeld CR, Browne R. The neonatal blood count in health and disease. I. Reference values for neutrophilic cells. *J Pediatr.* 1979;95(1):89–98.
40. Mouzinho A, Rosenfeld CR, Sanchez PJ, Risser R. Revised reference ranges for circulating neutrophils in very-low-birth-weight neonates. *Pediatrics.* 1994;94(1):76–82.
41. Engle WD, Rosenfeld CR, Mouzinho A, et al. Circulating neutrophils in septic preterm neonates: comparison of two reference ranges. *Pediatrics.* 1997;99(3):E10.
42. Arora HS, Asmar BI, Salimnia H, Agarwal P, Chawla S, Abdel-Haq N. Enhanced identification of group B streptococcus and *Escherichia coli* in young infants with meningitis using the biofire filmarray meningitis/encephalitis panel. *Pediatr Infect Dis J.* 2017.
43. Christensen RD, Brown MS, Hall DC, et al. Effect on neutrophil kinetics and serum opsonic capacity of intravenous administration of immune globulin to neonates with clinical signs of early-onset sepsis. *J Pediatr.* 1991;118(4 (Pt 1):606–614.
44. Christensen RD, Calhoun DA, Rimsza LM. A practical approach to evaluating and treating neutropenia in the neonatal intensive care unit. *Clin Perinatol.* 2000;27(3):577–601.
45. Ohlsson A, Lacy JB. Intravenous immunoglobulin for suspected or proven infection in neonates. *Cochrane Database Syst Rev.* 2015;3:CD001239.
46. Cairo MS, Worcester CC, Rucker RW, et al. Randomized trial of granulocyte transfusions versus intravenous immune globulin therapy for neonatal neutropenia and sepsis. *J Pediatr.* 1992;120(2 Pt 1):281–285.
47. Shaw CK, Thapalial A, Shaw P, et al. Intravenous immunoglobulins and haematopoietic growth factors in the prevention and treatment of neonatal sepsis: ground reality or glorified myths? *Int J Clin Pract.* 2007;61(3):482–487.
48. Benjamin DK Jr, DeLong ER, Steinbach WJ, et al. Empirical therapy for neonatal candidemia in very low birth weight infants. *Pediatrics.* 2003;112(3 Pt 1):543–547.
49. Struthers S, Underhill H, Albersheim S, et al. A comparison of two versus one blood culture in the diagnosis and treatment of coagulase-negative staphylococcus in the neonatal intensive care unit. *J Perinatol.* 2002;22(7):547–549.
50. Rubin LG, Sanchez PJ, Siegel J, et al. Evaluation and treatment of neonates with suspected late-onset sepsis: a survey of neonatologists' practices. *Pediatrics.* 2002;110(4):e42.
51. Cantey JB, Wozniak PS, Pruszynski JE, et al. Reducing unnecessary antibiotic use in the neonatal intensive care unit (SCOUT): a prospective interrupted time-series study. *Lancet Infect Dis.* 2016;16(10):1178–1184.
52. Bauer S, Eliakim A, Pomeranz A, et al. Urinary tract infection in very low birth weight preterm infants. *Pediatr Infect Dis J.* 2003;22(5):426–430.
53. Practice parameter. The diagnosis, treatment, and evaluation of the initial urinary tract infection in febrile infants and young children. American Academy of Pediatrics. Committee on Quality Improvement. Subcommittee on Urinary Tract Infection. *Pediatrics.* 1999;103(4 Pt 1):843–852.
54. Roberts KB. Urinary tract infection: clinical practice guideline for the diagnosis and management of the initial UTI in febrile infants and children 2 to 24 months. *Pediatrics.* 2011;128(3):595–610.
55. Sanchez PJ. Bacterial and fungal infections in the neonate: current diagnosis and therapy. *Adv Exp Med Biol.* 2004;549:97–103.
56. Sanchez PJ, Moallem M, Cantey JB, et al. Empiric therapy with vancomycin in the neonatal intensive care unit: let's "get smart" globally! *J Pediatr.* 2016;92(5):432–435.
57. Karlowicz MG, Buescher ES, Surka AE. Fulminant late-onset sepsis in a neonatal intensive care unit, 1988–1997, and the impact of avoiding empiric vancomycin therapy. *Pediatrics.* 2000;106(6):1387–1390.
58. Krediet TG, Jones ME, Gerards LJ, et al. Clinical outcome of cephalothin versus vancomycin therapy in the treatment of coagulase-negative staphylococcal septicemia in neonates: relation to methicillin resistance and mec A gene carriage of blood isolates. *Pediatrics.* 1999;103(3):E29.
59. Lawrence SL, Roth V, Slinger R, et al. Cloxacillin versus vancomycin for presumed late-onset sepsis in the Neonatal Intensive Care Unit and the impact upon outcome of coagulase negative staphylococcal bacteremia: a retrospective cohort study. *BMC Pediatr.* 2005;5:49.
60. Chiu CH, Michelow IC, Cronin J, et al. Effectiveness of a guideline to reduce vancomycin use in the neonatal intensive care unit. *Pediatr Infect Dis J.* 2011;30(4):273–278.
61. Thaden JT, Ericson JE, Cross H, et al. Survival benefit of empirical therapy for *Staphylococcus aureus* bloodstream infections in infants. *Pediatr Infect Dis J.* 2015;34(11):1175–1179.
62. Stoll BJ, Hansen N, Fanaroff AA, et al. Late-onset sepsis in very low birth weight neonates: the experience of the NICHD Neonatal Research Network. *Pediatrics.* 2002;110(2 Pt 1):285–291.
63. Garcia-Prats JA, Cooper TR, Schneider VF, et al. Rapid detection of microorganisms in blood cultures of newborn infants utilizing an automated blood culture system. *Pediatrics.* 2000;105(3 Pt 1):523–527.
64. Van Houten MA, Uiterwaal CS, Heesen GJ, et al. Does the empiric use of vancomycin in pediatrics increase the risk for gram-negative bacteremia? *Pediatr Infect Dis J.* 2001;20(2):171–177.
65. Healy CM, Hulten KG, Palazzi DL, et al. Emergence of new strains of methicillin-resistant *Staphylococcus aureus* in a neonatal intensive care unit. *Clin Infect Dis.* 2004;39(10):1460–1466.
66. Chuang YY, Huang YC, Lee CY, et al. Methicillin-resistant *Staphylococcus aureus* bacteraemia in neonatal intensive care units: an analysis of 90 episodes. *Acta Paediatr.* 2004;93(6):786–790.
67. Shane AL, Hansen NI, Stoll BJ, et al. Methicillin-resistant and susceptible *Staphylococcus aureus* bacteremia and meningitis in preterm infants. *Pediatrics.* 2012;129(4):e914–e922.

11

68. Haley RW, Cushion NB, Tenover FC, et al. Eradication of endemic methicillin-resistant *Staphylococcus aureus* infections from a neonatal intensive care unit. *J Infect Dis.* 1995; 171(3):614–624.

69. de Hoog M, Mouton JW, van den Anker JN. New dosing strategies for antibacterial agents in the neonate. *Semin Fetal Neonatal Med.* 2005;10(2):185–194.

70. Nestaas E, Bangstad HJ, Sandvik L, Wathne KO. Aminoglycoside extended interval dosing in neonates is safe and effective: a meta-analysis. *Arch Dis Child Fetal Neonatal Ed.* 2005;90(4): F294–F300.

71. Jackson GL, Sendelbach DM, Stehel EK, et al. Association of hypocalcemia with a change in gentamicin administration in neonates. *Pediatr Nephrol.* 2003;18(7):653–656.

72. de Man P, Verhoeven BA, Verbrugh HA, et al. An antibiotic policy to prevent emergence of resistant bacilli. *Lancet.* 2000;355(9208):973–978.

73. Acolet D, Ahmet Z, Houang E, et al. Enterobacter cloacae in a neonatal intensive care unit: account of an outbreak and its relationship to use of third generation cephalosporins. *J Hosp Infect.* 1994;28(4):273–286.

74. Bryan CS, John JF Jr, Pai MS, et al. Gentamicin vs cefotaxime for therapy of neonatal sepsis. Relationship to drug resistance. *Am J Dis Child (1960).* 1985; 139(11):1086–1089.

75. Clark RH, Bloom BT, Spitzer AR, Gerstmann DR. Empiric use of ampicillin and cefotaxime, compared with ampicillin and gentamicin, for neonates at risk for sepsis is associated with an increased risk of neonatal death. *Pediatrics.* 2006;117(1):67–74.

76. Bradley J, Nelson J. *2015 Nelson's Pediatric Antimicrobial Therapy.* 21st ed. Elk Grove Village, IL: American Academy of Pediatrics; 2015.

77. Ellis JM, Rivera L, Reyes G, et al. Cefepime cerebrospinal fluid concentrations in neonatal bacterial meningitis (May). *Ann Pharmacother.* 2007.

78. Capparelli E, Hochwald C, Rasmussen M, et al. Population pharmacokinetics of cefepime in the neonate. *Antimicrob Agents Chemother.* 2005;49(7):2760–2766.

79. Shah D, Narang M. Meropenem. *Indian Pediatr.* 2004;42:443–450.

80. Odio CM, Puig JR, Feris JM, et al. Prospective, randomized, investigator-blinded study of the efficacy and safety of meropenem vs. cefotaxime therapy in bacterial meningitis in children. Meropenem Meningitis Study Group. *Pediatr Infect Dis J.* 1999;18(7):581–590.

81. Arnold CJ, Ericson J, Cho N, et al. Cefepime and ceftazidime safety in hospitalized infants. *Pediatr Infect Dis J.* 2015;34(9):964–968.

82. Wong-Beringer A, Hindler J, Loeloff M, et al. Molecular correlation for the treatment outcomes in bloodstream infections caused by *Escherichia coli* and *Klebsiella pneumoniae* with reduced susceptibility to ceftazidime. *Clin Infect Dis.* 2002;34(2):135–146.

83. Patterson JE. Extended spectrum beta-lactamases: a therapeutic dilemma. *Pediatr Infect Dis J.* 2002;21(10):957–959.

84. Sinha AK, Kempley ST, Price E, et al. Early onset *Morganella morganii* sepsis in a newborn infant with emergence of cephalosporin resistance caused by depression of AMPC beta-lactamase production. *Pediatr Infect Dis J.* 2006;25(4):376–377.

85. Zerr DM, Weissman SJ, Zhou C, et al. The molecular and clinical epidemiology of extended-spectrum cephalosporin- and carbapenem-resistant enterobacteriaceae at 4 US pediatric hospitals. *J Pediatric Infect Dis Soc.* 2017.

86. Datta S, Roy S, Chatterjee S, et al. A five-year experience of carbapenem resistance in Enterobacteriaceae causing neonatal septicaemia: predominance of NDM-1. *PLoS One.* 2014;9(11): e112101.

87. Folgori L, Bielicki J, Heath PT, et al. Antimicrobial-resistant gram-negative infections in neonates: burden of disease and challenges in treatment. *Curr Opin Infect Dis.* 2017.

88. Kimura KWJ, Kurokawa H, Suzuki S, et al. Emergence of penicillin-resistant group B streptococci. Paper presented at: 46th Annual Interscience Conference on antimicrobial agents and chemotherapy (ICAAC™); 2006; San Francisco, CA.

89. Brook I. Anaerobic infections in the neonate. *Adv Pediatr.* 1994;41:369–383.

90. Cassell GH, Waites KB, Watson HL, et al. Ureaplasma urealyticum intrauterine infection: role in prematurity and disease in newborns. *Clin Microbiol Rev.* 1993;6(1):69–87.

91. Fernandez M, Moylett EH, Noyola DE, et al. Candidal meningitis in neonates: a 10-year review. *Clin Infect Dis.* 2000;31(2):458–463.

92. Frattarelli DA, Reed MD, Giacoia GP, et al. Antifungals in systemic neonatal candidiasis. *Drugs.* 2004;64(9):949–968.

93. Butler KM, Rench MA, Baker CJ. Amphotericin B as a single agent in the treatment of systemic candidiasis in neonates. *Pediatr Infect Dis J.* 1990;9(1):51–56.

94. Gurses N, Kalayci AG. Fluconazole monotherapy for candidal meningitis in a premature infant. *Clin Infect Dis.* 1996;23(3):645–646.

95. Black KE, Baden LR. Fungal infections of the CNS: treatment strategies for the immunocompromised patient. *CNS Drugs.* 2007;21(4):293–318.

96. Steinbach WJ, Benjamin DK. New antifungal agents under development in children and neonates. *Curr Opin Infect Dis.* 2005;18(6):484–489.

97. Santos RP, Sanchez PJ, Mejias A, et al. Successful medical treatment of cutaneous aspergillosis in a premature infant using liposomal amphotericin B, voriconazole and micafungin. *Pediatr Infect Dis J.* 2007;26(4):364–366.

98. Watt K, Manzoni P, Cohen-Wolkowiez M, et al. Triazole use in the nursery: fluconazole, voriconazole, posaconazole, and ravuconazole. *Curr Drug Metab.* 2013;14(2):193–202.

11

99. Odio CM, Araya R, Pinto LE, et al. Caspofungin therapy of neonates with invasive candidiasis. *Pediatr Infect Dis J*. 2004;23(12):1093–1097.

100. Heresi GP, Gerstmann DR, Reed MD, et al. The pharmacokinetics and safety of micafungin, a novel echinocandin, in premature infants. *Pediatr Infect Dis J*. 2006;25(12):1110–1115.

101. Manzoni P, Wu C, Tweddle L, et al. Micafungin in premature and non-premature infants: a systematic review of 9 clinical trials. *Pediatr Infect Dis J*. 2014;33(11):e291–e298.

101a. Lee EL, Robinson MJ, Thong ML, Puthucheary SD, Ong TH, Ng KK. Intraventricular chemotherapy in neonatal meningitis. *J Pediatr*. 1977;91(6):991–995.

102. McCracken GH Jr, Mize SG. A controlled study of intrathecal antibiotic therapy in gram-negative enteric meningitis of infancy. Report of the neonatal meningitis cooperative study group. *J Pediatr*. 1976;89(1):66–72.

103. McCracken GH Jr, Mize SG, Threlkeld N. Intraventricular gentamicin therapy in gram-negative bacillary meningitis of infancy. Report of the second neonatal meningitis cooperative study group. *Lancet*. 1980;1(8172):787–791.

104. McCracken GH Jr, Mustafa MM, Ramilo O, et al. Cerebrospinal fluid interleukin 1-beta and tumor necrosis factor concentrations and outcome from neonatal gram-negative enteric bacillary meningitis. *Pediatr Infect Dis J*. 1989;8(3):155–159.

105. Franz AR, Steinbach G, Kron M, et al. Reduction of unnecessary antibiotic therapy in newborn infants using interleukin-8 and C-reactive protein as markers of bacterial infections. *Pediatrics*. 1999;104(3 Pt 1):447–453.

106. Franz AR, Bauer K, Schalk A, et al. Measurement of interleukin 8 in combination with C-reactive protein reduced unnecessary antibiotic therapy in newborn infants: a multicenter, randomized, controlled trial. *Pediatrics*. 2004;114(1):1–8.

107. Perlman JM, Rollins N, Sanchez PJ. Late-onset meningitis in sick, very-low-birth-weight infants. Clinical and sonographic observations. *Am J Dis Child (1960)*. 1992; 146(11):1297–1301.

108. Faix RG, Donn SM. Association of septic shock caused by early-onset group B streptococcal sepsis and periventricular leukomalacia in the preterm infant. *Pediatrics*. 1985;76(3):415–419.

109. Perlman JM. White matter injury in the preterm infant: an important determination of abnormal neurodevelopment outcome. *Early Hum Dev*. 1998;53(2):99–120.

110. Brenner DJ. Estimating cancer risks from pediatric CT: going from the qualitative to the quantitative. *Pediatr Radiol*. 2002;32(4). 228–223; discussion 242–224.

111. Frush DP, Donnelly LF, Rosen NS. Computed tomography and radiation risks: what pediatric health care providers should know. *Pediatrics*. 2003;112(4):951–957.

112. Woodward LJ, Anderson PJ, Austin NC, et al. Neonatal MRI to predict neurodevelopmental outcomes in preterm infants. *N Engl J Med*. 2006;355(7):685–694.

113. Graham DR, Band JD. *Citrobacter diversus* brain abscess and meningitis in neonates. *JAMA*. 1981;245(19):1923–1925.

114. Doran TI. The role of *Citrobacter* in clinical disease of children: review. *Clin Infect Dis*. 1999;28(2): 384–394.

115. Oliveira CR, Morriss MC, Mistrot JG, et al. Brain magnetic resonance imaging of infants with bacterial meningitis. *J Pediatr*. 2014;165(1):134–139.

116. Lebel MH, Freij BJ, Syrogiannopoulos GA, et al. Dexamethasone therapy for bacterial meningitis. Results of two double-blind, placebo-controlled trials. *N Engl J Med*. 1988;319(15):964–971.

117. Schaad UB, Kaplan SL, McCracken GH Jr. Steroid therapy for bacterial meningitis. *Clin Infect Dis*. 1995;20(3):685–690.

118. Wald ER, Kaplan SL, Mason EO Jr, et al. Dexamethasone therapy for children with bacterial meningitis. Meningitis Study Group. *Pediatrics*. 1995;95(1):21–28.

119. Spreer A, Gerber J, Hanssen M, et al. Dexamethasone increases hippocampal neuronal apoptosis in a rabbit model of *Escherichia coli* meningitis. *Pediatr Res*. 2006;60(2):210–215.

120. Cotten CM, McDonald S, Stoll B, et al. The association of third-generation cephalosporin use and invasive candidiasis in extremely low birth-weight infants. *Pediatrics*. 2006;118(2):717–722.

121. Kaufman D, Boyle R, Hazen KC, et al. Fluconazole prophylaxis against fungal colonization and infection in preterm infants. *N Engl J Med*. 2001;345(23):1660–1666.

122. Manzoni P, Stolfi I, Pugni L, et al. A multicenter, randomized trial of prophylactic fluconazole in preterm neonates. *N Engl J Med*. 2007;356(24):2483–2495.

123. Benjamin DK Jr, Hudak ML, Duara S, et al. Effect of fluconazole prophylaxis on candidiasis and mortality in premature infants: a randomized clinical trial. *JAMA*. 2014;311(17):1742–1749.

124. Uko S, Soghier LM, Vega M, et al. Targeted short-term fluconazole prophylaxis among very low birth weight and extremely low birth weight infants. *Pediatrics*. 2006;117(4):1243–1252.

125. Salvatore CM, Chen TK, Toussi SS, et al. (1→3)-β-D-Glucan in cerebrospinal fluid as a biomarker for *candida* and *aspergillus* infections of the central nervous system in pediatric patients. *J Pediatric Infect Dis Soc*. 2016;5(3):277–286.

126. Vicetti Miguel CP, Mejias A, Ramilo O, et al. Cytomegalovirus meningitis in an infant with severe combined immunodeficiency. *J Pediatr*. 2016;173:235–237.

127. de Louvois J, Halket S, Harvey D. Neonatal meningitis in England and Wales: sequelae at 5 years of age. *Eur J Pediatr*. 2005;164(12):730–734.

128. Stoll BJ, Hansen NI, Adams-Chapman I, et al. Neurodevelopmental and growth impairment among extremely low-birth-weight infants with neonatal infection. *JAMA*. 2004;292(19):2357–2365.

129. Unhanand M, Mustafa MM, McCracken GH Jr, Nelson JD. Gram-negative enteric bacillary meningitis: a twenty-one-year experience. *J Pediatr*. 1993;122(1):15–21.

130. Edwards MS, Rench MA, Haffar AA, et al. Long-term sequelae of group B streptococcal meningitis in infants. *J Pediatr.* 1985;106(5):717–722.
131. Wald ER, Bergman I, Taylor HG, et al. Long-term outcome of group B streptococcal meningitis. *Pediatrics.* 1986;77(2):217–221.
132. Cantey JB, Ronchi A, Sanchez PJ. Spreading the benefits of infection prevention in the neonatal intensive care unit. *JAMA Pediatr.* 2015;169(12):1089–1091.

11

CHAPTER 12

Neonatal Herpes Simplex Virus, Congenital Cytomegalovirus, and Congenital Zika Virus Infections

Nazia Kabani and David W. Kimberlin

- After reading this chapter, readers will be familiar with the epidemiology of congenital infections such as CMV, HSV, and Zika virus.
- Risk factors for acquiring these infections are discussed.
- Clinical manifestations, diagnosis, treatment, and clinical outcomes are also discussed in detail.

Among the numerous viral pathogens that cause central nervous system (CNS) infections in the neonatal period, herpes simplex virus (HSV) and cytomegalovirus (CMV) are unique in their therapeutic management. Both have commercially available antiviral drugs that treat the virus, as well as evidence-based data documenting the benefit of antiviral therapy. Neonatal HSV infection primarily is acquired in the peripartum period, whereas congenital CMV infection is the most common viral infection acquired in utero. Utilization of antiviral therapy to improve disease outcomes is influenced by these differences, with antiviral therapy of neonatal HSV disease aimed primarily at improving mortality and antiviral therapy of congenital CMV infections targeting improvement in longer-term audiologic outcomes. Additionally, the extent of data and clinical experience differs between the two viruses, with antiviral treatment of neonatal HSV disease required in all cases, but antiviral management of congenital CMV infection an option rather than a requirement.

The studies conducted by the National Institute of Allergy and Infectious Diseases (NIAID) Collaborative Antiviral Study Group (CASG) over the past 30 years have defined the benefits and toxicities of antiviral treatment of neonatal HSV and congenital CMV. In conducting controlled investigations of these rare infections, the CASG also has characterized the natural history of infection with these viruses in neonates. These advances in our understanding of neonatal HSV and congenital CMV disease not only provide the foundation for advances in the management of these infections, but also establish the scope through which newly recognized congenital infections such as Zika are appreciated. Unlike HSV and CMV, which are transmitted person to person, Zika virus is unique among the viruses that cause congenital infections by being mosquito-borne. When a pregnant mother acquires a primary Zika infection, the virus can cross the placenta to infect the developing fetus, with devastating consequences, including microcephaly, tremendous brain abnormalities, and even fetal loss. While much about congenital Zika virus infection remains to be elucidated, what we know already draws heavily from existing knowledge of congenital CMV and even rubella disease. It is quite likely that treatment options for Zika, as they are developed, likewise will build on the expertise of the CASG and other groups of investigators with antiviral trial design and assessment.

Question 1: When Does Infection Occur?

Neonatal HSV Disease

HSV disease of the newborn is acquired during one of three distinct times: intrauterine (in utero), peripartum (perinatal), and postpartum (postnatal). Among infected infants, the time of transmission for the majority (~85%) of neonates is in the peripartum period.[1] An additional 10% of infected neonates acquire the virus postnatally, and the final 5% are infected with HSV in utero.[1]

Congenital CMV Infection

CMV infection also can occur at any of these three distinct times (intrauterine, peripartum, and postpartum). Congenital infection, though, is synonymous with in utero acquisition, and is clearly associated with long-term morbidity. In contrast, peripartum transmission can produce acute illness, but rarely if ever results in long-term sequelae. Infection of women both immediately before and during pregnancy puts the fetus at risk for congenital CMV infection.[2,3] In utero transmission occurs after primary maternal infection, as is the case with toxoplasmosis, rubella, and Zika (see later text), and also in recurrent infections, including reinfection with a different strain of the virus[4] or reactivation of latent virus.[5]

Congenital Zika Infection

Zika virus infection, although not common in the mainland United States, currently is very common in South America, Africa, and parts of Asia. Congenital Zika, like congenital CMV, is acquired most often in utero.[6] This happens when a pregnant woman acquires Zika for the first time from the bite of an infected mosquito. The resulting primary infection can cross the placenta and infect the developing fetus.[6]

Question 2: What Are the Risk Factors for Neonatal Infection?

Neonatal HSV Disease

The following five factors are known to influence transmission of HSV from mother to neonate:
1. Type of maternal infection (primary vs. recurrent)[7–11]
2. Maternal antibody status[11–14]
3. Duration of rupture of membranes[10]
4. Integrity of mucocutaneous barriers (e.g., use of fetal scalp electrodes)[11,15,16]
5. Mode of delivery (cesarean section vs. vaginal)[11]

Infants born to mothers who have a first episode of genital HSV infection near term are at much greater risk of developing neonatal herpes than are those whose mothers have recurrent genital herpes.[7–11] This increased risk is due both to lower concentrations of transplacentally passaged HSV-specific antibodies (which also are less reactive to expressed polypeptides) in women with primary infection,[13] and to the higher quantities of HSV that are shed for longer periods of time in the maternal genital tract when compared with women with recurrent genital HSV infection.[17]

The largest assessment of the influence of type of maternal infection on likelihood of neonatal transmission is a landmark study involving almost 60,000 women in labor who did not have clinical evidence of genital HSV infection, ~40,000 of whom had cultures performed within 48 hours of delivery (Fig. 12.1). Of these, 121 women were identified who both were asymptomatically shedding HSV and for whom sera were available for serologic analysis. In this large trial, 57% of infants delivered to women with first-episode primary infection developed neonatal HSV disease, compared with 25% of infants delivered to women with first-episode nonprimary infection and 2% of infants delivered to women with recurrent HSV disease (see Fig. 12.1).[11]

The duration of rupture of membranes and mode of deliver also appear to affect the risk for acquisition of neonatal infection. A small study published in 1971 demonstrated that cesarean delivery in a woman with active genital lesions can reduce the infant's risk of acquiring HSV if performed within 4 hours of rupture of membrane.[10] Based on this observation, it has been recommended for more than four decades that women with active genital lesions at the time of onset of labor be delivered by cesarean section.[18] It was not until 2003, however, that cesarean delivery was definitively proven to be effective in the prevention of HSV transmission to the neonate from a mother actively shedding virus from the genital tract.[11] Importantly,

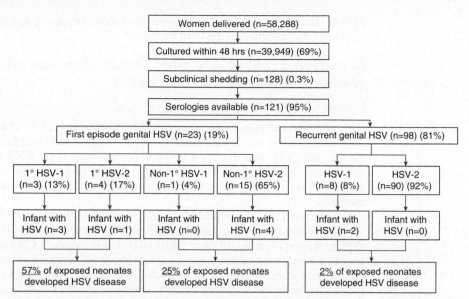

Fig. 12.1 Risk of neonatal herpes simplex virus *(HSV)* disease as a function of the type of maternal infection. *1°*, Primary infection. (Data from Brown ZA, Wald A, Morrow RA, et al. Effect of serologic status and cesarean delivery on transmission rates of herpes simplex virus from mother to infant. *JAMA.* 2003;289(2):203–209.)

neonatal infection has occurred despite cesarean delivery performed before rupture of membranes.[19,20]

Congenital CMV Infection

Intrauterine infection usually is the result of a susceptible woman acquiring infection from a child in the family or day care environment early during her gestation.[21–23] Multiple studies in Sweden and the United States have shown that the rate of CMV infection is much higher in children who attend day care than those who do not.[22,24–26] Many initially seronegative children become infected with CMV from their day care peers. CMV infection then is transmitted horizontally from child to child, most likely through saliva on hands and toys.[27,28] Infected children excrete large amounts of CMV for extended periods of time, exposing parents and other caregivers who may become pregnant.

Maternal shedding of virus directly correlates with the risk of perinatal infection. Infected breast milk and exposure to CMV in the genital tract lead to high rates of peripartum and postnatal CMV transmission.[29] Infants who breastfeed from CMV-seropositive women have an estimated rate of infection between 39% and 59%. The risk is greater when the maternal viral load is higher than 7×10^3 genome equivalents/mL. Excretion of the virus in breast milk is greatest between 2 weeks and 2 months after birth. Infected infants usually begin to excrete CMV between 3 weeks and 3 months after birth. Many of these infants excrete CMV chronically (for years), providing an opportunity to infect caretakers or others in contact with these children.

Congenital Zika Infection

Zika virus is acquired by a pregnant woman in one of three ways:
1. The bite of an infected mosquito to a nonimmune pregnant woman
2. Sexual transmission from a carrier to a pregnant woman
3. Transfusion of an infected blood product[30]

The prevalence of Zika virus currently is high in South America, particularly Brazil, owing to the high prevalence of the *Aedes aegypti* mosquito[30] and the high proportion of seronegative hosts. Other regions where Zika outbreaks have occurred include Africa, Southeast Asia, and the Pacific Islands. The greatest risk of serious sequelae for the fetus occurs in the first or second trimester, but has also been reported in the third trimester.[31] In a case series from Brazil, Zika virus caused adverse outcomes in 55% of infants when maternal infection occurred in the first trimester, in

12

52% of infants with maternal infection in the second trimester, and in 29% of infants with maternal infection in the third trimester.[6]

Question 3: What Are the Clinical Manifestations of Neonatal Infection and Disease?

Neonatal HSV Disease

HSV infections acquired either peripartum or postpartum can be classified as (1) disseminated disease involving multiple visceral organs, including lung, liver, adrenal glands, skin, eye, and the brain (disseminated disease); (2) CNS disease, with or without skin lesions (CNS disease); and (3) disease limited to the skin, eyes, and/or mouth (SEM disease). This classification system is predictive of both morbidity and mortality.[32–36]

Neonatal HSV disseminated disease is manifest by hepatitis that can be very severe, disseminated intravascular coagulopathy, and pneumonitis. The mean age at presentation (± standard error [SE]) is 11.4 ± 0.8 days.[33] CNS involvement is a common component of this category of infection, occurring in about 60% to 75% of infants with disseminated disease.[37] Although the presence of a vesicular rash can greatly facilitate the diagnosis of HSV infection, more than 40% of neonates with disseminated HSV disease will not have cutaneous vesicles at the time of illness presentation.[19,33,38,39] Events associated with disseminated neonatal HSV infection that can result in death relate primarily to the severe coagulopathy, liver dysfunction, and pulmonary involvement of the disease.

Clinical manifestations of neonatal HSV CNS disease include seizures (both focal and generalized), lethargy, irritability, tremors, poor feeding, temperature instability, and bulging fontanelle. The mean age at presentation (±SE) is 19.7 ± 1.6 days.[33] Between 60% and 70% of infants classified as having CNS disease have associated skin vesicles at any point in the disease course.[33,38] With CNS neonatal HSV disease, mortality is usually the product of devastating brain destruction, with resulting acute neurologic and autonomic dysfunction.

SEM disease is the most favorable of the presenting categories of neonatal HSV infection. By definition, infection in infants with SEM disease has not progressed to multiorgan, visceral involvement and does not involve the CNS. Presenting signs and symptoms can include skin vesicles in approximately 80% of patients, fever, lethargy, and/or conjunctivitis.[33] The mean age at presentation (±SE) is 12.0 ± 2.2 days.[33] There is a high degree of likelihood that, in the absence of antiviral therapy, SEM disease will progress to one of the more severe categories of neonatal HSV infection.[19]

Congenital CMV Infection

Congenital cytomegalovirus (CMV) infection is the most frequent known viral cause of mental retardation,[40] and is the leading nongenetic cause of neurosensory hearing loss in many countries including the United States.[41–43] It also is the most common congenital infection in humans, with approximately 1% of all live births in the United States involving CMV infection (~40,000 infants per year).[44] CMV can be acquired in utero during any trimester of pregnancy.

Of the fetuses infected, approximately 10% will be symptomatic at birth, and ~20% of these patients will die in the neonatal period; of the survivors, 90% will have significant neurologic sequelae.[45–50] The majority of these infants will have sensorineural hearing loss (SNHL), mental retardation, microcephaly, seizures, and/or paresis/paralysis.[42,51–54] These impairments frequently result in spastic quadriplegia requiring lifelong dependence on a wheelchair, along with cognitive and speech impairments that dramatically limit their ability to interact with and function in the world. Between 25% and 40% of all childhood SNHL is caused by intrauterine CMV infection.[55] Fetuses can be infected with CMV at any point throughout gestation. However, infections occurring earlier in gestation (first or early second trimesters) are more likely to result in severe forms of encephaloclastic injury.

Table 12.1 U.S. PUBLIC HEALTH IMPACT OF CONGENITAL CYTOMEGALOVIRUS INFECTION

	Estimated Number
No. of live births per year	4,000,000
Rate of congenital cytomegalovirus infection	1%
No. of infected infants	40,000
No. of infants symptomatic at birth (5%–7%)	2,800
No. with fatal disease (±12%)	336
No. with sequelae (90% of survivors)	2,160
No. of infants asymptomatic at birth (93%–95%)	37,200
No. with late sequelae (15%)	5,580
Total no. with sequelae or fatal outcome	8,076

From Dobbins JG, Stewart JA, Demmler GJ. Surveillance of congenital cytomegalovirus disease, 1990–1991. Collaborating Registry Group. *MMWR CDC Surveill Summ.* 1992;41(2):35–39.

Most infants (~90%) with congenital CMV infection have no detectable clinical abnormalities at birth (asymptomatic infection), and SNHL develops in about 10% of these children. Because most infants with congenital CMV have asymptomatic infection, approximately 70% of CMV-associated SNHL occurs in this group, even though the likelihood of sequelae in any given asymptomatically infected child is much lower than in a symptomatically infected child (Table 12.1).

CMV-associated SNHL is extremely variable with respect to the age of onset, laterality, degree of the deficit, and continued deterioration of the loss (progression) during early childhood.[41,52,54] About half of all children with CMV-associated SNHL have normal hearing at birth (delayed-onset SNHL) and therefore will not be detected by newborn hearing screening.[41] Delayed-onset SNHL, threshold fluctuations, and/or progressive loss of hearing are observed in both symptomatic and asymptomatic infection. The age of onset of delayed-onset SNHL can range from 6 to 197 months. However, the median age is 33 and 44 months for symptomatic and asymptomatic children, respectively.[41,52] Therefore neither routine physical examination in the nursery nor newborn hearing screening will identify the majority of children with CMV-associated SNHL at birth.

The natural history of congenitally acquired CMV infection is well described.[41,45,52,56–59] In contrast, outcomes of perinatally and postnatally acquired CMV infections are less well characterized. It is generally agreed that postnatal acquisition of CMV in term infants does not lead to symptomatology or disease.[60] In preterm infants, initial case reports suggested that perinatally and postnatally acquired CMV infections could produce severe disease.[61–66] Larger series and case-controlled trials more recently suggest that symptomatic disease in preterm infants is less common than asymptomatic infection, and long-term sequelae are rare.[67–71] Nevertheless, severe disseminated CMV disease can occur in premature infants, including life-threatening pneumonitis, hepatitis, and thrombocytopenia.[72]

Congenital Zika Infection

As with congenital CMV, congenital Zika infection can result in microcephaly, brain anomalies, and developmental delay.[73] In a review of 14 studies with radiologic assessment, the major findings in fetuses infected by Zika virus were ventriculomegaly in 33%, microcephaly in 24%, and intracranial calcifications in 27%.[73] There are multiple features of the congenital Zika virus syndrome, but the full spectrum of the syndrome is still under investigation.[74]

The principal clinical features of congenital Zika virus syndrome include microcephaly, facial disproportion, hypertonia/spasticity, hyperreflexia, and seizures.[74] Microcephaly is often a consequence of primary maternal infection in the first or second trimester. Microcephaly is defined by both the World Health Organization and the Centers for Disease Control and Prevention as an occipitofrontal circumference below the third percentile.[30] CNS abnormalities, positional abnormalities such

12

as arthrogryposis, hearing loss, and ocular abnormalities are also possible with congenital Zika infection. Finally, fetal loss, impaired fetal growth, and hydrops fetalis have also been reported in congenital Zika infection.[30]

Question 4: What Are the Treatments and Outcomes for HSV, CMV, and Zika Virus Infections in Neonates?

Neonatal HSV Disease

In the pre-antiviral era, 85% of patients with disseminated neonatal HSV disease died by 1 year of age, as did 50% of patients with CNS neonatal HSV disease (Table 12.2).[36] Evaluations of two different doses of vidarabine and of a lower dose of acyclovir (30 mg/kg per day for 10 days) documented that both of these antiviral drugs reduce mortality to comparable degrees,[34,36,75] with mortality rates at 1 year from disseminated disease decreasing to 54% and from CNS disease decreasing to 14% (see Table 12.2).[34] Despite its lack of therapeutic superiority, the lower dose of acyclovir quickly supplanted vidarabine as the treatment of choice for neonatal HSV disease because of its favorable safety profile and its ease of administration. Unlike acyclovir, vidarabine had to be administered over prolonged infusion times and in large volumes of fluid.

With utilization of a higher dose of acyclovir (60 mg/kg per day for 21 days), 12-month mortality is further reduced to 29% for disseminated neonatal HSV disease and to 4% for CNS HSV disease (Figs. 12.2 and 12.3, respectively).[32] Differences in mortality at 24 months among patients treated with the higher dose of acyclovir and the lower dose of acyclovir are statistically significant after stratification for disease category (CNS vs. disseminated; $P = .0035$; odds ratio = 3.3 with 95% confidence interval [CI] of 1.5–7.3).[32] Lethargy and severe hepatitis are associated with mortality among patients with disseminated disease, as are prematurity and seizures in patients with CNS disease.[33]

Table 12.2   MORTALITY AND MORBIDITY OUTCOMES AMONG 295 INFANTS WITH NEONATAL HSV INFECTION, EVALUATED BY THE NATIONAL INSTITUTES OF ALLERGY AND INFECTIOUS DISEASES COLLABORATIVE ANTIVIRAL STUDY GROUP BETWEEN 1974 AND 1997

Extent of Disease	Treatment			
	Placebo[36]	Vidarabine[34]	Acyclovir[34] (30 mg/kg per day)	Acyclovir[32] (60 mg/kg per day)
Disseminated disease	n = 13	n = 28	n = 18	n = 34
Dead	11 (85%)	14 (50%)	11 (61%)	10 (29%)
Alive	2 (15%)	14 (50%)	7 (39%)	24 (71%)
Normal	1 (50%)	7 (50%)	3 (43%)	15 (63%)
Abnormal	1 (50%)	5 (36%)	2 (29%)	3 (13%)
Unknown	0 (0%)	2 (14%)	2 (29%)	6 (25%)
Central nervous system infection	n = 6	n = 36	n = 35	n = 23
Dead	3 (50%)	5 (14%)	5 (14%)	1 (4%)
Alive	3 (50%)	31 (86%)	30 (86%)	22 (96%)
Normal	1 (33%)	13 (42%)	8 (27%)	4 (18%)
Abnormal	2 (67%)	17 (55%)	20 (67%)	9 (41%)
Unknown	0 (0%)	1 (3%)	2 (7%)	9 (41%)
Skin, eye, or mouth infection	n = 8	n = 31	n = 54	n = 9
Dead	0 (0%)	0 (0%)	0 (0%)	0 (0%)
Alive	8 (100%)	31 (100%)	54 (100%)	9 (100%)
Normal	5 (62%)	22 (71%)	45 (83%)	2 (22%)
Abnormal	3 (38%)	3 (10%)	1 (2%)	0 (0%)
Unknown	0 (0%)	6 (19%)	8 (15%)	7 (78%)

Adapted from Kimberlin DW. Advances in the treatment of neonatal herpes simplex infections. *Rev Med Virol.* 2001;11(3):157–163.

For neonates with disseminated or CNS neonatal HSV disease, improvements in morbidity rates with antiviral therapies have not been as dramatic as with mortality. In the pre-antiviral era, 50% of survivors of disseminated neonatal HSV infections were developing normally at 12 months of age (see Table 12.2).[36] With utilization of the higher dose of acyclovir for 21 days, this percentage has increased to 83% (Fig. 12.4).[32] In the case of CNS neonatal HSV disease, 33% of patients in the pre-antiviral era were developing normally at 12 months of age (see Table 12.2), whereas 31% of the recipients of the higher dose of acyclovir who develop normally at 12 months today (see Fig. 12.4).[32,36] A recent advance in outcomes from neonatal HSV CNS disease occurred with the determination by the CASG that oral acyclovir suppressive therapy for 6 months following acute parenteral treatment improves neurodevelopmental outcomes.[76] In this study involving infants with neonatal HSV with CNS involvement, Bayley developmental scores at 1 year of age were assessed in infants receiving 6 months of suppressive acyclovir therapy versus those receiving placebo.

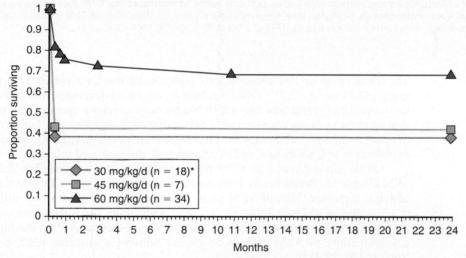

Fig. 12.2 Mortality in patients with disseminated neonatal herpes simplex virus disease. (From Kimberlin DW, Lin CY, Jacobs RF, et al. Safety and efficacy of high-dose intravenous acyclovir in the management of neonatal herpes simplex virus infections. *Pediatrics.* 2001;108(2):230–238.)

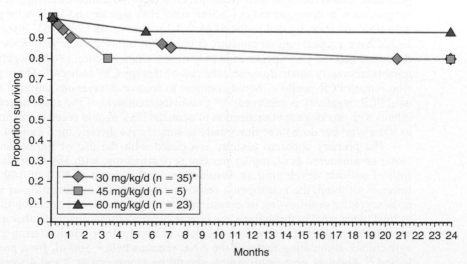

Fig. 12.3 Mortality in patients with central nervous system neonatal herpes simplex virus disease. (From Kimberlin DW, Lin CY, Jacobs RF, et al. Safety and efficacy of high-dose intravenous acyclovir in the management of neonatal herpes simplex virus infections. *Pediatrics.* 2001;108(2):230–238.)

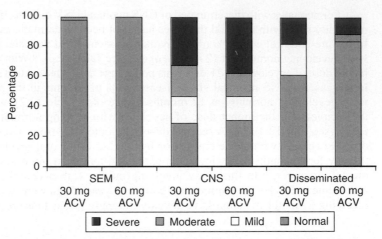

Fig. 12.4   Morbidity among patients with known outcomes after 12 months of life. *CNS*, Central nervous system; *SEM*, skin, eyes, and/or mouth. (Adapted from Kimberlin DW, Whitley RJ, Wan W, et al. Oral acyclovir suppression and neurodevelopment after neonatal herpes. *N Engl J Med.* 2011;365(14):1284–1292.)

The acyclovir group had a significantly higher mean Bayley score than the placebo group (88.24 vs. 68.12, $P = .046$),[77] indicating improved developmental outcomes in the suppression group (see Fig. 12.4). Suppressive acyclovir therapy also prevents skin recurrences in any classification of HSV disease.[77] Seizures at or before the time of initiation of antiviral therapy are associated with increased risk of morbidity both in patients with CNS disease and in patients with disseminated infection.[33]

Unlike disseminated or CNS neonatal HSV disease, morbidity following SEM disease has dramatically improved during the antiviral era. Before the use of antiviral therapies, 38% of SEM patients experienced developmental difficulties at 12 months of age (see Table 12.2).[36] With vidarabine and lower-dose acyclovir, these percentages were reduced to 12% and 2%, respectively.[34] In the high-dose acyclovir study, no SEM patients developed neurologic sequelae at 12 months of life (see Fig. 12.4).[32]

Infants with neonatal HSV disease should be treated with intravenous (IV) acyclovir at a dose of 60 mg/kg per day delivered intravenously in 3 divided daily doses.[32,78] The dosing interval of intravenous acyclovir may need to be increased in premature infants based on their creatinine clearance.[79] Duration of therapy is 21 days for patients with disseminated or CNS neonatal HSV disease and 14 days for patients with HSV infection limited to the SEM.[78] All patients with CNS HSV involvement should have a repeat lumbar puncture at the end of intravenous acyclovir therapy to determine that the CSF specimen is polymerase chain reaction (PCR)-negative in a reliable laboratory and to document the end-of-therapy CSF indices.[33] Those persons who remain PCR-positive should continue to receive intravenous antiviral therapy until PCR negativity is achieved.[33,80] Following treatment of the acute infection, all infants with any disease classification of neonatal HSV should receive oral acyclovir at 300 mg/m² per dose three times daily as suppressive therapy for 6 months.[71]

The primary apparent toxicity associated with the use of intravenous acyclovir administered at 60 mg/kg per day is neutropenia, with approximately one-fifth of patients developing an absolute neutrophil count (ANC) of 1000/μL or lower.[32] Although the neutropenia resolves either during continuation of intravenous acyclovir or following its cessation, it is prudent to monitor neutrophil counts at least twice weekly throughout the course of intravenous acyclovir therapy, with consideration given to decreasing the dose of acyclovir or administering granulocyte colony-stimulating factor if the ANC remains below 500/μL for a prolonged period.[32] Absolute neutrophil counts should be monitored at 2 and 4 weeks after starting oral suppressive therapy and then monthly thereafter while oral acyclovir is administered.[71]

Congenital CMV Infection

Administration of antiviral therapy with parenteral ganciclovir or oral valganciclovir beginning within the first month of life improves audiologic and developmental outcomes among patients with symptomatic congenital CMV disease.[76,81] From 1991 through 1999, 100 patients with symptomatic congenital CMV disease involving the CNS were enrolled on a pivotal CASG study. Patients were randomly assigned to ganciclovir treatment (6 mg/kg per dose administered intravenously every 12 hours for 6 weeks) or to no treatment.[81] Infants in the no-treatment arm were managed in a fashion identical to those receiving active drug. This study demonstrated that a relatively short duration of therapy of 6 weeks provides benefit in protection against worsening of hearing during the first 2 years of life. Denver developmental assessments were performed during the conduct of the ganciclovir study, and post hoc blinded analysis of the results demonstrated that patients receiving 6 weeks of intravenous ganciclovir experienced fewer developmental delays at 6 months and 12 months of age,[84] suggesting there may be a neurodevelopmental benefit to antiviral therapy as well.

Following this pivotal trial, the CASG conducted a phase I/II pharmacokinetic/pharmacodynamic investigation of oral valganciclovir in infants with symptomatic congenital CMV disease.[85] This study identified the oral dose of valganciclovir of 16 mg/kg per dose administered twice daily as that which reliably achieves the same ganciclovir blood concentrations as the previously studied intravenous ganciclovir dose of 6 mg/kg per dose administered every 12 hours. It was this dose that then was taken into a recently completed, large phase III trial of 6 weeks versus 6 months of oral valganciclovir for the treatment of infants with symptomatic congenital CMV disease.[76] Best-ear hearing outcomes at 6 months were similar for the groups ($P = .41$). Total-ear hearing was more likely to be improved or remain normal at 12 months in the 6-month group (73.4%) versus the 6-week group (57.1%) ($P = .01$). Benefit in total-ear hearing was maintained at 24 months (77.1% vs. 63.8%, respectively; $P = .04$). The 6-month group had higher Bayley-III Language Composite (84.6 ± 2.9 vs. 72.5 ± 2.9, $P < .01$) and Receptive Communication Scale (7.3 ± 0.5 vs. 5.2 ± 0.5, $P < .01$) neurodevelopmental scores at 24 months. Grade 3 or 4 neutropenia occurred in 19.3% during the first 6 weeks, and 21.3% (6-month group) versus 26.5% (6-week group) during the next 4.5 months of treatment ($P = .64$). As a consequence of this study, the standard duration of treatment of infants with symptomatic congenital CMV disease now is 6 months.[86] Antiviral therapy must be started within the first month of life when used to affect hearing and developmental outcomes in this population. Antiviral therapy now is being studied in the asymptomatic congenital CMV population as well, but there currently are not data to justify its use in that group.

Congenital Zika Infection

There currently are no antiviral therapeutic options for congenital Zika infection. All management is supportive.[87] Medical management of seizures, spasticity, and hearing loss are all routine parts of newborn follow-ups of infants affected by congenital Zika infection.[87] Further studies and investigations are currently underway to look for potential vaccines or treatments.

Question 5: Do All Infants With HSV and CMV Infections Have to Be Treated?

Neonatal HSV Disease

Yes. Neonatal HSV disease has significant mortality and morbidity, and all affected infants require parenteral acyclovir therapy.

Congenital CMV Infection

No. Antiviral therapy administered for 6 months improves audiologic and developmental outcomes for infants with symptomatic congenital CMV disease with or without CNS involvement. However, the toxicities from the therapy are not inconsequential, and the degree of benefit is modest. Therefore antiviral therapy should be considered for the management of symptomatic congenital CMV disease,[86] but managing physicians and families could opt to not treat in some cases.[86]

Congenital Zika Infection

Not applicable. With no current treatment, antiviral therapy of congenital Zika infection is not feasible at this time. However, multiple follow-up visits and medical management of sequelae are necessary parts of the syndrome management and treatment.[87]

Question 6: What Is the Appropriate Diagnostic Approach to an Infant in Whom HSV, CMV, or Congenital Zika Infection Is Suspected?

Neonatal HSV Disease

For diagnosis of neonatal HSV infection, the following specimens should be obtained: (1) swabs of the mouth, nasopharynx, conjunctivae, and rectum ("surface cultures") for HSV culture; (2) specimens of skin vesicles and CSF for HSV culture and PCR; (3) whole blood for HSV PCR; and (4) whole blood for alanine aminotransferase.[78] Positive cultures obtained from any of the surface sites more than 12 to 24 hours after birth indicate viral replication, and therefore are suggestive of infant infection rather than merely contamination after intrapartum exposure. As with any PCR assay, false-negative and false-positive results can occur. The presence of red blood cells in spinal fluid historically has been associated with HSV CNS infections. The data suggesting this association are older and reflect a time when the hemorrhagic encephalitis produced by HSV was more advanced at the time of diagnosis. As a consequence of enhanced appreciation for HSV CNS infections and of rapid diagnostic testing such as PCR, most CNS HSV infections today do not have a significant amount of blood in the CSF. Whole blood PCR may be of benefit in the diagnosis of neonatal HSV disease, but its use should not supplant the standard workup of such patients (which includes surface cultures and CSF PCR); no data exist to support use of serial blood PCR assay to monitor response to therapy. Rapid diagnostic techniques also are available, such as direct fluorescent antibody staining of vesicle scrapings or enzyme immunoassay detection of HSV antigens. These techniques are as specific but slightly less sensitive than culture. Typing HSV strains differentiates between HSV-1 and HSV-2 isolates. Radiographs and clinical manifestations can suggest HSV pneumonitis, and elevated transaminase values can suggest HSV hepatitis; both are seen commonly in neonatal HSV disseminated disease. Histologic examination of lesions for the presence of multinucleated giant cells and eosinophilic intranuclear inclusions typical of HSV (e.g., with Tzanck test) has low sensitivity and should not be performed.

Serologic diagnosis of neonatal HSV infection is not of great clinical value. The presence of transplacentally acquired maternal IgG confounds the assessment of the neonatal antibody status during acute infection, especially given the large proportions of the adult American population who are HSV-1- and HSV-2-seropositive. Serial antibody assessment may be useful in the very specific circumstance of a mother who has a primary infection late in gestation and transfers very little or no antibody to the fetus. In general, however, serologic studies play no role in the diagnosis of neonatal HSV disease.

Congenital CMV Infection

Proof of congenital infection requires isolation of CMV from urine, stool, respiratory tract secretions, or CSF obtained within 2 to 4 weeks of birth.[86] The sensitivity of CMV DNA detection by PCR of dried blood spots is low,[88] limiting use of this type of specimen for widespread screening for congenital CMV. A positive PCR result from a neonatal dried blood spot confirms congenital infection, but a negative result does not rule out congenital infection. Saliva PCR is emerging as the gold standard approach to the diagnosis of congenital CMV infection.[89] Differentiation between intrauterine and perinatal infection is difficult later than 2 to 4 weeks of age unless clinical manifestations of the former, such as chorioretinitis or intracranial calcifications, are present.

Congenital Zika Infection

Proof of congenital Zika virus infection requires suspicion for Zika clinically as well as knowledge of confirmed Zika infection in the mother. Confirmation by laboratory evidence of maternal infection is accomplished by positive real-time reverse transcription (rRT)-PCR findings in any clinical specimen or positive Zika virus IgM with confirmatory neutralizing antibody titers from the mother.[87]

The infant should have samples collected within 2 days of birth. These samples include serum and urine for Zika virus ribonucleic acid (RNA) via rRT-PCR and serum Zika virus IgM enzyme-linked immunosorbent assay. CSF testing can be done for these as well but are not required for the diagnosis of Zika.[87] A false-positive IgM test result can be ruled out by performing the plaque reduction neutralization test (PRNT). This test measures virus-specific neutralizing antibodies. A false-negative rRT result is possible and does not exclude infection because viremia can be transient.[90] A positive IgM test rest with a negative rRT result would suggest Zika infection. However, if both are negative congenital infection can be excluded.

Question 7: How Should You Monitor the Response to Treatment?

Neonatal HSV Disease

The primary measure of responsiveness to therapy is clinical improvement in the patient. All patients with CNS HSV involvement should have a repeat lumbar puncture at the end of intravenous acyclovir therapy to determine that the CSF specimen is PCR-negative in a reliable laboratory, and to document the end-of-therapy CSF indices.[33] Those persons who remain PCR-positive should continue to receive intravenous antiviral therapy until PCR negativity is achieved.[33,80] There are no data correlating clearance or persistence of HSV DNA in blood with clinical outcomes. Therefore serial blood PCR measurements of HSV DNA in blood are not recommended to establish response to antiviral therapy or to guide determinations regarding the appropriate time to discontinue therapy.

Congenital CMV Infection

Although great deal of work is being performed in this area, at the current time there are no biomarkers that are clearly established for predicting audiologic outcomes in infants with congenital CMV infection.[58,59,91–94] Therefore treatment duration should be based on the period established in the most recent controlled study (6 months) rather than on other measures of possible response to therapy such as serial blood PCR measurements of CMV DNA.

Congenital Zika Infection

Because there is no current treatment for Zika virus, management of patients with Zika infection is purely supportive through medical management of individual symptoms.

Question 8: What Are the Biggest Gaps in Our Current Understanding of the Natural History, Diagnosis, and Management of These Infections?

Neonatal HSV Disease

The duration of parenteral therapy for neonatal HSV disease is well established at 14 (SEM disease) or 21 (CNS or disseminated disease) days. The CASG's randomized controlled trial of oral acyclovir suppression following parenteral therapy proved that such additional treatment improves outcomes further, suggesting that subclinical viral reactivation is occurring in the brain of affected infants. Understanding the full scope of this treatment is a major unmet need at this time. Additional gaps in our knowledge of neonatal HSV disease relate to detection of HSV DNA in whole blood, both for diagnosis of infection and for assessment of treatment efficacy over time.

Congenital CMV Infection

There is a tremendous unmet need in the identification of biomarkers (either host or virus) that will predict who is at highest risk of sequelae from congenital CMV infection, especially asymptomatic infection. While a large treatment study conducted by the CASG in infants with asymptomatic congenital CMV infection is just now getting underway, more targeted therapeutic approaches in patients with the highest risks of detrimental outcomes would be ideal.

Congenital Zika Infection

Unlike CMV and HSV, there is a tremendous amount of information currently unknown about Zika. This lack is likely due to the very recent nature of the Zika epidemic in the Americas, the lack of large clinical studies or case studies on the topic, and the geographic areas affected by Zika transmission. Even the exact definition of congenital Zika virus syndrome is still under development as more cases with different manifestations continue to be recognized.

Conclusions

An impressive amount of knowledge has been amassed over the past three decades about the pathogenesis, diagnosis, and treatment of congenital CMV infection and neonatal HSV disease. Management recommendations have been standardized and broadly implemented. The degree of distance traveled in our knowledge of neonatal HSV and congenital CMV infections can be seen in the very new Zika virus pandemic. Over time, we undoubtedly will increase our understanding of the extent and pathogenesis of congenital Zika infections, and hopefully we will have a therapeutic drug or effective vaccine to manage and prevent infections from affecting the most vulnerable among us—namely, neonates and infants. Frontiers will continue to be advanced as new therapeutic options and modalities are identified.

REFERENCES

1. Whitley RJ, Roizman B. Herpes simplex virus infections. *Lancet*. 2001;357:1513–1518.
2. Schopfer K, Lauber E, Krech U. Congenital cytomegalovirus infection in newborn infants of mothers infected before pregnancy. *Arch Dis Child*. 1978;53:536–539.
3. Stagno S, Reynolds DW, Huang ES, et al. Congenital cytomegalovirus infection. *N Engl J Med*. 1977;296:1254–1258.
4. Boppana SB, Rivera LB, Fowler KB, et al. Intrauterine transmission of cytomegalovirus to infants of women with preconceptional immunity. *N Engl J Med*. 2001;344:1366–1371.
5. Stagno S, Pass RF, Dworsky ME, et al. Maternal cytomegalovirus infection and perinatal transmission. *Clin Obstet Gynecol*. 1982;25:563–576.
6. Brasil P, Pereira JP Jr, Moreira ME, et al. Zika virus infection in pregnant women in Rio de Janeiro. *N Engl J Med*. 2016;375:2321–2334.
7. Brown ZA, Benedetti J, Ashley R, et al. Neonatal herpes simplex virus infection in relation to asymptomatic maternal infection at the time of labor. *N Engl J Med*. 1991;324:1247–1252.
8. Brown ZA, Vontver LA, Benedetti J, et al. Effects on infants of a first episode of genital herpes during pregnancy. *N Engl J Med*. 1987;317:1246–1251.
9. Corey L, Wald A. Genital herpes. In: Holmes KK, Sparling PF, Mardh PA, et al., eds. *Sex Transm Dis*. 3rd ed. New York: McGraw-Hill; 1999:285–312.
10. Nahmias AJ, Josey WE, Naib ZM, et al. Perinatal risk associated with maternal genital herpes simplex virus infection. *Am J Obstet Gynecol*. 1971;110:825–837.
11. Brown ZA, Wald A, Morrow RA, et al. Effect of serologic status and cesarean delivery on transmission rates of herpes simplex virus from mother to infant. *JAMA*. 2003;289:203–209.
12. Yeager AS, Arvin AM. Reasons for the absence of a history of recurrent genital infections in mothers of neonates infected with herpes simplex virus. *Pediatrics*. 1984;73:188–193.
13. Prober CG, Sullender WM, Yasukawa LL, et al. Low risk of herpes simplex virus infections in neonates exposed to the virus at the time of vaginal delivery to mothers with recurrent genital herpes simplex virus infections. *N Engl J Med*. 1987;316:240–244.

14. Yeager AS, Arvin AM, Urbani LJ, et al. Relationship of antibody to outcome in neonatal herpes simplex virus infections. *Infect Immun*. 1980;29:532–538.
15. Parvey LS, Ch'ien LT. Neonatal herpes simplex virus infection introduced by fetal-monitor scalp electrodes. *Pediatrics*. 1980;65:1150–1153.
16. Kaye EM, Dooling EC. Neonatal herpes simplex meningoencephalitis associated with fetal monitor scalp electrodes. *Neurology*. 1981;31:1045–1047.
17. Whitley RJ. Herpes simplex viruses. In: Fields BN, Knipe DM, Howley PM, et al., eds. *Fields Virology*. 3rd ed. Philadelphia: Lippincott-Raven Publishers; 1996:2297–2342.
18. Anonymous. ACOG practice bulletin. Management of herpes in pregnancy. Number 8 October 1999. Clinical management guidelines for obstetrician-gynecologists. *Int J Gynaecol Obstet*. 2000;68:165–173.
19. Whitley RJ, Corey L, Arvin A, et al. Changing presentation of herpes simplex virus infection in neonates. *J Infect Dis*. 1988;158:109–116.
20. Peng J, Krause PJ, Kresch M. Neonatal herpes simplex virus infection after cesarean section with intact amniotic membranes. *J Perinatol*. 1996;16:397–399.
21. Taber LH, Frank AL, Yow MD, et al. Acquisition of cytomegaloviral infections in families with young children: a serological study. *J Infect Dis*. 1985;151:948–952.
22. Pass RF, August AM, Dworsky M, et al. Cytomegalovirus infection in day-care center. *N Engl J Med*. 1982;307:477–479.
23. Pass RF, Hutto C, Ricks R, et al. Increased rate of cytomegalovirus infection among parents of children attending day-care centers. *N Engl J Med*. 1986;314:1414–1418.
24. Adler SP. The molecular epidemiology of cytomegalovirus transmission among children attending a day care center. *J Infect Dis*. 1985;152:760–768.
25. Hutto C, Ricks R, Garvie M, et al. Epidemiology of cytomegalovirus infections in young children: day care vs. home care. *Pediatr Infect Dis*. 1985;4:149–152.
26. Pass RF, Little EA, Stagno S, et al. Young children as a probable source of maternal and congenital cytomegalovirus infection. *N Engl J Med*. 1987;316:1366–1370.
27. Hutto C, Little EA, Ricks R, et al. Isolation of cytomegalovirus from toys and hands in a day care center. *J Infect Dis*. 1986;154:527–530.
28. Faix RG. Survival of cytomegalovirus on environmental surfaces. *J Pediatr*. 1985;106:649–652.
29. Stagno S, Reynolds DW, Pass RF, et al. Breast milk and the risk of cytomegalovirus infection. *N Engl J Med*. 1980;302:1073–1076.
30. Rasmussen SA, Jamieson DJ, Honein MA, et al. Zika virus and birth defects—reviewing the evidence for causality. *N Engl J Med*. 13 April 2016;374:1981–1987.
31. Pacheco O, Beltran M, Nelson CA, et al. Zika virus disease in Colombia—preliminary report. *N Engl J Med*. 2016;15:15.
32. Kimberlin DW, Lin CY, Jacobs RF, et al. Safety and efficacy of high-dose intravenous acyclovir in the management of neonatal herpes simplex virus infections. *Pediatrics*. 2001;108:230–238.
33. Kimberlin DW, Lin CY, Jacobs RF, et al. Natural history of neonatal herpes simplex virus infections in the acyclovir era. *Pediatrics*. 2001;108:223–229.
34. Whitley R, Arvin A, Prober C, et al. A controlled trial comparing vidarabine with acyclovir in neonatal herpes simplex virus infection. *N Engl J Med*. 1991;324:444–449.
35. Whitley R, Arvin A, Prober C, et al. Predictors of morbidity and mortality in neonates with herpes simplex virus infections. *N Engl J Med*. 1991;324:450–454.
36. Whitley RJ, Nahmias AJ, Soong SJ, et al. Vidarabine therapy of neonatal herpes simplex virus infection. *Pediatrics*. 1980;66:495–501.
37. Whitley RJ. Herpes simplex virus infections. In: Remington JS, Klein JO, eds. *Infectious Diseases of the Fetus and Newborn Infants*. 3rd ed. Philadelphia: WB Saunders Company; 1990:282–305.
38. Sullivan-Bolyai JZ, Hull HF, Wilson C, et al. Presentation of neonatal herpes simplex virus infections: implications for a change in therapeutic strategy. *Pediatr Infect Dis*. 1986;5:309–314.
39. Arvin AM, Yeager AS, Bruhn FW, et al. Neonatal herpes simplex infection in the absence of mucocutaneous lesions. *J Pediatr*. 1982;100:715–721.
40. Elek SD, Stern H. Development of a vaccine against mental retardation caused by cytomegalovirus infection in utero. *Lancet*. 1974;1:1–5.
41. Fowler KB, McCollister FP, Dahle AJ, et al. Progressive and fluctuating sensorineural hearing loss in children with asymptomatic congenital cytomegalovirus infection. *J Pediatr*. 1997;130:624–630.
42. Harris S, Ahlfors K, Ivarsson S, et al. Congenital cytomegalovirus infection and sensorineural hearing loss. *Ear & Hearing*. 1984;5:352–355.
43. Fowler KB, Dahle AJ, Boppana SB, et al. Newborn hearing screening: will children with hearing loss caused by congenital cytomegalovirus infection be missed? *J Pediatr*. 1999;135:60–64.
44. Demmler GJ. Infectious Diseases Society of America and Centers for Disease Control. Summary of a workshop on surveillance for congenital cytomegalovirus disease. *Rev Infect Dis*. 1991;13:315–329.
45. Stagno S, Whitley RJ. Herpesvirus infections of pregnancy. Part I: cytomegalovirus and Epstein-Barr virus infections. *N Engl J Med*. 1985;313:1270–1274.
46. McCracken GH Jr, Shinefield HM, Cobb K, et al. Congenital cytomegalic inclusion disease. A longitudinal study of 20 patients. *Am J Dis Child*. 1969;117:522–539.
47. Pass RF, Stagno S, Myers GJ, et al. Outcome of symptomatic congenital cytomegalovirus infection: results of long-term longitudinal follow-up. *Pediatrics*. 1980;66:758–762.
48. Weller TH. The cytomegaloviruses: ubiquitous agents with protean clinical manifestations. I. *N Engl J Med*. 1971;285:203–214.

49. Weller TH, Hanshaw JB. Virologic and clinical observations on cytomegalic inclusion disease. *N Engl J Med*. 1962;266:1233–1244.
50. Conboy TJ, Pass RF, Stagno S, et al. Early clinical manifestations and intellectual outcome in children with symptomatic congenital cytomegalovirus infection. *J Pediatr*. 1987;111:343–348.
51. Ahlfors K, Ivarsson SA, Harris S. Report on a long-term study of maternal and congenital cytomegalovirus infection in Sweden. Review of prospective studies available in the literature. *Scand J Infect Dis*. 1999;31:443–457.
52. Dahle AJ, Fowler KB, Wright JD, et al. Longitudinal investigation of hearing disorders in children with congenital cytomegalovirus. *J Am Acad Audiol*. 2000;11:283–290.
53. Williamson WD, Desmond MM, LaFevers N, et al. Symptomatic congenital cytomegalovirus. Disorders of language, learning, and hearing. *Am J Dis Child*. 1982;136:902–905.
54. Williamson WD, Percy AK, Yow MD, et al. Asymptomatic congenital cytomegalovirus infection. Audiologic, neuroradiologic, and neurodevelopmental abnormalities during the first year. *Am J Dis Child*. 1990;144:1365–1368.
55. Morton CC, Nance WE. Newborn hearing screening—a silent revolution. *N Engl J Med*. 2006;354:2151–2164.
56. Boppana SB, Fowler KB, Vaid Y, et al. Neuroradiographic findings in the newborn period and long-term outcome in children with symptomatic congenital cytomegalovirus infection. *Pediatrics*. 1997;99:409–414.
57. Boppana SB, Pass RF, Britt WJ, et al. Symptomatic congenital cytomegalovirus infection: neonatal morbidity and mortality. *Pediatr Infect Dis J*. 1992;11:93–99.
58. Fowler KB, Boppana SB. Congenital cytomegalovirus (CMV) infection and hearing deficit. *J Clin Virol*. 2006;35:226–231.
59. Rivera LB, Boppana SB, Fowler KB, et al. Predictors of hearing loss in children with symptomatic congenital cytomegalovirus infection. *Pediatrics*. 2002;110:762–767.
60. Stronati M, Lombardi G, Di Comite A, et al. Breastfeeding and cytomegalovirus infections. *J Chemother*. 2007;19(suppl 2):49–51.
61. Vochem M, Hamprecht K, Jahn G, et al. Transmission of cytomegalovirus to preterm infants through breast milk. *Pediatr Infect Dis J*. 1998;17:53–58.
62. Maschmann J, Hamprecht K, Dietz K, et al. Cytomegalovirus infection of extremely low-birth weight infants via breast milk. *Clin Infect Dis*. 2001;33:1998–2003.
63. Takahashi R, Tagawa M, Sanjo M, et al. Severe postnatal cytomegalovirus infection in a very premature infant. *Neonatology*. 2007;92:236–239.
64. Vancikova Z, Kucerova T, Pelikan L, et al. Perinatal cytomegalovirus hepatitis: to treat or not to treat with ganciclovir. *J Paediatr Child Health*. 2004;40:444–448.
65. Bradshaw JH, Moore PP. Perinatal cytomegalovirus infection associated with lung cysts. *J Paediatr Child Health*. 2003;39:563–566.
66. Hsu ML, Cheng SN, Huang CF, et al. Perinatal cytomegalovirus infection complicated with pneumonitis and adrenalitis in a premature infant. *J Microbiol Immunol Infect*. 2001;34:297–300.
67. Neuberger P, Hamprecht K, Vochem M, et al. Case-control study of symptoms and neonatal outcome of human milk-transmitted cytomegalovirus infection in premature infants. *J Pediatr*. 2006;148:326–331.
68. Kothari A, Ramachandran VG, Gupta P. Cytomegalovirus infection in neonates following exchange transfusion. *Indian J Pediatr*. 2006;73:519–521.
69. Mussi-Pinhata MM, Yamamoto AY, do Carmo Rego MA, et al. Perinatal or early-postnatal cytomegalovirus infection in preterm infants under 34 weeks gestation born to CMV-seropositive mothers within a high-seroprevalence population. *J Pediatr*. 2004;145:685–688.
70. Yasuda A, Kimura H, Hayakawa M, et al. Evaluation of cytomegalovirus infections transmitted via breast milk in preterm infants with a real-time polymerase chain reaction assay. *Pediatrics*. 2003;111:1333–1336.
71. Vollmer B, Seibold-Weiger K, Schmitz-Salue C, et al. Postnatally acquired cytomegalovirus infection via breast milk: effects on hearing and development in preterm infants. *Pediatr Infect Dis J*. 2004;23:322–327.
72. Hamprecht K, Maschmann J, Jahn G, et al. Cytomegalovirus transmission to preterm infants during lactation. *J Clin Virol*. 2008;41:198–205.
73. Vouga M, Baud D. Imaging of congenital Zika virus infection: the route to identification of prognostic factors. *Prenat Diagn*. 2016;36:799–811.
74. Costello A, Dua T, Duran P, et al. Defining the syndrome associated with congenital Zika virus infection. *Bull World Health Organ*. 2016;94:406–406A.
75. Whitley RJ, Yeager A, Kartus P, et al. Neonatal herpes simplex virus infection: follow-up evaluation of vidarabine therapy. *Pediatrics*. 1983;72:778–785.
76. Kimberlin DW, Jester PM, Sanchez PJ, et al. Valganciclovir for symptomatic congenital cytomegalovirus disease. *N Engl J Med*. 2015;372:933–943.
77. Kimberlin DW, Whitley RJ, Wan W, et al. Oral acyclovir suppression and neurodevelopment after neonatal herpes. *N Engl J Med*. 2011;365:1284–1292.
78. American Academy of Pediatrics: Herpes simplex. In: Kimberlin DW, Brady MT, Jackson MA, et al., eds. *Red Book: 2015 Report of the Committee on Infectious Diseases*. 30th ed. Elk Grove Village, IL: American Academy of Pediatrics; 2015:432–445.
79. Englund JA, Fletcher CV, Balfour HH Jr. Acyclovir therapy in neonates. *J Pediatr*. 1991;119:129–135.

80. Kimberlin DW, Lakeman FD, Arvin AM, et al. Application of the polymerase chain reaction to the diagnosis and management of neonatal herpes simplex virus disease. *J Infect Dis*. 1996;174:1162–1167.
81. Kimberlin DW, Lin CY, Sanchez PJ, et al. Effect of ganciclovir therapy on hearing in symptomatic congenital cytomegalovirus disease involving the central nervous system: a randomized, controlled trial. *J Pediatr*. 2003;143:16–25.
82. Deleted in review.
83. Deleted in review.
84. Oliver SE, Cloud GA, Sanchez PJ, et al. Neurodevelopmental outcomes following ganciclovir therapy in symptomatic congenital cytomegalovirus infections involving the central nervous system. *J Clin Virol*. 2009;46(suppl 4):S22–S26.
85. Kimberlin DW, Acosta EP, Sanchez PJ, et al. Pharmacokinetic and pharmacodynamic assessment of oral valganciclovir in the treatment of symptomatic congenital cytomegalovirus disease. *J Infect Dis*. 2008;197:836–845.
86. American Academy of Pediatrics: Cytomegalovirus infection. In: Kimberlin DW, Brady MT, Jackson MA, et al., eds. *Red Book: 2015 Report of the Committee on Infectious Diseases*. 30th ed. Elk Grove Village, IL: American Academy of Pediatrics; 2015:317–322.
87. Russell K, Oliver SE, Lewis L, et al. Update: Interim Guidance for the Evaluation and Management of Infants with Possible Congenital Zika Virus Infection—United States. *MMWR Morb Mortal Wkly Rep*. 2016;65:870–878.
88. Boppana SB, Ross SA, Novak Z, et al. Dried blood spot real-time polymerase chain reaction assays to screen newborns for congenital cytomegalovirus infection. *JAMA*. 2010;303:1375–1382.
89. Boppana SB, Ross SA, Shimamura M, et al. Saliva polymerase-chain-reaction assay for cytomegalovirus screening in newborns. *N Engl J Med*. 2011;364:2111–2118.
90. Rabe IB, Staples JE, Villanueva J, et al. Interim guidance for interpretation of Zika virus antibody test results. *MMWR Morb Mortal Wkly Rep*. 2016;65:543–546.
91. Noyola DE, Demmler GJ, Williamson WD, et al. Cytomegalovirus urinary excretion and long term outcome in children with congenital cytomegalovirus infection. Congenital CMV Longitudinal Study Group. *Pediatr Infect Dis J*. 2000;19:505–510.
92. Rosenthal LS, Fowler KB, Boppana SB, et al. Cytomegalovirus shedding and delayed sensorineural hearing loss: results from longitudinal follow-up of children with congenital infection. *Pediatr Infect Dis J*. 2009;28:515–520.
93. Boppana SB, Fowler KB, Pass RF, et al. Congenital cytomegalovirus infection: association between virus burden in infancy and hearing loss. *J Pediatr*. 2005;146:817–823.
94. Ross SA, Novak Z, Fowler KB, et al. Cytomegalovirus blood viral load and hearing loss in young children with congenital infection. *Pediatr Infect Dis J*. 2009;28:588–592.

12

CHAPTER 13

Neonatal Hypotonia

Adele D'Amico and Enrico Bertini

- Neonatal hypotonia can be caused by diseases of the central and/or peripheral nervous systems.
- A systematic collection of family, pregnancy, and prenatal and birth clinical data is helpful for diagnostic workup.
- Accurate clinical examination, including neurologic assessment, is needed to address the differential diagnosis and to avoid needless or invasive diagnostic tests.
- Generalized hypotonia associated with muscle weakness and preserved social orientation suggests a neuromuscular disorder.
- Spinal muscular atrophy type 1 and congenital myotonic dystrophy represent the most common neuromuscular causes of "floppy infant syndrome."

Neonatal hypotonia, also defined as "floppy infant syndrome," represents a diagnostic challenge for both the experienced neonatologist and pediatric neurologist. Hypotonia is a manifestation reflecting either a disorder of the central nervous system (CNS), the peripheral nervous system (PNS), or both (Box 13.1) and thus the differential diagnosis is very broad. More than 600 conditions are reported in the Online Mendelian Inheritance in Man (OMIM) compendium as being associated with early-onset hypotonia. Moreover, transitory hypotonic posturing and behavior can be part of the normal variability in the premature infant, typically accompanying acute illness or systemic illnesses.[1] Based on clinical estimates of large series of patients, hypotonia of central origin accounts for about 66% to 88% of cases, with PNS involvement or unknown causes accounting for the remaining cases.[2]

Improving the methodology in decision making to detect causes of hypotonia is important to avoid needless or invasive diagnostic tests, to offer an effective clinical assessment and suitable genetic counseling to the family, and finally to inform about prognosis and future medical intervention.

In this chapter, we analyze the stepwise diagnostic approach to the investigation of neonatal hypotonia and discuss the differential diagnosis of hypotonia, summarizing the most common neuromuscular disorders that manifest principally with hypotonia or early-onset weakness.

Clinical History Collection

A detailed family, pregnancy, prenatal, and birth clinical history should be conducted first to collect important information than can help in the diagnostic process. The family history should include any other family members with hypotonia, muscle diseases, or genetic disorders and should explore for parental consanguinity. A family history of neurologic or neuromuscular conditions has been reported in about 50% of hypotonic infants,[3] and parental consanguinity increases the risk of autosomal recessive disorders.

Box 13.1 DISORDERS OF THE CENTRAL OR PERIPHERAL NERVOUS SYSTEM LEADING TO NEONATAL HYPOTONIA

Central nervous system involvement
Systemic diseases
Congenital heart disease
Sepsis
Inborn errors of metabolism
Maternal infection
Syndromic central hypotonia
Hypoxic-ischemic encephalopathy
Chromosomal defects
Lemli-Opitz syndrome
Prader-Willi syndrome
Cerebro-occulo-facial syndrome
Coffin-Lowry syndrome
Angelman syndrome
Sotos syndrome
Joubert syndrome
Marfan syndrome
Osteogenesis imperfecta
Nonsyndromic central hypotonia
Cerebral malformation
Schizencephaly
Lissencephaly
Holoprosencephaly
Delayed myelination
Congenital ataxia
Peripheral nervous system involvement
Spinal muscular atrophy
Metabolic myopathies (Pompe disease)
Peripheral neuropathies
Congenital myasthenic syndromes
Congenital myopathies
Botulism
Spinal injury or other horn cell diseases
Central and peripheral nervous system involvement
Congenital muscular dystrophies
Congenital myotonic dystrophy
Metabolic diseases (mitochondrial disorders)
Congenital myasthenic syndromes

The prenatal and perinatal history should include the mother's description of fetal movements; polyhydramnios or oligohydramnios; any maternal illness or maternal exposure to infectious agents, drugs, or alcohol; abnormal fetal presentation; the need for respiratory support; feeding difficulties; and seizures. The developmental history in infants older than a few months should include the age when major milestones are attained. Intrauterine growth restriction associated with oligohydramnios may suggest a CNS involvement related to poor maternal nutrition or chromosomal/genetic syndromes. A history of seizures, head growth failure, and global developmental delay are also evocative of brain involvement.[4] Conversely, a clinical history of maternal polyhydramnios, reduced fetal movement, breech presentation, respiratory distress, swallowing problems, and poor suck at birth are strong indicators of a neuromuscular disorder.[5–7]

Clinical Evaluation

The general physical examination of a floppy infant may reveal organomegaly, abnormalities of the genitalia, skin changes, dysmorphic features, contractures, or skeletal abnormalities that are suggestive of genetic syndromic disease, including some connective disorders such as Marfan and Ehlers-Danlos syndromes, because hyperlaxity of the ligaments can also manifest as hypotonia.[8,9]

Neurologic Examination of the Hypotonic Infant

In the newborn and infant, there is an overlapping significance between tone versus strength and between hypotonia versus weakness. Clinical assessment of a floppy infant should include the evaluation of muscle tone, primitive reflexes, deep tendon reflexes, placing reactions, resting postures in prone and supine positions, antigravity movements, and visual following / alertness. Moreover, because there is a higher prevalence of cognitive delay in infants with central hypotonia, a standardized assessment of cognitive development and observational assessment of the infant's affective behavior development are important as well.

A clinical diagnosis of hypotonia is based on three features: (1) bizarre and unusual distribution of tone, (2) diminished resistance to passive movements, and (3) excessive range of joint movements.[10] Muscle tone can be further evaluated by performing simple maneuvers such as "pull to sit," the "scarf sign," and "ventral suspension."

The "**pull to sit**" maneuver evaluates axial tone of the neck and back and appendicular tone of the shoulder and arms. It also tests strength to some extent because the normal response from the infant being tested is to resist pulling on the arms and shoulders.[11] The hypotonic infant tends to have significant head lag when pulled to the seated position and does not keep the head erect when sitting.

The "**scarf sign**" is observed as an infant's arm is pulled across the chest to the opposite shoulder and there is minimal resistance. Normally, the elbow can be brought to the midline of the infant's chin and chest. In the hypotonic infant, the elbow can easily be brought well beyond the midline before encountering resistance.

On **ventral suspension**, the normal term infant will keep the arms and legs flexed and will be able to lift the head above the horizontal position for a few seconds. A floppy infant "slips through" at the shoulder and assumes the position of a rag doll.

Once the infant has clearly been identified as hypotonic, it is important to complete the neurologic examination to understand the neuroanatomic site of the lesion and to determine whether hypotonia is accompanied by weakness because the presence of a profound muscle weakness suggests the involvement of the PNS.[12] The assessment of muscle strength of infants can be limited to inspection.

At clinical inspection, a weak infant assumes a frog-leg position. Spontaneous antigravity movements of limbs may be absent or decreased, although social interaction is preserved. Other clinical indicators of weakness are weak cry, poor suck, poor swallowing ability, and a paradoxical breathing pattern (intercostal muscles paralyzed with intact diaphragm). Normal head circumference may also suggest the isolated involvement of PNS. Pronounced head lag on traction response and inverted-U posture at ventral suspension are indicative of weakness of axial and trunk muscles.

Conversely, an infant affected by a CNS disorder general manifests global developmental delay and visual contact, consciousness, and social interactions are generally poor. Early-onset strabismus is highly evocative of a CNS origin of hypotonia. Significant axial and trunk hypotonia with relative sparing of limb tone is often observed. Tendon reflexes are brisk together with sustained ankle clonus and extensor plantar response and persistence of primitive reflexes. Abnormal head size, microcephaly or macrocephaly, seizures, and dysmorphia are also additional useful indicators of CNS involvement.

Central hypotonia can be related to systemic diseases (e.g., cardiac failure, sepsis, or inborn errors of metabolism) or to genetic syndromic and nonsyndromic diseases. Finally, mixed signs of central and peripheral hypotonia can be observed in several diseases involving both the CNS and PNS (e.g., congenital muscular dystrophy and congenital myotonic dystrophy as reported in Box 13.1). Differential clinical features and distinct patterns of weakness are very useful for the differential diagnosis as reported in Table 13.1.

Diagnostic Investigation

Hypotonia can be related to disorders that affect any level of the nervous system. A clinical history and physical examination of the brain, cerebellum, brainstem, spinal cord, peripheral nerves, neuromuscular junction, and muscle should guide the investigations.

The initial laboratory evaluation of a floppy infant is directed to rule out systemic disorders. Routine tests should include blood and urine cultures; serum electrolytes; liver

Table 13.1   DISTINCT PATTERNS OF WEAKNESS AND DIFFERENTIAL CLINICAL FEATURES
AIDING DIFFERENTIAL DIAGNOSIS OF NEONATAL HYPOTONIA

Pattern of Weakness	
Central Hypotonia	**Peripheral Hypotonia**
Increased tendon reflexes	Poor antigravity movements
Extensor plantar response	Hypo- to areflexia
Sustained ankle clonus	Selective motor delay
Global developmental delay	Preserved social interaction
Microcephaly	Weak cry
Seizures	Respiratory distress
Differential Clinical Signs	
Spinal muscular atrophy	Generalized weakness with sparing of the diaphragm and facial muscles tongue fasciculations
Pompe diseases	Generalized weakness with sparing of the diaphragm and facial muscles enlargement of the tongue Cardiomegaly Increased creatine phosphokinase levels in blood
Congenital myopathy	Bulbar and oculomotor muscles involvement
Myasthenic syndrome	Respiratory weakness
Myotonic dystrophy	
Botulism	
Peripheral neuropathy	Distal muscle group involvement, distal contractures
Congenital muscular dystrophy	Structural brain and eye abnormalities contractures

function tests; determination of ammonia, glucose, and creatinine levels; and a complete blood cell count. When a metabolic disorder is suspected, an immediate search for disorders of energy metabolism, amino acid metabolism, fatty acid metabolism, and urea cycle function should be undertaken if the child shows signs of metabolic decompensation because metabolic disorders may be more easily suspected and detected during a metabolic crisis than in the intercritical period. Screening for toxoplasmosis; other (congenital syphilis and viruses), rubella, cytomegalovirus, and herpes (TORCH) screening; and urine drug screening should be undertaken to exclude maternal infection or drug exposure. Brain imaging in parallel with metabolic screening are appropriate if a CNS disorder is suspected. The presence of particular dysmorphic features may prompt karyotyping, array comparative genomic hybridization (CGH), methylation study for chromosome 15q11.2 deletion (Prader-Willi/Angelman syndrome), or other specific molecular tests.

When a neuromuscular disorder is suspected, a creatine phosphokinase (CPK) test may be useful; however, it must be noted that most congenital myopathies (CMs) are associated with a normal CPK level and that a transitory high CPK level in newborns can be observed in fetal asphyxia or following a vaginal delivery, especially if complicated by forceps, vacuum, and breech presentation. Persistent high CPK values are highly suggestive of a muscular dystrophy, whereas in anterior horn cell disease the CPK level is generally normal or mildly increased.[13] If spinal muscular atrophy 1 is suspected, current guidelines suggest a prompt request for molecular genetic testing to rule out a survival motor neuron (SMN) defect, because treatment options should follow shortly. Electromyography and nerve conduction studies are useful diagnostic tests if a neuromuscular junction defect or neuropathy is suspected, whereas a muscle biopsy is required to investigate a myopathy or a metabolic myopathy (e.g., mitochondrial disease).

Muscle ultrasound is noninvasive and very useful for the assessment of a floppy infant. It can be used as a first screening option. Screening results are normal in children with hypotonia of cerebral origin, Prader-Willi syndrome, ligamentous laxity, or other "nonneuromuscular" causes.[14]

Finally, some conditions warrant specific testing, such as echocardiogram in Pompe disease or brain magnetic resonance imaging (MRI) in congenital muscular dystrophy, to support the diagnosis. A schematic approach to the diagnosis of a floppy infant is shown in Fig. 13.1.

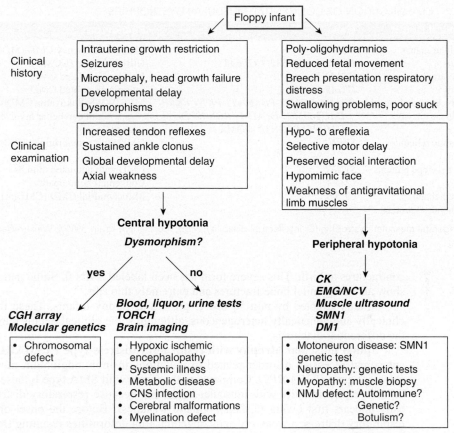

Fig. 13.1   Schematic diagnostic approach and algorithm to neonatal hypotonia.

Most Common Neuromuscular Disorders Presenting With Congenital Hypotonia

Spinal Muscular Atrophies

Spinal muscular atrophies (SMAs) are hereditary disorders characterized by degeneration of motor neurons in the spinal cord and brainstem, resulting in progressive muscle weakness and atrophy. The most common form of SMA is caused by decreased levels of the SMN protein. This autosomal recessive condition results from mutations or homozygous deletions involving the *SMN1* gene on chromosome 5q13. 5q13 related SMAs are classified into three clinical groups based on maximal motor achievement.[15] Non-5q SMAs are genetically heterogeneous, clinically diverse, and rare compared with 5q SMAs associated with mutations in a variety of different genes.[16]

SMA type I, the most severe form, represents the primary genetic cause of death in children younger than 2 years of age, affecting 1 in 6000 to 1 in 10,000 live births.[17] Typically infants with SMA type I have onset of clinical signs before 6 months of age. They show progressive proximal weakness, poor head control, profound hypotonia that causes them to assume a frog-leg posture when lying and to slip through on vertical suspension, and areflexia. The intercostal muscles weakness with relative sparing of the diaphragm produces a bell-shaped chest and a paradoxical breathing pattern. Infants with SMA type I classically exhibit tongue fasciculations and have difficulty swallowing with risk for aspiration, and they fail to thrive. Cognition is normal and affected infants' bright expression contrasts with their generalized weakness and poor movements.

In the most severe forms, decreased intrauterine movements suggest prenatal onset of the disease and infants tend to present with severe weakness and joint

Table 13.2 CLASSIFICATION OF CONGENITAL MUSCULAR DYSTROPHIES

Biochemical Defect	Gene	Phenotype
Extracellular matrix proteins	*LAMA2* *COL6A1, COL6A2, COL6A3*	Merosin deficiency CMD (MDC1A) Ullrich disease (UCMC)
External sarcolemmal proteins	*ITGA7* *ITGA9*	Integrin a7-related CMD Integrin a9-related CMD
Dystroglycan and glycosyl-transferase enzymes	*POMT1-POMT2-POMGnT1-FKTN-FKRP-DAG1-DMP2-DPM3-LARGE-ISPD-GMPPB-* B3GNT1 *-POMK*	MEB-WWS-Fukuyama CMD with or without cerebellar involvement and ID
Endoplasmic reticulum protein	*SEPN1*	CMD with spinal rigidity (RSMD1)
Nuclear envelope proteins	*SYNE1* *LMNA*	CMD with adducted thumbs Congenital laminopathy
Sarcolemmal and mitochondrial protein	*CHKB*	Mitochondrial CMD (CMDmt)

CMD, Congenital muscular dystrophy; *ID*, intellectual disability; *MEB*, muscle-eye-brain, *WWS*, Walker-Warburg syndrome.

contractures at birth. This severe form has been labeled SMN 0. Some patients may show also congenital bone fractures and extremely thin ribs.[18]

Infants affected by non-5q SMAs present as floppy infants. These forms are clinically and genetically heterogeneous, although some clinical details may help in the differential diagnosis.

Spinal muscular atrophy with respiratory distress type 1 (SMARD1) is an autosomal recessive disorder related to mutations in immunoglobulin mu-binding protein 2 gene *(IGHMBP2)*. Compared with infants with SMA type I, these patients do not present initially with muscular hypotonia because respiratory distress typically appears first owing to diaphragmatic weakness. Before the onset of a frank respiratory distress, a weak cry and congenital foot deformities resulting from early involvement of distal muscles of the lower limbs may have been present. Later the upper limbs become involved and muscle weakness rapidly progresses to generalized and symmetric weakness of limb and trunk muscles. Early involvement of the diaphragm and predominance of distal muscle weakness clearly distinguishes SMARD1 from SMA type I.[19]

Myopathies

The congenital muscular dystrophies (CMDs) and the CMs constitute the two most important groups of congenital-onset muscle disease. The CMDs are defined as early-onset muscle disorders in which the muscle biopsy result is compatible with the presence of a dystrophic process without histologic evidence of another neuromuscular disease. Conversely, CMs are nondystrophic myopathies with characteristic histologic and histochemical findings, although overlapping of criteria between these two groups of diseases group may occur, thereby blurring the boundaries between these conditions.[20]

Congenital Muscular Dystrophies

CMDs are clinically and genetically heterogeneous neuromuscular disorders with onset at birth or in early infancy and in which the muscle biopsy shows dystrophic features. Recent classification of CMDs is based on combined clinical, genetic, and pathologic data,[21] as reported in Table 13.2.

All these genetic forms share some clinical features, such as congenital hypotonia and weakness, contractures, difficulty swallowing, and respiratory distress at birth. Therefore the integration of accurate clinical, morphologic, and genetic data is mandatory to address a differential diagnosis. Fig. 13.2 shows some examples.

Congenital contractures, hip dislocation, and excessive laxity are evocative of Ullrich congenital muscular dystrophy, whereas eye abnormalities, retinal dysplasia, anterior chamber malformation, and congenital cataract are highly suggestive of an α-dystroglycanopathy (ADG-RD), defined as muscle-eye-brain disease and

α-Dystroglycan

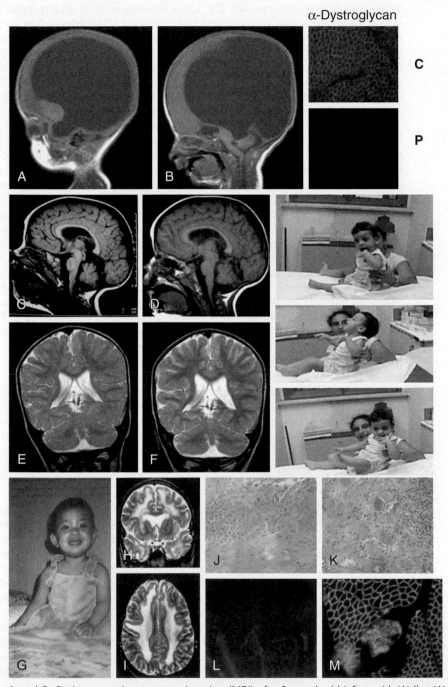

Fig. 13.2 A and B, Brain magnetic resonance imaging (MRI) of a 3-month-old infant with Walker-Warburg syndrome correlated to α-dystroglycanopathy related to a novel homozygous p.W495R mutation (c.1483T>C) in the *LARGE* gene; the child also had coarctation of the aorta with persistent ductus arteriosus. On the *right panel,* histopathology shows absent immunofluorescence *(lower panel)* for anti-mouse α-DG (VIA4-1, Upstate Biotechnology, Lake Placid, NY) in patient *P* versus control C. C to F, Brain MRI of a 2-year-old girl with neonatal hypotonia, developmental delay, and early cerebellar hypoplasia (C and E, MRI performed at age 1 year; D and F, MRI performed at age 2 years, demonstrating a nonprogressive cerebellar hypoplasia); The creatine phosphokinase level was 720 U/L; the patient had a homozygous c.860G>A (p.Arg287Gln) mutation in *GMPPB* (GDP-mannose pyrophosphorylase B) (Carss et al.[35]). On the *right panel,* clinical features of the girl with biallelic mutations in *GMPPB* show unsteadiness in the sitting position and antigravity weakness of head flexors. G to M, Clinical, MRI, and histopathologic features of a 2-year-old girl with a homozygous mutation in *LAMA2* (merosin). The girl was able to sit but not able to stand up; brain MRI showed typical diffuse hyperintensities of the white matter (H, I). Muscle histopathology showed prominent fibrosis (J) and inflammatory changes (K). Immunofluorescence labeling using an 80-kDa anti-merosin antibody showed absent signal in the subject's muscle and intramuscular nerve structures (L) compared with control (M).

Walker-Warburg syndrome (see Fig 13.2). Prominent axial and respiratory weaknesses are suggestive of CMD related to *SEPN1* or *LMNA* defects. The most important tools to address these differential diagnoses, beyond a careful family history and the physical examination, are CPK assessment, brain MRI, and muscle biopsy.[22] The CPK level can be normal or only mildly elevated in CDM associated with defects in the *SEPN1* and *COL6* genes, while it is consistently elevated in *LAMA2*-related disorders (RDs), and most of the time in ADG-RD. Brain MRI is essential to identify structural brain abnormalities observed in *LAMA2*-RD and ADG-RD.

The *LAMA2* defect is associated with typical findings on brain MRI, including high signal in the white matter on T2-weighted and fluid attenuation inversion recovery (FLAIR) images (see Fig. 13.2). The internal capsule, corpus callosum, and other dense fiber tracts are usually spared, but there may be subcortical cysts. Once evident, white matter changes do not require serial imaging. In a smaller percentage (about 5%) of patients, imaging shows more obvious structural brain abnormalities, including a particular type of occipital cortical dysgenesis with a subcortical band of heterotopia and cerebellar hypoplasia.[20,23] The MRI hallmark of CNS involvement in ADG-RD is represented by the cobblestone complex, ranging from complete lissencephaly (type II) to more focal pachygyria or polymicrogyria. As in *LAMA*-RD, an occipital cortical dysplasia and an underlying heterotopic band of neurons can be observed. Characteristic infratentorial findings include midbrain hypoplasia, pontocerebellar hypoplasia, abnormalities of cerebellar foliation, and cerebellar cysts. In addition, MRI may also show hydrocephalus and occipital encephalocele.[24] Seizures may occur in patients with *LAMA2* defects and in ADG-RD, including those with no obvious evidence for a cortical malformation on imaging.

Congenital Myopathies

CMs are a heterogeneous group of inherited muscle disorders, divided into subtypes based on the predominant histopathologic findings. Hypotonia and muscle weakness, with neonatal/childhood onset, are the most typical signs at presentation, but additional clinical features together with histopathologic findings may help in the differential diagnosis. The major forms of CM are (1) nemaline myopathy, (2) core myopathies (including central core disease and multi-minicore disease), (3) centronuclear myopathies, (4) myosin storage myopathy, and (5) congenital fiber-type disproportion.[25]

CMs manifest with typical signs of floppy infant (hypotonia and weakness) that clearly overlap with other neuromuscular diseases, as well as Prader-Willi syndrome. However, certain patterns of clinical findings may address the differential diagnosis. Prominent facial weakness with extraocular involvement and bulbar muscles are typical features of CMs. The severity of weakness and disability varies widely, from floppy infant to infants with subtle weakness that first manifests only during childhood with delayed motor milestones. There is usually reduced muscle bulk. Weakness is often generalized or more prominent in limb-girdle and proximal limb muscles, although some CMs have prominent axial and/or respiratory muscle weakness or weakness of ankle dorsiflexion. Respiratory insufficiency is common and the most severely affected infants require continuous ventilation for survival. The distinct clinical features of the different forms of CMs are reported in Table 13.3.

Pompe Disease

The first metabolic disease that can be easily mistaken for a spinal muscular atrophy or CM is Pompe disease, a lysosomal storage disorder caused by a deficiency of the enzyme acid α-glucosidase. The onset of symptoms can occur at any point in life. The classical infantile form of Pompe disease (IPD) presents with severe generalized hypotonia, respiratory problems, and cardiomegaly as the most common symptoms in the first months of life. Affected infants may exhibit hypertrophic tongue, feeding problems, and hepatomegaly.[26] The electrocardiogram shows a short PR interval, high QRS amplitude, and left ventricular hypertrophy.[27] The diagnosis is supported by an increased CPK value, generally less than 10 times the upper limit of normal. The muscle biopsy shows large vacuoles with a high glycogen content (positive

Table 13.3   CLINICAL FEATURES OF CONGENITAL MYOPATHIES USEFUL IN DIFFERENTIAL
DIAGNOSIS

Clinical Features	Congenital Myopathy	Gene
Facial weakness, ptosis, extraocular muscles involvement, bulbar dysfunction	Nemaline myopathy Centronuclear myopathy	*(NEB, ACTA1)* *MTM1-RYR1-DNM2*
Ophthalmoplegia	Myotubular myopathy Myosin 2 defect	*MTM1* *MYH2*
Facial dysmorphism (dolichocephaly, long face)	Myotubular myopathy Severe RYR1-related myopathies	*MTM1* *RYR1*
Predominant axial hypotonia and respiratory involvement	Selenoprotein-related diseases	*SEPN1*
Severe congenital hypotonia	Nemaline myopathy Myotubular myopathy Severe RYR1-related myopathies	*ACTA1, LMOD3, KLHL40,* *CFL2, MTM1* *RYR1*
Fetal akinesia	Nemaline myopathy Severe RYR1-related myopathies	*ACTA1, LMOD3, KLHL40* *RYR1*

13

periodic acid–Schiff staining) and strong reactivity for acid phosphatase, identifying them as secondary lysosomes. If IPD is suspected, the diagnosis can quickly be confirmed by acid α-glucosidase activity following dried blood spot testing.[28] Because IPD responds well to enzyme replacement therapy, this treatment should be promptly initiated for a better prognosis.[29]

Congenital Myotonic Dystrophy

Congenital myotonic dystrophy occurs in 15% to 25% of infants born to affected mothers, who can be asymptomatic or only mildly symptomatic. Pregnancy is usually complicated by poor fetal movements and polyhydramnios. Clinical features include neonatal hypotonia, respiratory distress, clubfoot, poor suck and swallow, and myopathic facies.

Myotonia is absent in the neonatal period and the creatine phosphokinase value is usually normal. Therefore this form is often erroneously defined as CM. Muscle biopsy shows nonspecific abnormalities consisting of increased variability in fiber size, with type I fiber atrophy in some cases.[30] The genetic defect in myotonic dystrophy has been identified as an expansion of a trinucleotide CTG repeat located in the 3′ untranslated region of a gene encoding for a serine-threonine protein kinase, also known as myotonin protein kinase.[31] The CTG copy number increases during consecutive generations, explaining the phenomenon of genetic anticipation (i.e., increasing severity of the disease phenotype and/or earlier onset in successive generations) in families with myotonic dystrophy.[32] The mother of a hypotonic neonate should always be examined, even if she appears to be asymptomatic, and the examiner should look closely for evidence of myotonia, weakness of distal muscles and neck flexors, or premature manifestation of cataracts.

Neuromuscular Junction Defects

Defects in neuromuscular transmission presenting as congenital hypotonia can be caused by genetic defects, can occur as a transitory phenomenon in 10% to 15% of infants born to women who have myasthenia, or can be related to botulism intoxication.

Congenital myasthenic syndromes are transmitted via autosomal recessive inheritance and are very rare (Table 13.4). Many infants require assisted ventilation at birth. Arthrogryposis may be present, as well as ptosis and generalized weakness. The infants are able to be weaned from mechanical ventilation within weeks, but persistent episodes of weakness and apnea may occur. The transitory myasthenic syndrome, however, is due to the passive placental transfer of antibodies against the acetylcholine receptor protein from a myasthenic mother.[33] The duration of symptoms averages 18 days, recovery is complete, and the severity of symptoms correlates with the newborn's antibody concentration. Difficulty in feeding and

Table 13.4 CLASSIFICATION OF CONGENITAL MYASTHENIC SYNDROMES: PATTERN OF INHERITANCE AND MOLECULAR TARGETS[a]

Defect	Deficiency	Mode of Inheritance
Presynaptic defects	Chat deficiency	AR
	SNAP25 deficiency	AD
	Synaptotagmin-2 deficiency	AD
Acetylcholine receptor defect	Primary deficiency	AR
	Slow-channel syndrome	AD
	(*CHRNA1, CHRNB, CHRND, CHRNE, CHRNG* genes)	AR
	Fast-channel syndrome (*CHRNA, CHRND, CHRND, CHRNE* genes)	
Synaptic basal lamina defects	Acetylcholinesterase deficiency (*ColQ* gene)	AR
	β_2-Laminin deficiency	
End-plate development and maintenance congenital defects	Agrin deficiency	AR
	MuSK deficiency	AR
	LRP4 deficiency	AR
	Dok-7 deficiency	AR
	Rapsyn deficiency	AR
	COL13A1 gene mutations	AR
Metabolic and mitochondrial disorders	Congenital disorders of glycosylation *SLC25A1* gene	AR
	mutations	AR

[a]The table shows the classification of congenital myasthenic syndromes based on pattern of inheritance and molecular targets at the neuromuscular junction.
AD, Autosomal dominant; *AR*, autosomal recessive.

generalized hypotonia are the major clinical features. The diagnosis is established by the patient's response to an intravenous or subcutaneous injection of edrophonium chloride (weight under 75 lbs, 0.1 mL or 1 mg IV; weight above 75 lbs, 2 mg IV). Ptosis and oculomotor paresis are the only functions that can be tested reliably.

Infantile botulism is characterized clinically by the acute onset of descending weakness, involvement of cranial nerves, ptosis and unreactive pupils, constipation, and rarely, respiratory insufficiency. Diagnosis in based on the isolation of the organism and toxin from stool culture.[34]

REFERENCES

1. Carboni P, Pisani F, Crescenzi A, et al. Congenital hypotonia with favorable outcome. *Pediatr Neurol.* 2002;26(5):383–386.
2. Kim C-T, Strommen JA, Johns JS. Neuromuscular rehabilitation and electrodiagnosis. 4. Pediatric issues. *Arch Phys Med Rehabil.* 2005;86(suppl 1):S28–S32.
3. Birdi K, Prasad AN, Prasad C, et al. The floppy infant: retrospective analysis of clinical experience (1990–2000) in a tertiary care facility. *J Child Neurol.* 2005;20:803–808.
4. Prasad AN, Prasad C. The floppy infant: contribution of genetic and metabolic disorders. *Brain Dev.* 2003;25(7):457–476. Review.
5. Hageman AT, Gabreëls FJ, Liem KD, et al. Congenital myotonic dystrophy; a report on thirteen cases and a review of the literature. *J Neurol Sci.* 1993;115(1):95–101. Review.
6. Das S, Dowling J, Pierson CR. X-linked centronuclear myopathy. 2002 February 25 [updated 2011 Oct 6]. In: Pagon RA, Adam MP, Ardinger HH, et al., eds. GeneReviews® [Internet].
7. Kizilates SU, Talim B, Sel K, et al. Severe lethal spinal muscular atrophy variant with arthrogryposis. *Pediatr Neurol.* 2005;32(3):201–214.
8. Yeowell HN, Steinmann B. Ehlers-Danlos syndrome, kyphoscoliotic form. 2000 February 2 [updated 2013 Jan 24]. In: Pagon RA, Adam MP, Ardinger HH, et al., eds. GeneReviews® [Internet].
9. Punetha J, Kesari A, Hoffman EP, et al. Novel Col12A1 variant expands the clinical picture of congenital myopathies with extracellular matrix defects. *Muscle Nerve.* 2017;55(2):277–281.
10. Dubowitz V. *The Floppy Infant 2nd ed.* Philadelphia, PA: JB Lippincott; 1980:1–9.
11. Bodensteiner JB. The evaluation of the hypotonic infant. *Semin Pediatr Neurol.* 2008;15(1):10–20. Review.
12. Harris SR. Congenital hypotonia: clinical and developmental assessment. *Dev Med Child Neurol.* 2008;50(12):889–892.
13. Amato M, Nagel R, Hüppi P. [Creatine-kinase MM in the perinatal period]. *Klin Padiatr.* 1991;203(5):389–394.

14. Heckmatt JZ, Pier N, Dubowitz V. Real-time ultrasound imaging of muscles. *Muscle Nerve.* 1988;11(1):56–65.
15. Dubowitz V. Chaos in the classification of SMA: a possible resolution. *Neuromuscul Disord.* 1995;5(1):3–5.
16. Darras BT. Non-5q spinal muscular atrophies: the alphanumeric soup thickens. *Neurology.* 2011;77(4): 312–314.
17. Hendrickson BC, Donohoe C, Akmaev VR, et al. Differences in SMN1 allele frequencies among ethnic groups within North America. *J Med Genet.* 2009;46(9):641–644.
18. D'Amico A, Mercuri E, Tiziano FD, Bertini E. Spinal muscular atrophy. *Orphanet J Rare Dis.* 2011;6:71. Review.
19. Grohmann K, Varon R, Stolz P, et al. Infantile spinal muscular atrophy with respiratory distress type 1 (SMARD1). *Ann Neurol.* 2003;54(6):719–724.
20. Bönnemann CG, Wang CH, Quijano-Roy S, et al. Members of international standard of care committee for congenital muscular dystrophies. Diagnostic approach to the congenital muscular dystrophies. *Neuromuscul Disord.* 2014;24(4):289–311.
21. Mercuri E, Muntoni F. The ever-expanding spectrum of congenital muscular dystrophies. *Ann Neurol.* 2012;72(1):9–17.
22. Bertini E, D'Amico A, Gualandi F, Petrini S. Congenital muscular dystrophies: a brief review. *Semin Pediatr Neurol.* 2011;18(4):277–288.
23. Philpot J, Cowan F, Pennock J, et al. Merosin-deficient congenital muscular dystrophy: the spectrum of brain involvement on magnetic resonance imaging. *Neuromuscul Disord.* 1999;9(2):81–85.
24. Clement E, Mercuri E, Godfrey C, et al. Brain involvement in muscular dystrophies with defective dystroglycan glycosylation. *Ann Neurol.* 2008;64(5):573–582.
25. North KN, Wang CH, Clarke N, et al. International Standard of Care Committee for Congenital Myopathies. Approach to the diagnosis of congenital myopathies. *Neuromuscul Disord.* 2014; 24(2):97–116.
26. Hebert K, Haritos D, Kannikeswaran N. A floppy baby. *Pediatr Emerg Care.* 2015;31(6):419–421.
27. Bulkley BH, Hutchins GM. Pompe's disease presenting as hypertrophic myocardiopathy with Wolff-Parkinson-White syndrome. *Am Heart J.* 1978;92:246.
28. Kishnani PS, Steiner RD, Bali D, et al. Pompe disease diagnosis and management guideline. *Genet Med.* 2006;8:267–288.
29. Chien YH, Hwu WL, Lee NC. Pompe disease: early diagnosis and early treatment make a difference. *Pediatr Neonatol.* 2013;54(4):219–227.
30. Ho G, Cardamone M, Farrar M. Congenital and childhood myotonic dystrophy: current aspects of disease and future directions. *World J Clin Pediatr.* 2015;4(4):66–80.
31. Brook JD, McCurrach ME, Harley HG, et al. Molecular basis of myotonic dystrophy: expansion of a trinucleotide (CTG) repeat at the 3' end of a transcript encoding a protein kinase family member. *Cell.* 1992;68:799.
32. Suthers GK, Huson SM, Davies KE. Instability versus predictability: the molecular diagnosis of myotonic dystrophy. *J Med Genet.* 1992;29:761.
33. Jovandaric MZ, Despotovic DJ, Jesic MM, Jesic MD. Neonatal outcome in pregnancies with autoimmune myasthenia gravis. *Fetal Pediatr Pathol.* 2016;35(3):167–172.
34. Tseng-Ong L, Mitchell WG. Infant botulism: 20 years' experience at a single institution. *J Child Neurol.* 2007;22(12):1333–1337.
35. Carss KJ, Stevens E, Foley AR, et al. Mutations in GDP-mannose pyrophosphorylase B cause congenital and limb-girdle muscular dystrophies associated with hypoglycosylation of α-dystroglycan. *Am J Hum Genet.* 2013:29–41.

13

CHAPTER 14

Amplitude-Integrated EEG and Its Potential Role in Augmenting Management Within the NICU

Lauren C. Weeke, Mona C. Toet, and Linda S. de Vries

14

- aEEG is easy to apply and interpret at the bedside.
- The aEEG background pattern is a reliable marker for encephalopathy in full-term infants and for brain maturation in preterm infants and can therefore be used for prognostication.
- Electrographic seizures detected with the aEEG should always be confirmed on the real EEG.
- Factors influencing the aEEG such as interelectrode spacing, medication, and common artifacts should be considered when interpreting the aEEG.

Interest in the neonatal brain has increased considerably during the past decades. This is in part due to better diagnostic methods in the acute and subacute stage. The presence and extent of structural lesions of the brain is provided by imaging techniques such as ultrasound and magnetic resonance imaging (MRI). Information about cerebral metabolism can also be obtained during the same examination using MR spectroscopy. Near-infrared spectroscopy (NIRS) allows noninvasive monitoring of brain oxygenation and cerebral hemodynamics.

Electroencephalography (EEG) or amplitude-integrated EEG (aEEG) provides information about brain function. It may detect epileptic discharges and signs of hypoxic-ischemic encephalopathy (HIE). Today aEEG is used routinely in an increasing number of neonatal intensive care units (NICUs). The extent of EEG monitoring in the NICU has been evaluated by analyzing 210 surveys (124 from Europe and 54 from the United States). Ninety percent of the respondents had access to either EEG or aEEG monitoring; 51% had both. The EEG was mainly interpreted by neurophysiologists (72%), whereas aEEG was usually interpreted by the neonatologist (80%). However, as many as 31% of the respondents reported that they were not confident in their ability to interpret aEEG/EEG.[1]

Amplitude-Integrated EEG

Maynard originally constructed the cerebral function monitor (CFM) in the late 1960s for continuous monitoring. Prior developed the clinical application, mainly for adult patients during anesthesia and intensive care, after cardiac arrest, during status epilepticus, and after heart surgery.[2]

The term aEEG is currently preferred to denote a method for encephalographic monitoring, whereas CFM is used to refer to a specific type of equipment. The EEG signal for the single-channel aEEG is usually recorded from one pair of parietally placed electrodes (corresponding to P3 and P4 according to the international EEG 10-20 classification, ground Fz). Two-channel EEG (F3-P3 and F4-P4 or C3-P3 and C4-P4, ground Fz according to the international EEG 10-20 classification) is now predominantly used and will provide information about hemispheric asymmetry, which may be especially helpful in children with a unilateral brain lesion.[3] In the two-channel

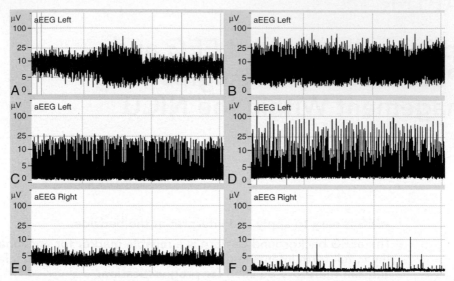

Fig. 14.1 A, Continuous normal voltage pattern with sleep-wake cycling. B, Discontinuous normal voltage pattern. C, Dense burst suppression. D, Sparse burst suppression pattern. E, Continuous low-voltage pattern. *aEEG*, Amplitude-integrated electroencephalogram; F, flat trace pattern.

recording the F3-P3 and F4-P4 position is preferred for assessment of the background pattern, opposed to the short electrode distance of the C3-P3 and C4-P4 position, which will affect the background pattern but is better for seizure detection.[4]

The signal is amplified and passed through an asymmetric band-pass filter that strongly prefers higher frequencies over lower ones and suppresses activity below 2 Hz and above 15 Hz to minimize artifacts from sources such as sweating, movement, muscle activity, and electrical interference. Additional processing includes rectification (negative waves become positive), smoothing, and considerable time compression. The signal is displayed on a semilogarithmic scale at slow speed (6 cm/hr) at the bedside. A second tracing continuously displays the original EEG from either one or two channels. The electrode impedance is continuously recorded but not necessarily displayed; there will be an alarm when the impedance is high, often as the result of a loose electrode. The bandwidth (BW) in the output reflects variations in minimum and maximum EEG amplitude, both of which depend on the maturity and severity of illness of the newborn. Because the semilogarithmic scale is used to plot the output, changes in background activity of very low amplitude (<5 µV) are enhanced.

Assessment of aEEG Background Pattern

The aEEG traces are assessed visually based on pattern recognition and classified into the following five categories in full-term infants[5]:

1. The continuous normal voltage (CNV) pattern is a continuous trace with a voltage between 10 and 25 (–50) µV (Fig. 14.1A)
2. The discontinuous normal voltage (DNV) pattern is a discontinuous trace, in which the lower margin is predominantly below 5 µV (no burst suppression [BS]) (Fig. 14.1B)
3. The discontinuous background pattern (BS); periods of low amplitude (inactivity) intermixed with bursts of higher amplitude (usually >25 µV; BS) (Fig. 14.1C and D)
4. The continuous background pattern of very low voltage (around or below 5 µV) sometimes has bursts of higher (but <25 µV) amplitude (continuous low voltage [CLV]) (Fig. 14.1E)
5. Very low voltage, mainly inactive tracing with activity below 5 µV (flat trace [FT]) (Fig. 14.1F)

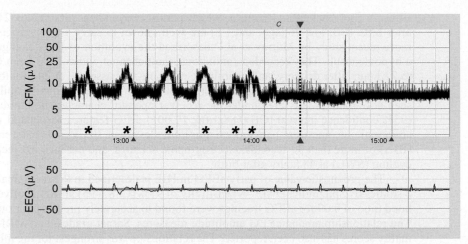

Fig. 14.2 The patient was born at full term via an emergency cesarean section. Sinusoidal cardiotocography was seen. Arterial umbilical pH was 6.70, and the first arterial lactate level was 30 mmol/L. Upper panel, drift of the baseline with seizures (indicated by *). Lower panel, real EEG shows electrocardiogram artifact. The loading dose of lidocaine was given at point *C*. *CFM*, Cerebral function monitor; *EEG*, electroencephalogram.

Another classification according to al Naqeeb[6] uses absolute values for background patterns:
- Normal: upper margin greater than 10 μV; lower margin less than 5 μV
- Moderately abnormal: upper margin greater than 10 μV; lower margin less than 5 μV
- Severely abnormal: upper margin less than 10 μV; lower margin less than 5 μV

We prefer the pattern recognition criteria because the background pattern may be influenced by the so-called drift of the baseline (Fig. 14.2). This drift is especially common in infants with very poor background activity, where the lower margin is lifted upward by a high-frequency external signal such as the ECG signal.[7]

When these two aEEG scoring systems were compared in the same dataset containing comparable normothermia and hypothermia-treated infants,[8] it was noted that the pattern recognition method was superior for early outcome prediction in a subgroup of patients with HIE. The appearance of the aEEG trace is influenced by several factors, including interference from the electrocardiogram, muscle activity, and interelectrode distance.[9] Interobserver agreement was slightly lower using the voltage criteria compared with the pattern recognition method. However, both methods are equally good in determining the background pattern compared with the use of standard EEG.[4] The voltage classification system is easier to use for clinicians with little experience in reading aEEG, but one should always try to assess the underlying pattern. It has been shown that a BS pattern may be read as a normal voltage pattern when a drift of the baseline is bringing the lower margin above 5 μV.[10] When this artifact is not recognized, the background pattern may be misclassified and as a consequence hypothermia may not be offered to eligible infants, for example (see Fig. 14.2).

Comparison With Standard EEG

Background Pattern

Several studies investigating simultaneous use of aEEG and standard EEG have been performed to compare the two techniques. A good correlation between the aEEG background pattern and standard EEG background activity was seen in full-term infants with moderate to severe neonatal encephalopathy.[11–14]

Prognostic Value of aEEG in HIE: Noncooled Situation

The value of the background pattern in the prediction of neurodevelopmental outcome in infants with HIE was already well established with the use of the standard

EEG. A poor background pattern, which persists beyond the first 12 to 24 hours after birth (BS, low voltage, and FT) are well known to carry a poor prognosis. A more recent study by Murray et al.[15] described the evolution of EEG changes after a hypoxic insult. They recorded continuous, multichannel, video EEG from 6 hours to 72 hours after delivery, and neurologic outcome was assessed at 24 months in 44 infants. Of those, 20 (45%) had an abnormal outcome. The best predictive ability was seen at 6 hours of age (area under the receiver operator characteristic curve: 0.958 (95% confidence interval [CI] 0.88-1.04; P .001). EEG features associated with an abnormal outcome were background amplitude less than 30 μV, interburst intervals (IBIs) of more than 30 seconds, electrographic seizures, and absence of sleep-wake cycling (SWC) at 48 hours after birth.

The prognostic value of early aEEG in HIE is described in the meta-analysis of 8 studies by Spitzmiller et al.[16] A sensitivity of 91% (CI 87–95) and a negative likelihood ratio of 0.09 for aEEG tracings were found to accurately predict poor outcome. The relationship among aEEG amplitude measures, Sarnat grades, and MRI abnormality scores has also been reported. The relationship was strongest for the minimum amplitude measures in both hemispheres. A minimum amplitude of less than 4 μV was useful in predicting severe MRI abnormalities.[17]

Both positive and negative predictive values were slightly lower when aEEG was assessed at 3 instead of 6 hours after birth, but they were still considered sufficiently high to use this technique for early selection in hypothermia or other intervention studies. Combining a neurologic examination with aEEG performed less than 12 hours after birth further increased predictive accuracy from 75% to 85%.[18]

Recovery of the background pattern within 24 hours after perinatal asphyxia with a poor background activity (BS, FT, and CLV) has been reported in 20% of the cases.[19] Of these infants, 60% survived with a mild disability or were normal at follow-up. The patients who did not recover either died in the neonatal period or survived with a severe disability.

Another way of looking at recovery of the background pattern is to assess the presence, quality, and time of onset of SWC (see also Figs. 14.1A, 14.8A, and 14.9C). The presence, time of onset, and quality of SWC reflect the severity of the hypoxic-ischemic insult to which newborns have been exposed. The time of onset of SWC was shown to predict neurodevelopmental outcome based on whether SWC returns before 36 hours (good outcome) or after 36 hours (bad outcome). Therefore we recommend continuous monitoring for at least 48 hours or until a normal SWC pattern is established.[20]

Prognostic Value of aEEG in HIE: Cooled Situation

Del Rio and colleagues[21] recently performed a systematic review investigating and comparing the prognostic value of aEEG in cooled and noncooled infants with HIE. Seven studies have reported on the predictive value of aEEG in cooled infants (Table 14.1).[8,22–27] All found the predictive value, especially the specificity, of aEEG to be poor at 6 to 24 hours after birth. However, from 36 hours onward both the sensitivity and specificity were above 80% and comparable to the predictive value of aEEG in the normothermic situation.

The appearance of SWC in cooled infants with HIE has been addressed in several studies.[8,26,28] Researchers found that the onset of SWC may be markedly delayed in term neonates with moderate to severe HIE treated with hypothermia, but when SWC returns within 36 hours the majority of infants will have a normal outcome.[26,28] However, when SWC is never achieved, this predicts a poor outcome with a positive predictive value of 0.73.[8,26] Therefore SWC is an important additional tool for assessing recovery in term infants with moderate to severe HIE treated with hypothermia.

Care should be taken when antiepileptic drugs (AEDs) are given for seizures in infants who have not recovered their background pattern within 24 to 48 hours. High blood levels of AED as the result of altered metabolism and accumulation under hypothermia may influence the background pattern of the aEEG.

Table 14.1 STUDIES INVESTIGATING THE PREDICTIVE VALUE OF AEEG IN HYPOTHERMIA-TREATED INFANTS

Study (Year of Publication)	Normo-thermia (n)	Hypothermia (n)	Follow-Up (mo)	6 hours		24 hours		36 hours		48 hours	
				Sensitivity, % (95% CI)	Specificity, % (95% CI)	Sensitivity, % (95% CI)	Specificity, % (95% CI)	Sensitivity, % (95% CI)	Specificity, % (95% CI)	Sensitivity, % (95% CI)	Specificity, % (95% CI)
Hallberg et al.[22] (2010)	0	23	12	100 (54–100)	31 (11–59)	100 (54–100)	76 (50–93)	100 (54–100)	82 (57–96)	80 (28–99)	100 (80–100)
Thoresen et al.[8] (2010)	31	43	18	100 (80–100)	62 (41–80)	94 (71–100)	73 (52–88)	88 (64–99)	96 (80–100)	82 (57–96)	100 (87–100)
Ancora et al.[23] (2013)	0	12	≥12	100 (40–100)	50 (16–84)	75 (19–99)	25 (3–65)	NR	NR	NR	NR
Shankaran et al.[24] (2011)	51	57	18	100 (86–100)	30 (16–49)	NR	NR	NR	NR	NR	NR
Gucuyener et al.[25] (2012)	0	10	8–24	100 (16–100)	38 (9–76)	NR	NR	NR	NR	NR	NR
Cseko et al.[26] (2013)	0	70	18–24	100 (87–100)	40 (25–56)	95 (76–100)	74 (50–93)	95 (74–100)	83 (68–93)	82 (57–96)	93 (80–98)
Azzopardi[27] (2014)	158	156	18	97 (89–100)	31 (21–42)	NR	NR	NR	NR	NR	NR

aEEG, Amplitude-integrated electroencephalogram; CI, confidence interval; HT, hypothermia; NR, not reported; NT, normothermia.

14

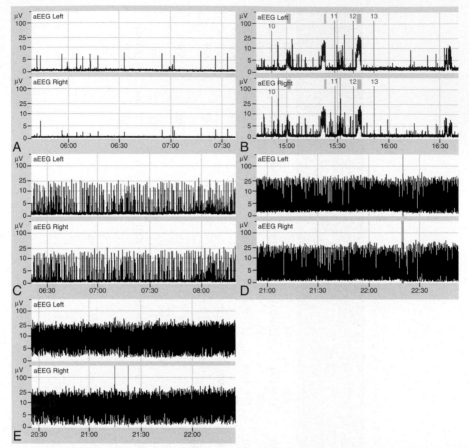

Fig. 14.3 The patient was born at 40 weeks' gestation and weighed 3150 g at birth. An emergency cesarean section was performed for suspected fetal compromise with bradycardia on the cardiotocogram because of a nuchal cord. Apgar scores were 1, 0, 0 at 1, 5, and 10 minutes. The infant was resuscitated for 15 minutes with intravenous adrenalin given once. The umbilical cord pH was 7.25, and base excess was −3.5. the first arterial lactate concentration was 26.4 mmol/L. The infant was cooled for 72 hours at 33.5°C. Seizures were treated with phenobarbital, midazolam, and lidocaine. Magnetic resonance imaging on day 4 showed severe abnormalities in the basal ganglia and thalami. The infant died on day 5 after redirection of care. A, Cooling was started at 3 hours after birth. B, Amplitude-integrated electroencephalogram (aEEG) at 18 hours after birth during cooling shows a flat trace pattern with seizures (indicated by the *pink bars*). *10,* care; *11,* x-ray; *12 + 13,* midazolam is given. C, A sparse burst suppression pattern is seen 36 hours after birth (during cooling). D, A dense burst suppression is seen 48 hours after birth. E, A discontinuous normal voltage pattern is seen 72 hours after birth.

aEEG and Seizures

Seizure Detection

A multichannel video EEG study by Murray et al.[29] showed that only one-third of neonatal EEG seizures display clinical signs on simultaneous video recordings. Two-thirds of these clinical manifestations were not recognized or were misinterpreted by experienced neonatal staff with very low interobserver agreement.[30] These findings show that clinical diagnosis is not sufficient for the recognition and management of neonatal seizures and underline the importance of EEG monitoring in infants at risk of developing seizures.

A rapid rise of both the lower and the upper margins of the aEEG tracing is suggestive of an ictal discharge (Fig. 14.3B). Seizures can be recognized as single seizures, repetitive seizures, and as status epilepticus (see also Fig. 14.10C). The latter usually resembles a sawtooth pattern. Correct interpretation is greatly improved by simultaneous reading of the raw EEG, which is now available on most digital aEEG monitors (see Fig. 14.9A).

Multichannel video EEG is the gold standard for neonatal seizure detection,[31] but it is not always readily available or feasible in the NICU. The advantages of limited channel aEEG compared with multichannel EEG are the easy application and interpretation that can be done in real time by NICU personnel. This can reduce the time to diagnosis and treatment of seizures significantly. However, owing to the nature of the aEEG technique it is not surprising that very brief seizure activity as well as focal seizure activity may be missed. This was also shown by Shellhaas et al.[32] in a large dataset of 125 multichannel EEGs with 851 neonatal seizures. They found that 94% of the multichannel EEGs detected one or more seizures on the C3–C4 channel, which is often used for aEEG. Thus multichannel EEG remains the gold standard for quantification of seizure burden. Rakshasbhuvankar and colleagues[33] recently reviewed 10 studies to answer the question of whether aEEG is as accurate as multichannel EEG in the detection of seizures.

Detection of individual seizures using aEEG was difficult (12%–38%)[34,35] without access to the real EEG, especially when the seizures were infrequent, brief, or of low amplitude. There were no false-positive findings among control records. Infants with focal seizures, however, usually develop more widespread ictal discharges, which will be identified by limited channel aEEG. In addition, 81% of the neonatal seizures originated from central temporal or midline vertex electrodes, which can potentially be picked up by the aEEG electrodes.[11] An important study is the one from Shah et al.,[36] showing that the combination of two-channel aEEG with the real EEG signal detected the majority (76%) of electrical seizures in at-risk newborns. Use of aEEG in combination with the real EEG signal was clearly better in seizure detection than use of aEEG alone (27%–44%). In a review by Evans and colleagues,[12] 44 studies with aEEG and simultaneous multichannel EEG were analyzed. Sensitivity for the presence of seizures by aEEG was 80% and specificity was 50%. Several seizures were overdiagnosed by aEEG as well as by standard EEG (63% vs. 45.5%, respectively). The specificity of aEEG for seizure detection was higher in neonates undergoing EEG for suspected seizures. On the other hand, monitoring for seizures with limited channel aEEG (two channels with access to the real EEG) can be accurately interpreted, compares favorably to multichannel EEG, and is associated with a trend toward reduced seizure burden.[37] It is important to use at least two channels, especially in infants with suspected unilateral brain lesions.[3]

Sometimes the aEEG shows a seizure pattern, but the two-channel real EEG is not conclusive. This could be due to multifocal epileptiform activity. The only way to check this is to perform a multichannel EEG (Fig. 14.4).

Since the increased use of continuous monitoring, it has become apparent that subclinical seizures are common and occur especially following administration of the first AED. This so-called uncoupling or electroclinical dissociation has been reported by several groups and was found in 50% to 60% of the children studied. The aEEG can play an important role in the detection of these subclinical seizures.[38,39]

Even status epilepticus is not uncommon and occurred in 18% of 56 full-term infants admitted with neonatal seizures recorded with aEEG.[40,41] The duration of status epilepticus may influence prognosis as well. In a group of 48 infants with HIE and aEEG-detected status epilepticus, there was a significant difference in background pattern, as well as in duration of the status epilepticus between infants with a poor outcome, compared with those with a good outcome. The background pattern at the onset of status epilepticus appeared to be the main predictor of outcome in all neonates with status epilepticus. The background pattern also proved to be an independent predictor of seizures in a group of 90 infants with HIE treated with therapeutic hypothermia.[42] The incidence of seizures did not change after the introduction of therapeutic hypothermia, but the overall seizure burden was reduced.[43] However, status epilepticus is not uncommon in infants with HIE treated with hypothermia; status epilepticus was observed in 10% to 23% of infants.[44–46] A high seizure burden and status epilepticus have been related to more severe brain injury on MRI in hypothermia-treated infants.[44,45,47,48]

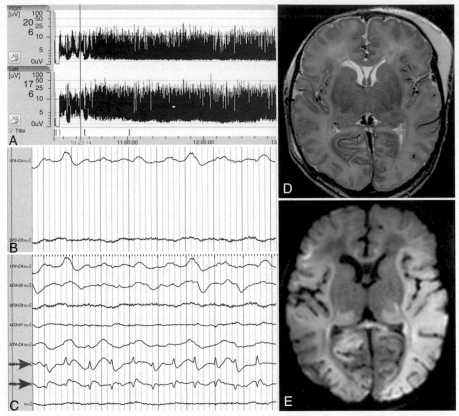

Fig. 14.4 Labor was induced at 42 weeks gestational age. The infant's birth weight was 4100 g. There was shoulder dystocia during labor. Apgar scores were 2 and 5 after 1 and 5 minutes, respectively. The infant was resuscitated for 4 minutes. Umbilical pH was 6.98 and base excess was −18. The infant was not cooled but started to have seizures within 12 hours after birth. He was treated initially with phenobarbital and was transferred to the neonatal intensive care unit. He subsequently needed ventilatory support and was treated with phenobarbital, lidocaine, and midazolam. Cranial ultrasound performed within 24 hours after birth showed diffuse echogenicities in the subcortical white matter and basal ganglia. Magnetic resonance imaging showed extensive cortical gray matter and subcortical white matter abnormalities in the entire left hemisphere and in large areas of the right hemisphere together with the thalami. A, Amplitude-integrated electroencephalogram at 25 hours after birth was performed for suspected seizures, but findings from the two-channel aEEG and real electroencephalogram (B) were not conclusive. C, Multichannel electroencephalogram showed epileptic activity over the vertex (red arrows). D, Axial T2-weighted image. E, Axial diffusion-weighted image.

Should We Treat Subclinical Seizures?

There is no consensus whether clinical events without an EEG correlate should be treated or how aggressively to treat electrographic-only seizures.[49,50] Although human data are scarce, several studies do suggest an adverse effect of both clinical and subclinical seizures on neurodevelopmental outcome. Neonatal seizures have been reported to predispose patients to later problems with regard to cognition, behavior, and development of postneonatal epilepsy.[51–53] Two previous aEEG studies have shown that infants treated for both clinical and subclinical seizures had a lower incidence of postneonatal epilepsy (8%–9%) compared with those treated only for clinical seizures (20%–50%).[54–57] It was of interest that in the study by Brunquell[53] the infants with subtle seizures and generalized tonic seizures had a significantly higher prevalence of postneonatal epilepsy ($P = .04$ and $P = .01$, respectively), cognitive impairment ($P = .02$; $P = .007$), and cerebral palsy ($P = .03$; $P = .002$) compared with patients with other seizure types. Subtle seizures were, in addition, more likely to be associated with abnormalities on neurologic examination at follow-up ($P = .03$). Prolonged seizures can increase brain temperature and thus increase metabolic demands.[58] Prolonged seizures cause progressive cerebral hypoxia and increase local cerebral blood flow and may steal perfusion from injured brain regions.[59] In a study by Miller et al. of term newborns with HIE, brain injury was independently associated with the severity of seizures.[52] They performed MRI and proton magnetic resonance spectroscopy (MRS) in 90 full-term infants. EEG-confirmed seizures developed in 33 (37%), and the seizures were scored based on frequency and severity, EEG findings, and AED use. Multivariable linear regression tested the independent association of seizure severity with impaired cerebral metabolism measured by lactate/choline and compromised neuronal integrity measured by N-acetylaspartate/choline in the basal nuclei and the intervascular boundary zones. Seizure severity was associated with increased lactate/choline in both the intervascular boundary zone ($P < .001$) and the basal nuclei ($P = .011$) when controlling for potential confounders of MRI abnormalities and extent of resuscitation at birth. Seizure severity was independently associated with diminished N-acetylaspartate/choline in the intervascular boundary zone ($P = .034$).

The same group was able to show an independent effect of clinical neonatal seizures and their treatment on neurodevelopment in 77 children who were born at term and were at risk for hypoxic-ischemic brain injury, and had brain MRI performed in the newborn period.[60] About one-third of the children (25/77) had clinically detected neonatal seizures. Neonatal MRIs were classified for anatomic distribution and severity of acute injury. The severity of brain injury was assessed using high-resolution newborn MRI, and outcome was assessed at age 4 years, using the Full-Scale Intelligence Quotient (FSIQ) of the Wechsler Preschool and Primary Scale of Intelligence–Revised, as well as a neuromotor score. After controlling for severity of injury on MRI, the children with neonatal seizures had worse motor and cognitive outcomes compared with those without seizures. The children with severe seizures had a lower FSIQ than those with mild or moderate seizures ($P < .001$). The major limitation of these two important studies is the reliance on clinical evaluation for classification of seizure diagnosis and severity.

In the randomized controlled trial of van Rooij et al.[61] the seizure burden was very high in both groups (treatment of subclinical seizures vs. treatment of clinical seizures only), but the burden was higher in the treatment of clinical seizures only group. It was of interest to see that there was a significant correlation between the duration of seizure patterns and the severity of brain injury on MRI in the blinded group, but not in the group treated for clinical as well as subclinical seizures. More recently, another randomized controlled trial showed that infants treated for electrographic seizures alone had fewer seizures, a lower seizure burden. and a shorter time to treatment than infants treated for clinical seizures only. These authors also confirmed that seizure burden was associated with brain injury scores and showed in addition that high seizure burden was associated with poorer outcome at 18 to 24 months.[47]

Adequate and fast detection of electrographic seizures is important to reduction of the seizure burden. However, it is difficult to constantly monitor real-time EEG. On some digital aEEG machines seizure detection algorithms are available, which may help in detecting seizures.[62] More recently, attempts have been made to develop neonatal seizure detection algorithms for multichannel EEG.[63] The performance of this seizure detection algorithm was not altered by the presence of a depressed EEG background activity caused by phenobarbital administration.[64]

aEEG in Preterm Infants

In parallel with multichannel EEG, aEEG background activity is more discontinuous in preterm infants. Normative values for aEEG background activity at different gestational ages have been published.[65] A scoring system for evaluation of brain maturation in preterm infants has also been developed.[66] Zhang et al. described reference values for aEEG amplitude obtained for 274 infants with a wide range of postmenstrual ages (PMAs) (30–55 weeks).[67] The normative amplitudes of aEEG margins, especially of the lower margin in quiet sleep, were recommended as a source of reference data for the identification of potentially abnormal aEEG results. The upper and lower margins of the aEEGs in both active and quiet sleep clearly rose after the neonatal period. The BW, defined as the graphic distance between the upper and lower margins, decreased almost monotonically throughout the PMA range from 30 to 55 weeks. The lower margin of the aEEG was positively correlated with PMA, with a larger rank correlation coefficient during quiet sleep (r = 0.89) than during active sleep (r = 0.49).

Studies with automated quantification of aEEG characteristics in premature infants by use of digital equipment have also been reported. Niemarkt et al. describe a method where the upper margin amplitude (UMA), lower margin amplitude (LMA), and BW were quantitatively calculated using a special software system.[68] In addition, the relative duration of discontinuous background pattern (discontinuous background defined as activity with LMA <5 µV, expressed as a percentage) was calculated. Analyses of the first-week recordings demonstrated a strong positive correlation between gestational age (GA) and LMA, while the percentage of discontinuous pattern decreased significantly. Longitudinally, all infants showed an increase of LMA. They found that GA and postnatal age (PA) both contributed independently and equally to LMA and the percentage of discontinuous pattern. They also found a strong correlation between postmenstrual age (GA + PA) and LMA and the percentage of discontinuous pattern, respectively. They conclude that LMA and percentage of discontinuous pattern are simple quantitative measures of neurophysiologic development and may be used to evaluate neurodevelopment in infants.

Other groups studied IBI duration or burst duration as a measure of discontinuity (or maturation). Palmu et al. described the characteristics of activity bursts in the early preterm EEG to assess interrater agreement of burst detection by visual inspection, and to determine the performance of an automated burst detector that uses a nonlinear energy operator (NLEO).[69] They conclude that visual detection of bursts from the early preterm EEG is comparable, albeit not identical, between raters. The original automated detector underestimates the amount of burst occurrence but can be readily improved to yield results comparable to visual detection. More recently Koolen et al. developed an automated burst detection method based on line length, which had a sensitivity and specificity above 84 and even performed well with a limited number of channels.[70] The same group also developed a quantitative measure of discontinuity called the suppression curve, which proved to be a reliable measure of preterm brain maturation.[71] Further clinical studies are warranted to assess the optimal descriptors of burst detection for monitoring and prognostication. Validation of a burst detector may offer an evidence-based platform for further development of brain monitors in very preterm babies.

SWC can be clearly identified in the aEEG from around 30 weeks' gestation, but also at 25 to 26 weeks GA a cyclical pattern resembling SWC can be seen in stable infants (Fig. 14.5). Effects from common medications (e.g., surfactant, morphine, and diazepam) and elevated carbon dioxide blood levels can be readily seen as a deterioration of the aEEG background pattern in preterm infants.[72–76]

Early prediction of outcome based on aEEG is a more complicated issue in preterm infants than in full-term infants. A predominantly discontinuous background pattern can be considered normal in most infants younger than 30 weeks' gestation. In the most immature infants, factors other than initial brain function may influence long-term neurodevelopmental outcome (e.g., bronchopulmonary dysplasia and late-onset sepsis), which makes prediction of outcome from the early EEG less certain. Nevertheless, several EEG and aEEG studies have shown early background depression to correlate with the severity of a periventricular-intraventricular hemorrhage.[77] The prognostic value of aEEG in premature infants was assessed by Klebermass et al., who compared the prognostic value of aEEG and cranial ultrasound.[78] Specificity was 73% for assessment within the first and increased to 95% in the second week of life, whereas sensitivity remained approximately the same 87% (first week) to 83% (second week).

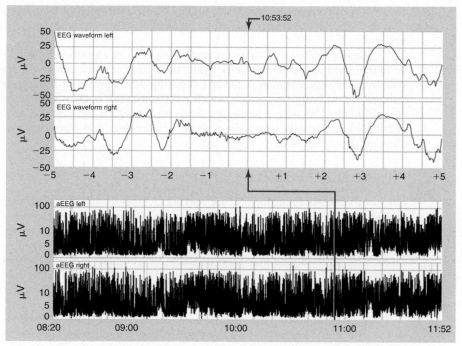

Fig. 14.5   Preterm infant born at 25+2 weeks gestational age with a birth weight of 860 g. An emergency cesarean section was performed because of fetal bradycardia. Apgar score: 5 and 8 after 1 and 5 minutes. The infant was supported with nasal CPAP and was on caffeine during the first few days after delivery. Cranial ultrasound examination was normal. Day 3, two-channel recording shows normal background pattern for this age with some cycling.

Cranial ultrasound showed a specificity of 86% within the first and second week, sensitivity also remained the same (74% and 75%). This group concluded that the aEEG also has a predictive value for later outcome in preterm infants and can be used as an early prognostic tool. West et al. evaluated 76 infants younger than 29 weeks' gestation with two-channel EEG within 48 hours of delivery and a Bayley-II at 18 months corrected age.[79] The analyzed segments of EEG were obtained around 24 hours (median; range 3–48 hours) of age. The neurophysiologist's assessment was a better predictor of adverse outcome than quantitative continuity measures defined as percentage of time above 25μV (positive predictive value 95% CI 75 [54%–96%] versus 41 [22%–60%] at 25-μV threshold, negative predictive value 88% [80%–96%] versus 84% [74%–94%], and positive likelihood ratio 9.0 [3.2–24.6] versus 2.0 [1.2–3.6]). All infants with definite seizures identified by the neurophysiologist had poor outcomes. They conclude that modified bedside EEG has potential to assist with identification of extremely preterm infants at risk for adverse neurodevelopmental outcomes. However, analysis by a neurophysiologist performed better than the currently available continuity analyses.

In analogy of amplitude depression after severe asphyxia in term infants, ter Horst et al. related a neonatal acute physiology score (Score for Neonatal Acute Physiology II [SNAP-II] as an acute reflection of severity of illness) in preterm infants with aEEG scores.[80] The aEEGs were assessed by pattern recognition, by calculating a Burdjalov score, and by calculating the mean values of the 5th, 50th, and 95th centiles of the aEEG amplitudes. Illness severity was determined within the first 24 hours of life. They recorded aEEGs in 38 infants with a mean GA of 29.7 weeks (26.0–31.8 weeks) during the first 5 days of life. They found that severity of illness as measured by the SNAP-II and low blood pressure had a negative effect on the aEEGs of preterm infants. These findings were confirmed by two recent studies relating the SNAP-II and hemodynamic parameters to the Burdjalov score and aEEG amplitudes.[81,82]

Epileptic seizure activity in preterm infants can be identified in a manner similar to that used in full-term infants. Epileptic seizure activity, often without clinical symptoms, is very common in the aEEG during development of intracerebral hemorrhages. Identifying seizure activity on a discontinuous background pattern can be very difficult. With access to the real EEG on the digital devices this problem can be handled more easily, especially with the seizure detection algorithm available on some devices (Fig. 14.6).

Pitfalls and Artifacts

The simultaneous recording of the real EEG, present on digital devices, helps in the identification of artifacts that are quite common during long-term recordings.[83] Hagmann et al. have shown that 12% of their 200 hours of recordings was affected by artifacts.[84] This was due to electrical interference in 55% of cases, which could be either ECG artifact (39%) or fast activity (>50 Hz, 61%) and to movement artifact in the remaining 45%. They state that the dual facility (aEEG with simultaneous real EEG) is crucial for the correct interpretation of the aEEG.

Inappropriate electrode position can also lead to aEEG recordings with artifact or drift of the baseline as noted earlier in this chapter. Some apparently normal aEEGs in infants with severe encephalopathy have electrocardiographic artifacts that could explain a drift of a severely depressed baseline to a baseline within the normal voltage range (see Fig. 14.2). It is very important to recognize this so-called drift of the baseline because the interpretation of aEEG background patterns is used for selection for therapeutic hypothermia. In a study by Sarkar et al.,

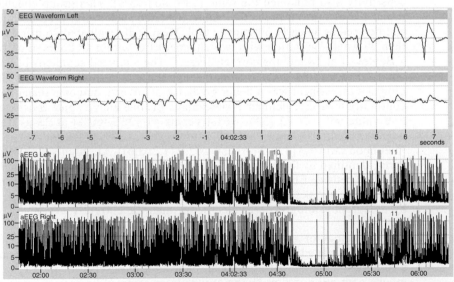

Fig. 14.6   Preterm infant born at 28+5 weeks gestational age with a birth weight of 1065 g, unexplained preterm delivery. Apgar score: 5 and 9 after 1 and 5 minutes. Cranial ultrasound revealed a bilateral IVH grade 2 with parenchymal involvement on the left. Therefore a two-channel aEEG recording was obtained. No clinical seizures were observed. The aEEG at 52 hours after birth showed subclinical seizures, which were picked up by the seizure detection algorithm and visible in the aEEG. There was no posthemorrhagic ventricular dilatation. Three loading doses (10 mg-kg) of phenobarbital, lidocaine, and clonazepam were given. The infant died on day 6 after redirection of care. A discontinuous pattern without cycling at 29 weeks postmenstrual age with a sudden depression of the aEEG after administration of clonazepam. On day 3 subclinical seizures picked up by the seizure detection algorithm (*pink squares*) and the aEEG (abrupt, transient rise of the lower border).

54 infants with moderate or severe HIE were evaluated with aEEG for selection for hypothermic neuroprotection.[85] Seven encephalopathic infants with a normal aEEG who were not cooled were subsequently shown to have abnormalities on their MRI. They concluded that there was a poor correlation between early aEEG and short-term adverse outcome with a sensitivity of 54.8% and a negative predictive value of only 44%. All of these normal aEEGs, however, had electrocardiographic artifacts that could explain the drift of the baseline (personal communication). Retrospectively, these patients would have been eligible for the cooling study on the basis of their background pattern.

Medication can also affect the background pattern. AEDs can lead to a temporary decrease in amplitude on the aEEG recording, although this does not influence prognosis.[15,18] Other drugs such as morphine can have a similar effect.[75] We therefore recommend the use of pattern recognition, taking the values of upper and lower margins into account as well.

Seizure-Like Artifacts

Any movement or handling of the infant, such as a ventilation artifact resulting in a sudden increase of the baseline of the aEEG recording, can mimic seizure activity on the aEEG (Fig. 14.7). The simultaneously recorded real EEG signal can help to interpret aEEG traces more accurately.[83] In addition, marking events on the aEEG recording by nursing staff is extremely important.

aEEG in Other Clinical Conditions

Continuous monitoring of EEG is also useful in neonates with congenital heart disease (CHD), especially after surgery with cardiac arrest. [86] Only a few studies describe the role of the aEEG in this condition, some in combination with NIRS.[87–89] In a study by ter Horst et al., the aEEG data obtained before surgery were described in neonates with CHD.[90] The first 72 hours after starting prostaglandin E_1 therapy were used for analysis. The background patterns were mildly abnormal in 45% of the infants and severely abnormal at some point during the recording in 14% of the infants. A severely abnormal aEEG and epileptiform activity were associated with more profound acidosis. The authors conclude that the

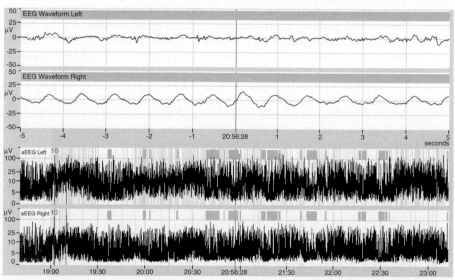

Fig. 14.7 Preterm infant born at 27+1 weeks gestational age with a birth weight of 1020 g, ventilated because of infant respiratory distress syndrome. This patient had a normal cranial ultrasound examination. At 2 years of age the infant had a cognition composite score of 115 and a motor composite score of 127 on the Bayley-III. Two-channel recording showing several seizure detection alerts because of a rhythmic pattern. This turned out to be an artifact as the waveform pattern on the real EEG form the right hemisphere synchronizes with the ventilator settings while the infant was lying on its right side.

majority of infants with CHD had an abnormal aEEG before surgery. aEEG helped to identify epileptiform activity and was a useful tool to evaluate brain function before surgery in CHD.

The same group also studied aEEG during neonatal sepsis with or without meningitis.[91] Their aim was to investigate the longitudinal course and prognostic value of aEEG in infants with neonatal sepsis or meningitis with a gestation of 34 to 42 weeks. They found that low-voltage background pattern, SWC, and epileptiform activity on the aEEG are helpful to predict neurologic outcome in infants with neonatal sepsis or meningitis. Others looked at the effect of sepsis on the aEEG in extremely premature infants.[92] Monthly aEEG was performed from 28 weeks until 36 weeks PMA in 108 premature infants born before 28 weeks' gestation. Additional aEEG recordings were performed during the first episode of sepsis. They found that sepsis was associated with acute EEG changes, as indicated by BS, but not with a decrease in aEEG maturation score.

A sudden rise of arterial partial pressure of carbon dioxide ($PaCO_2$) levels can result in a sudden drop in aEEG amplitude (Fig. 14.8).[76] Wikström et al. performed an observational study in 32 infants with a GA of 22 to 27 weeks.[93] They performed simultaneous single-channel EEG and repeated blood gas/plasma glucose analyses during the first 3 days (n = 247 blood samples with corresponding EEG). IBIs and EEG power were averaged at the time of each blood sample. They found a linear relationship between $PaCO_2$ and IBI: increasing $PaCO_2$ was associated with longer IBIs. One day after birth, a 1-kPa increase in $PaCO_2$ was associated with a 16% increase in IBI in infants who survived the first week without severe brain injury. EEG power was highest at a $PaCO_2$ value of 5.1 kPa and was attenuated both at higher and lower $PaCO_2$ values. In addition, these researchers found that plasma glucose levels, corrected for carbon dioxide effects, were also associated with IBI. Lowest IBI appeared at a plasma glucose level of 4.0 mmol/L, and there was a U-shaped relationship between plasma glucose level and EEG with increasing discontinuity at glucose concentrations above and below 4.0 mmol/L. Both carbon dioxide and plasma glucose levels influenced EEG activity in extremely preterm infants, and values considered to be within normal physiologic ranges were associated with the best EEG background. Increasing EEG discontinuity occurred at carbon dioxide levels frequently applied in lung protection strategies; in addition, moderate hyperglycemia was associated with measurable EEG changes. Extreme fluctuations in $PaCO_2$ and a higher maximum $PaCO_2$ have been associated with worse neurodevelopmental outcome in very low-birth-weight preterm infants.[94] The association between fluctuations in $PaCO_2$ could be mediated through the induction of brain damage such as intracranial hemorrhage and periventricular leukomalacia.[95,96]

Severe hyperbilirubinemia (Fig. 14.9) may also lead to aEEG background depression with or without seizures. aEEG can be used in congenital metabolic disorders, resulting in hyperammonemia and seizures (Fig. 14.10).[97] Deterioration of background patterns, abnormal SWC patterns, and seizures have been described and can be recognized in various metabolic diseases.[98]

aEEG can be of use in genetic disorders associated with neonatal epilepsy as well. For example, neonatal seizures associated with mutations in the *KCNQ2* gene result in a specific aEEG pattern (Fig. 14.11).[99,100] The interictal background activity in infants with genetic disorders and neonatal seizures is usually normal (as seen in Fig. 14.11 and as was described in infants with neonatal seizures and mutations in the *SLC13A5* gene).[100]

Gaps in Knowledge

As with all (new) techniques, there is a learning curve for aEEG. From the paper by Boylan et al.,[1] we know that the aEEG is mainly assessed by neonatologists, 30% of whom are not confident in their ability to interpret it. So training is essential.

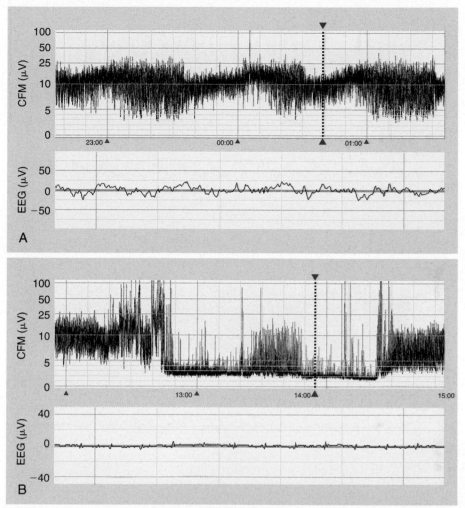

Fig. 14.8 Full-term infant who was discharged home after a normal vaginal delivery with good Apgar scores. The infant was admitted to the neonatal intensive care unit on the second day after birth because of a group B streptococcal septicemia. The patient needed High Frequency Oscillation because of pulmonary hypertension and required inotropes to maintain a normal blood pressure. A, On day 7 a normal background pattern (continuous normal voltage) was seen with clear sleep-wake cycling. B, On day 7 there was a sudden drop in amplitude to an almost flat trace. During this period of low amplitude, there was a sudden rise in $PaCO_2$ up to 130 mm Hg caused by an obstructed endotracheal tube. The amplitude-integrated electroencephalogram pattern normalized again when the $PaCO_2$ normalized. *CFM*, Cerebral function monitor; *EEG*, electroencephalogram.

We need to be aware that EEG remains the gold standard. So if one is not sure about the assessment of the aEEG, a multichannel EEG should always be performed. Therefore it is very important for the practitioner to have a good relationship with the neurophysiology department of his or her hospital. Furthermore, we recommend performing a multichannel EEG during office hours at least once during an aEEG recording of several days. Several centers are now using continuous multichannel recording, with a two-channel display for the neonatologist, but with remote access for the neurophysiologist for all channels.

The aEEG assessment of the preterm infant is different and more difficult to interpret than the aEEG assessment of a term infant. With digital equipment and advanced techniques increasingly available, quantitative assessment of IBI and the use of automated burst detectors will be performed more often.[50] Still, more research should be done in this field.

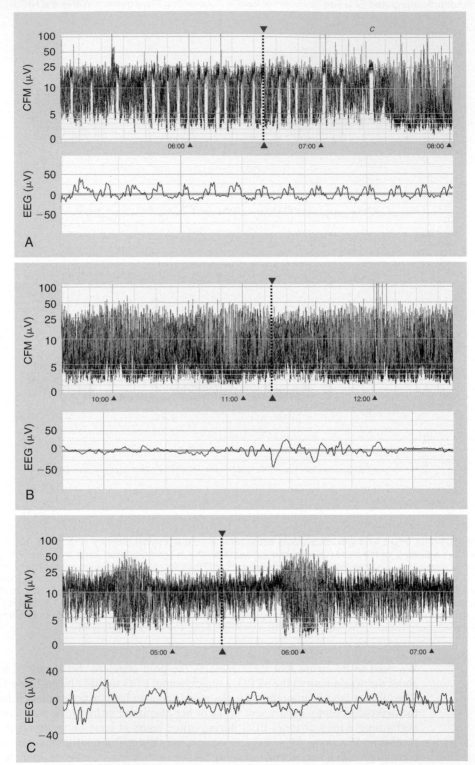

Fig. 14.9 Full-term infant of Chinese origin, born at 37 + 2 weeks gestational age. The infant developed severe hyperbilirubinemia with a blood level of 588 μmol/L on day 5. He developed seizures at a referring hospital where they started amplitude-integrated electroencephalogram (aEEG) monitoring. Following a loading dose of phenobarbital (20 mg/kg) he was referred to the neonatal intensive care unit. Brainstem auditory evoked potentials were abnormal, and magnetic resonance imaging showed clear signal intensity changes in the globus pallidus. Exchange transfusion and phototherapy were performed. Further evaluation revealed a G6PD-deficiency. The infant developed an auditory neuropathy, but motor and cognitive function were in the normal range at the age of 7 years. A, Epileptiform activity at the referring hospital on an aEEG *(top panel)*. The lower panel shows epileptiform activity on the real EEG. A loading dose of phenobarbital was given at point *C*. B, Day 5 EEG on admission (after phenobarbital). A discontinuous normal voltage pattern without seizures was seen. C, Day 6 aEEG (1 day after admission) shows continuous normal voltage pattern with sleep-wake cycling. *CFM*, Cerebral function monitor; *EEG*, electroencephalogram.

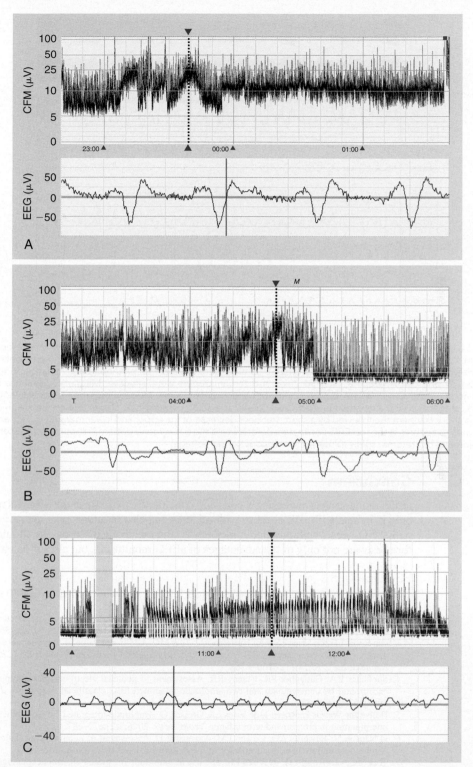

Fig. 14.10   Full-term infant born at home after an uncomplicated pregnancy and delivery. The infant was admitted to the hospital on day 2 because of a low body temperature and an incident after oral feeding. The infant developed seizures with apneas, needed ventilation, and was referred to a neonatal intensive care unit. He was treated with phenobarbital, midazolam, lidocaine, and pyridoxine because of refractory seizures. Serum ammonia level was elevated on admission and increased linearly (1245—3293—3293—8700—4719 μmol/L). He was subsequently diagnosed to have a urea cycle defect (ornithine transcarbamylase deficiency) and died on day 4. A, Seizures were noted on admission. B, Repetitive seizures were observed the day after admission. After a loading dose of midazolam (at M), a sparse burst suppression pattern was seen. C, Several hours after the repetitive seizures shown in B, status epilepticus on a flat background pattern is seen. CFM, Cerebral function monitor; EEG, electroencephalogram.

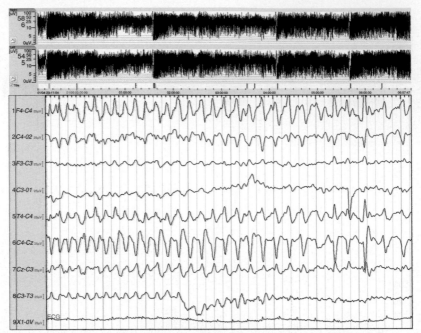

Fig. 14.11   Full-term infant born after an uncomplicated pregnancy and delivery. On day 2 the infant developed clinical seizures. On day 3 the infant was admitted to the neonatal intensive care unit where seizures were confirmed on amplitude-integrated electroencephalogram (aEEG). Seizures were treated with phenobarbital, midazolam, lidocaine, levetiracetam, and carbamazepine. Only lidocaine and carbamazepine were effective. Magnetic resonance imaging showed no structural abnormalities, but on proton MR spectroscopy, a low *N*-acetyl aspartate peak was noted. The infant was diagnosed with a mutation in the *KCNQ2* gene. The aEEG on admission shows four seizures with a typical pattern: a short, transient rise followed by a short, transient decrease of the upper and lower margin *(upper panel)*. This corresponds to seizures in the real EEG *(lower panel)*. Afterwards the background pattern is suppressed (discontinuous normal voltage) but returns rapidly to normal (continuous normal voltage).

Conclusion

aEEG monitoring is increasingly considered the standard of care in the neonatal unit, not only in infants with HIE or those with seizures, but also in infants who are seriously ill with CHD, sepsis with or without meningitis, and metabolic diseases. We should therefore be aware not only of the advantages of aEEG monitoring, but also of its pitfalls.

REFERENCES

1. Boylan G, Burgoyne L, Moore C, O'Flaherty B, Rennie J. An international survey of EEG use in the neonatal intensive care unit. *Acta Paediatr*. 2010;99(8):1150–1155.
2. Prior PF, Maynard DE, Sheaff PC, et al. Monitoring cerebral function: clinical experience with new device for continuous recording of electrical activity of brain. *Br Med J*. 1971;2(5764):736–738.
3. van Rooij LG, de Vries LS, van Huffelen AC, Toet MC. Additional value of two-channel amplitude integrated EEG recording in full-term infants with unilateral brain injury. *Arch Dis Child Fetal Neonatal Ed*. 2010;95(3):F160–F168.
4. Shellhaas RA, Gallagher PR, Clancy RR. Assessment of neonatal electroencephalography (EEG) background by conventional and two amplitude-integrated EEG classification systems. *J Pediatr*. 2008;153(3):369–374.
5. Hellström-Westas L, Rosén I, de Vries LS, Greisen G. Amplitude-integrated EEG classification and interpretation in preterm and term infants. *NeoReviews*. 2006;7(2):e72–e87.
6. al Naqeeb N, Edwards AD, Cowan FM, Azzopardi D. Assessment of neonatal encephalopathy by amplitude-integrated electroencephalography. *Pediatrics*. 1999;103(6 Pt 1):1263–1271.
7. Toet MC, van Rooij LG, de Vries LS. The use of amplitude integrated electroencephalography for assessing neonatal neurologic injury. *Clin Perinatol*. 2008;35(4):665–678, v.
8. Thoresen M, Hellstrom-Westas L, Liu X, de Vries LS. Effect of hypothermia on amplitude-integrated electroencephalogram in infants with asphyxia. *Pediatrics*. 2010;126(1):e131–e139.
9. Quigg M, Leiner D. Engineering aspects of the quantified amplitude-integrated electroencephalogram in neonatal cerebral monitoring. *J Clin Neurophysiol*. 2009;26(3):145–149.
10. de Vries LS, Toet MC. How to assess the aEEG background. *J Pediatr*. 2009;154(4):625–626.
11. Toet MC, van der Meij W, de Vries LS, Uiterwaal CS, van Huffelen KC. Comparison between simultaneously recorded amplitude integrated electroencephalogram (cerebral function monitor) and standard electroencephalogram in neonates. *Pediatrics*. 2002;109(5):772–779.

12. Evans E, Koh S, Lerner J, Sankar R, Garg M. Accuracy of amplitude integrated EEG in a neonatal cohort. *Arch Dis Child Fetal Neonatal Ed.* 2010;95(3):F169–F173.
13. Bennet L, Fyfe KL, Yiallourou SR, Merk H, Wong FY, Horne RS. Discrimination of sleep states using continuous cerebral bedside monitoring (amplitude-integrated electroencephalography) compared to polysomnography in infants. *Acta Paediatr.* 2016;105(12):e582–e587.
14. Meledin I, Abu TM, Gilat S, et al. Comparison of amplitude-integrated EEG and conventional EEG in a cohort of premature infants. *Clin EEG Neurosci.* 2017;48(2):146–154.
15. Murray DM, Boylan GB, Ryan CA, Connolly S. Early EEG findings in hypoxic-ischemic encephalopathy predict outcomes at 2 years. *Pediatrics.* 2009;124(3):e459–e467.
16. Spitzmiller RE, Phillips T, Meinzen-Derr J, Hoath SB. Amplitude-integrated EEG is useful in predicting neurodevelopmental outcome in full-term infants with hypoxic-ischemic encephalopathy: a meta-analysis. *J Child Neurol.* 2007;22(9):1069–1078.
17. Shah DK, Lavery S, Doyle LW, Wong C, McDougall P, Inder TE. Use of 2-channel bedside electroencephalogram monitoring in term-born encephalopathic infants related to cerebral injury defined by magnetic resonance imaging. *Pediatrics.* 2006;118(1):47–55.
18. Shalak LF, Laptook AR, Velaphi SC, Perlman JM. Amplitude-integrated electroencephalography coupled with an early neurologic examination enhances prediction of term infants at risk for persistent encephalopathy. *Pediatrics.* 2003;111(2):351–357.
19. van Rooij LG, Toet MC, Osredkar D, van Huffelen AC, Groenendaal F, de Vries LS. Recovery of amplitude integrated electroencephalographic background patterns within 24 hours of perinatal asphyxia. *Arch Dis Child Fetal Neonatal Ed.* 2005;90(3):F245–F251.
20. Osredkar D, Derganc M, Paro-Panjan D, Neubauer D. Amplitude-integrated electroencephalography in full-term newborns without severe hypoxic-ischemic encephalopathy: case series. *Croat Med J.* 2006;47(2):285–291.
21. Del Rio R, Ochoa C, Alarcon A, Arnaez J, Blanco D, Garcia-Alix A. Amplitude integrated electroencephalogram as a prognostic tool in neonates with hypoxic-ischemic encephalopathy: a systematic review. *PLoS One.* 2016;11(11):e0165744.
22. Hallberg B, Grossmann K, Bartocci M, Blennow M. The prognostic value of early aEEG in asphyxiated infants undergoing systemic hypothermia treatment. *Acta Paediatr.* 2010;99(4):531–536.
23. Ancora G, Maranella E, Grandi S, et al. Early predictors of short term neurodevelopmental outcome in asphyxiated cooled infants. a combined brain amplitude integrated electroencephalography and near infrared spectroscopy study. *Brain Dev.* 2013;35(1):26–31.
24. Shankaran S, Pappas A, McDonald SA, et al. Predictive value of an early amplitude integrated electroencephalogram and neurologic examination. *Pediatrics.* 2011;128(1):e112–e120.
25. Gucuyener K, Beken S, Ergenekon E, et al. Use of amplitude-integrated electroencephalography (aEEG) and near infrared spectroscopy findings in neonates with asphyxia during selective head cooling. *Brain Dev.* 2012;34(4):280–286.
26. Cseko AJ, Bango M, Lakatos P, Kardasi J, Pusztai L, Szabo M. Accuracy of amplitude-integrated electroencephalography in the prediction of neurodevelopmental outcome in asphyxiated infants receiving hypothermia treatment. *Acta Paediatr.* 2013;102(7):707–711.
27. Azzopardi D. Predictive value of the amplitude integrated EEG in infants with hypoxic ischaemic encephalopathy: data from a randomised trial of therapeutic hypothermia. *Arch Dis Child Fetal Neonatal Ed.* 2014;99(1):F80–F82.
28. Takenouchi T, Rubens EO, Yap VL, Ross G, Engel M, Perlman JM. Delayed onset of sleep-wake cycling with favorable outcome in hypothermic-treated neonates with encephalopathy. *J Pediatr.* 2011;159(2):232–237.
29. Murray DM, Boylan GB, Ali I, Ryan CA, Murphy BP, Connolly S. Defining the gap between electrographic seizure burden, clinical expression and staff recognition of neonatal seizures. *Arch Dis Child Fetal Neonatal Ed.* 2008;93(3):F187–F191.
30. Malone A, Ryan CA, Fitzgerald A, Burgoyne L, Connolly S, Boylan GB. Interobserver agreement in neonatal seizure identification. *Epilepsia.* 2009;50(9):2097–2101.
31. Shellhaas RA, Chang T, Tsuchida T, et al. The American clinical neurophysiology society's guideline on continuous electroencephalography monitoring in neonates. *J Clin Neurophysiol.* 2011;28(6):611–617.
32. Shellhaas RA, Clancy RR. Characterization of neonatal seizures by conventional EEG and single-channel EEG. *Clin Neurophysiol.* 2007;118(10):2156–2161.
33. Rakshasbhuvankar A, Paul S, Nagarajan L, Ghosh S, Rao S. Amplitude-integrated EEG for detection of neonatal seizures: a systematic review. *Seizure.* 2015;33:90–98.
34. Shellhaas RA, Soaita AI, Clancy RR. Sensitivity of amplitude-integrated electroencephalography for neonatal seizure detection. *Pediatrics.* 2007;120(4):770–777.
35. Bourez-Swart MD, van RL, Rizzo C, et al. Detection of subclinical electroencephalographic seizure patterns with multichannel amplitude-integrated EEG in full-term neonates. *Clin Neurophysiol.* 2009;120(11):1916–1922.
36. Shah DK, Mackay MT, Lavery S, et al. Accuracy of bedside electroencephalographic monitoring in comparison with simultaneous continuous conventional electroencephalography for seizure detection in term infants. *Pediatrics.* 2008;121(6):1146–1154.
37. Lawrence R, Mathur A, Nguyen The Tich, Zempel J, Inder T. A pilot study of continuous limited-channel aEEG in term infants with encephalopathy. *J Pediatr.* 2009;154(6):835–841.
38. Boylan GB, Rennie JM, Pressler RM, Wilson G, Morton M, Binnie CD. Phenobarbitone, neonatal seizures, and video-EEG. *Arch Dis Child Fetal Neonatal Ed.* 2002;86(3):F165–F170.
39. Scher MS, Alvin J, Gaus L, Minnigh B, Painter MJ. Uncoupling of EEG-clinical neonatal seizures after antiepileptic drug use. *Pediatr Neurol.* 2003;28(4):277–280.

14

40. van Rooij LG, de Vries LS, Handryastuti S, et al. Neurodevelopmental outcome in term infants with status epilepticus detected with amplitude-integrated electroencephalography. *Pediatrics*. 2007;120(2):e354–e363.

41. Pisani F, Cerminara C, Fusco C, Sisti L. Neonatal status epilepticus vs recurrent neonatal seizures: clinical findings and outcome. *Neurology*. 2007;69(23):2177–2185.

42. Rothman SM, Glass HC, Chang T, Sullivan JE, Bonifacio SL, Shellhaas RA. Risk factors for EEG seizures in neonates treated with hypothermia: a multicenter cohort study. *Neurology*. 2014;83(19):1773–1774.

43. Boylan GB, Kharoshankaya L, Wusthoff CJ. Seizures and hypothermia: importance of electroencephalographic monitoring and considerations for treatment. *Semin Fetal Neonatal Med*. 2015;20(2):103–108.

44. Glass HC, Nash KB, Bonifacio SL, et al. Seizures and magnetic resonance imaging-detected brain injury in newborns cooled for hypoxic-ischemic encephalopathy. *J Pediatr*. 2011;159(5):731–735.

45. Nash KB, Bonifacio SL, Glass HC, et al. Video-EEG monitoring in newborns with hypoxic-ischemic encephalopathy treated with hypothermia. *Neurology*. 2011;76(6):556–562.

46. Wusthoff CJ, Dlugos DJ, Gutierrez-Colina A, et al. Electrographic seizures during therapeutic hypothermia for neonatal hypoxic-ischemic encephalopathy. *J Child Neurol*. 2011;26(6):724–728.

47. Srinivasakumar P, Zempel J, Trivedi S, et al. Treating EEG seizures in hypoxic ischemic encephalopathy: a randomized controlled trial. *Pediatrics*. 2015;136(5):e1302–e1309.

48. Shah DK, Wusthoff CJ, Clarke P, et al. Electrographic seizures are associated with brain injury in newborns undergoing therapeutic hypothermia. *Arch Dis Child Fetal Neonatal Ed*. 2014;99(3):F219–F224.

49. Sankar R, Painter MJ. Neonatal seizures: after all these years we still love what doesn't work. *Neurology*. 2005;64(5):776–777.

50. Silverstein FS, Jensen FE. Neonatal seizures. *Ann Neurol*. 2007;62(2):112–120.

51. McBride MC, Laroia N, Guillet R. Electrographic seizures in neonates correlate with poor neurodevelopmental outcome. *Neurology*. 2000;55(4):506–513.

52. Miller SP, Weiss J, Barnwell A, et al. Seizure-associated brain injury in term newborns with perinatal asphyxia. *Neurology*. 2002;58(4):542–548.

53. Brunquell PJ, Glennon CM, DiMario FJ Jr, Lerer T, Eisenfeld L. Prediction of outcome based on clinical seizure type in newborn infants. *J Pediatr*. 2002;140(6):707–712.

54. Hellstrom-Westas L, Blennow G, Lindroth M, Rosen I, Svenningsen NW. Low risk of seizure recurrence after early withdrawal of antiepileptic treatment in the neonatal period. *Arch Dis Child Fetal Neonatal Ed*. 1995;72(2):F97–F101.

55. Toet MC, Groenendaal F, Osredkar D, van Huffelen AC, de Vries LS. Postneonatal epilepsy following amplitude-integrated EEG-detected neonatal seizures. *Pediatr Neurol*. 2005;32(4):241–247.

56. Clancy RR, Legido A. Postnatal epilepsy after EEG-confirmed neonatal seizures. *Epilepsia*. 1991;32(1):69–76.

57. Ronen GM, Buckley D, Penney S, Streiner DL. Long-term prognosis in children with neonatal seizures: a population-based study. *Neurology*. 2007;69(19):1816–1822.

58. Yager JY, Armstrong EA, Jaharus C, Saucier DM, Wirrell EC. Preventing hyperthermia decreases brain damage following neonatal hypoxic-ischemic seizures. *Brain Res*. 2004;1011(1):48–57.

59. Boylan GB, Panerai RB, Rennie JM, Evans DH, Rabe-Hesketh S, Binnie CD. Cerebral blood flow velocity during neonatal seizures. *Arch Dis Child Fetal Neonatal Ed*. 1999;80(2):F105–F110.

60. Glass HC, Glidden D, Jeremy RJ, Barkovich AJ, Ferriero DM, Miller SP. Clinical neonatal seizures are independently associated with outcome in Infants at risk for hypoxic-ischemic brain injury. *J Pediatr*. 2009;155(3):318–323.

61. van Rooij LG, Toet MC, van Huffelen AC, et al. Effect of treatment of subclinical neonatal seizures detected with aEEG: randomized, controlled trial. *Pediatrics*. 2010;125(2):e358–e366.

62. Navakatikyan MA, Colditz PB, Burke CJ, Inder TE, Richmond J, Williams CE. Seizure detection algorithm for neonates based on wave-sequence analysis. *Clin Neurophysiol*. 2006;117(6):1190–1203.

63. Mathieson SR, Stevenson NJ, Low E, et al. Validation of an automated seizure detection algorithm for term neonates. *Clin Neurophysiol*. 2016;127(1):156–168.

64. Mathieson SR, Livingstone V, Low E, Pressler R, Rennie JM, Boylan GB. Phenobarbital reduces EEG amplitude and propagation of neonatal seizures but does not alter performance of automated seizure detection. *Clin Neurophysiol*. 2016;127(10):3343–3350.

65. Olischar M, Klebermass K, Kuhle S, et al. Reference values for amplitude-integrated electroencephalographic activity in preterm infants younger than 30 weeks' gestational age. *Pediatrics*. 2004;113(1 Pt 1):e61–e66.

66. Burdjalov VF, Baumgart S, Spitzer AR. Cerebral function monitoring: a new scoring system for the evaluation of brain maturation in neonates. *Pediatrics*. 2003;112(4):855–861.

67. Zhang D, Liu Y, Hou X, et al. Reference values for amplitude-integrated EEGs in infants from preterm to 3.5 months of age. *Pediatrics*. 2011;127(5):e1280–e1287.

68. Niemarkt HJ, Andriessen P, Peters CH, et al. Quantitative analysis of amplitude-integrated electroencephalogram patterns in stable preterm infants, with normal neurological development at one year. *Neonatology*. 2010;97(2):175–182.

69. Palmu K, Wikstrom S, Hippelainen E, Boylan G, Hellstrom-Westas L, Vanhatalo S. Detection of 'EEG bursts' in the early preterm EEG: visual vs. automated detection. *Clin Neurophysiol*. 2010;121(7):1015–1022.

70. Koolen N, Jansen K, Vervisch J, et al. Line length as a robust method to detect high-activity events: automated burst detection in premature EEG recordings. *Clin Neurophysiol*. 2014;125(10):1985–1994.

71. Dereymaeker A, Koolen N, Jansen K, et al. The suppression curve as a quantitative approach for measuring brain maturation in preterm infants. *Clin Neurophysiol*. 2016;127(8):2760–2765.
72. Shany E, Benzaquen O, Friger M, Richardson J, Golan A. Influence of antiepileptic drugs on amplitude-integrated electroencephalography. *Pediatr Neurol*. 2008;39(6):387–391.
73. Hellstrom-Westas L, Bell AH, Skov L, Greisen G, Svenningsen NW. Cerebroelectrical depression following surfactant treatment in preterm neonates. *Pediatrics*. 1992;89(4 Pt 1):643–647.
74. Bell AH, Greisen G, Pryds O. Comparison of the effects of phenobarbitone and morphine administration on EEG activity in preterm babies. *Acta Paediatr*. 1993;82(1):35–39.
75. Young GB, da Silva OP. Effects of morphine on the electroencephalograms of neonates: a prospective, observational study. *Clin Neurophysiol*. 2000;111(11):1955–1960.
76. Weeke LC, Dix LML, Groenendaal F, et al. Severe hypercapnia causes reversible depression of aEEG background activity in neonates: an observational study. *Arch Dis Child Fetal Neonatal Ed*. 2017;102(5):F383–F388.
77. Hellstrom-Westas L, Klette H, Thorngren-Jerneck K, Rosen I. Early prediction of outcome with aEEG in preterm infants with large intraventricular hemorrhages. *Neuropediatrics*. 2001;32(6):319–324.
78. Klebermass K, Olischar M, Waldhoer T, Fuiko R, Pollak A, Weninger M. Amplitude-integrated EEG pattern predicts further outcome in preterm infants. *Pediatr Res*. 2011;70(1):102–108.
79. West CR, Harding JE, Williams CE, Nolan M, Battin MR. Cot-side electroencephalography for outcome prediction in preterm infants: observational study. *Arch Dis Child Fetal Neonatal Ed*. 2011;96(2):F108–F113.
80. ter Horst HJ, Jongbloed-Pereboom M, van Eykern LA, Bos AF. Amplitude-integrated electroencephalographic activity is suppressed in preterm infants with high scores on illness severity. *Early Hum Dev*. 2011;87(5):385–390.
81. Shah D, Paradisis M, Bowen JR. Relationship between systemic blood flow, blood pressure, inotropes, and aEEG in the first 48 h of life in extremely preterm infants. *Pediatr Res*. 2013;74(3):314–320.
82. Shibasaki J, Toyoshima K, Kishigami M. Blood pressure and aEEG in the 96 h after birth and correlations with neurodevelopmental outcome in extremely preterm infants. *Early Hum Dev*. 2016;101:79–84.
83. de Vries NK, ter Horst HJ, Bos AF. The added value of simultaneous EEG and amplitude-integrated EEG recordings in three newborn infants. *Neonatology*. 2007;91(3):212–216.
84. Hagmann CF, Robertson NJ, Azzopardi D. Artifacts on electroencephalograms may influence the amplitude-integrated EEG classification: a qualitative analysis in neonatal encephalopathy. *Pediatrics*. 2006;118(6):2552–2554.
85. Sarkar S, Barks JD, Donn SM. Should amplitude-integrated electroencephalography be used to identify infants suitable for hypothermic neuroprotection? *J Perinatol*. 2008;28(2):117–122.
86. Clancy RR, Sharif U, Ichord R, et al. Electrographic neonatal seizures after infant heart surgery. *Epilepsia*. 2005;46(1):84–90.
87. Toet MC, Flinterman A, Laar I, et al. Cerebral oxygen saturation and electrical brain activity before, during, and up to 36 hours after arterial switch procedure in neonates without pre-existing brain damage: its relationship to neurodevelopmental outcome. *Exp Brain Res*. 2005;165(3):343–350.
88. Latal B, Wohlrab G, Brotschi B, Beck I, Knirsch W, Bernet V. Postoperative Amplitude-Integrated Electroencephalography Predicts Four-Year Neurodevelopmental Outcome in Children with Complex Congenital Heart Disease. *J Pediatr*. 2016;178:55–60.
89. Algra SO, Schouten AN, Jansen NJ, et al. Perioperative and bedside cerebral monitoring identifies cerebral injury after surgical correction of congenital aortic arch obstruction. *Intensive Care Med*. 2015;41(11):2011–2012.
90. ter Horst HJ, Mud M, Roofthooft MT, Bos AF. Amplitude integrated electroencephalographic activity in infants with congenital heart disease before surgery. *Early Hum Dev*. 2010;86(12):759–764.
91. ter Horst HJ, van Olffen M, Remmelts HJ, de Vries H, Bos AF. The prognostic value of amplitude integrated EEG in neonatal sepsis and/or meningitis. *Acta Paediatr*. 2010;99(2):194–200.
92. Helderman JB, Welch CD, Leng X, O'Shea TM. Sepsis-associated electroencephalographic changes in extremely low gestational age neonates. *Early Hum Dev*. 2010;86(8):509–513.
93. Wikström S, Lundin F, Ley D, et al. Carbon dioxide and glucose affect electrocortical background in extremely preterm infants. *Pediatrics*. 2011;127(4):e1028–e1034.
94. McKee LA, Fabres J, Howard G, Peralta-Carcelen M, Carlo WA, Ambalavanan N. PaCO$_2$ and neurodevelopment in extremely low birth weight infants. *J Pediatr*. 2009;155(2):217–221.
95. Kaiser JR, Gauss CH, Williams DK. The effects of hypercapnia on cerebral autoregulation in ventilated very low birth weight infants. *Pediatr Res*. 2005;58(5):931–935.
96. Greisen G, Munck H, Lou H. May hypocarbia cause ischaemic brain damage in the preterm infant? *Lancet*. 1986;2(8504):460.
97. Olischar M, Shany E, Aygun C, et al. Amplitude-integrated electroencephalography in newborns with inborn errors of metabolism. *Neonatology*. 2012;102(3):203–211.
98. Theda C. Use of amplitude integrated electroencephalography (aEEG) in patients with inborn errors of metabolism—a new tool for the metabolic geneticist. *Mol Genet Metab*. 2010;100(suppl 1):S42–S48.
99. Hellstrom-Westas L, de Vries LS. *An Amplitude Integrated EEGs in the Newborn*. 2nd ed. London: Informa Healthcare; 2008.
99a. Vilan A, Mendes Ribeiro J, Striano P, et al. A distinctive ictal amplitude-integrated electroencephalography pattern in newborns with neonatal epilepsy associated with KCNQ2 mutations. *Neonatology*. 2017;112(4):387–393.
100. Weeke LC, Brilstra E, Braun KP, et al. Punctate white matter lesions in full-term infants with neonatal seizures associated with SLC13A5 mutations. *Eur J Paediatr Neurol*. 2017;21(2):396–403.

14

CHAPTER 15

Congenital Heart Disease: An Important Cause of Brain Injury and Dysmaturation

Torin J.A. Glass, Michael Seed, and Vann Chau

- Transposition of great arteries and hypoplastic left heart syndromes are two of the most common indications for neonatal cardiac surgery. These forms of congenital heart disease (CHD) are also the most often studied in relation to neurodevelopmental outcome.

- Despite medical progress and better survival, infants with CHD continue to sustain high rates of brain injury and neurodevelopmental impairments.

- Advanced magnetic resonance imaging (MRI) techniques, such as diffusion tensor imaging and MR spectroscopy, suggest that neonates with CHD show MRI evidence of brain microstructural and metabolic dysmaturation, which make them at higher risk of brain injury typically seen in preterm newborns.

- This primary issue of maturation arrest rather than cellular loss highlights the potential for brain recovery from injury.

- The failure to improve neurodevelopmental outcomes through modifications of cardiopulmonary bypass calls for a paradigm shift toward fetal, preoperative, and postoperative interventions aimed at improving brain health of infants with CHD.

Congenital heart disease (CHD) affects 8 per 1000 live births,[1–6] with up to 50% of these children requiring heart surgery.[7] Variation is primarily due to different diagnostic tools to detect CHD.[4,7] Interestingly, a recent systemic review and meta-analysis showed that since 1930, the reported total CHD prevalence increased substantially worldwide.[8] The highest reported total CHD birth prevalence was found in Asia (9.3 per 1000 live births) and the lowest in Africa (1.9 per 1000 live births).[8] The increase in reported prevalence over time may be partly due to changes in diagnostic methods and screening modalities rather than representing a true increase. Nonetheless, higher survival of preterm newborns, the increase in maternal age, and longer life expectancy of adults with CHD, all known risk factors for CHD may contribute to this higher prevalence over time. Certain clinical factors are associated with CHD and their presence should raise clinical suspicion. These factors include prematurity,[2] family history,[9,10] maternal chronic conditions (such as diabetes mellitus, hypertension, obesity, phenylketonuria, thyroid disorders, systemic connective tissue disorders, and epilepsy),[11,12] maternal consumption of certain drugs,[13] and fetal exposures to alcohol,[14] tobacco,[15,16] and congenital infections.[17]

Most forms of CHD are amenable to surgical repair with low mortality, However, developmental deficits are very common.[18] The system-wide cost associated with CHD accounts for almost half of the economic burden of all birth defects. Before brain magnetic resonance imaging (MRI) was used more routinely, children with CHD were not suspected to have such a high rate of brain injury. Indeed, brain lesions are often clinically silent in the neonatal period, partly because of pharmacological sedation and paralysis in the early postoperative period. Neuroimaging, particularly with advanced MRI techniques, now enables us to better understand the impacts on brain maturation of cardiac malformations as well as their surgical repair and other therapeutic interventions have. Neuromonitoring tools are also playing a more active role in improving care and outcomes in this population.

Fetal Brain Injury and Maturation

In the fetus with CHD, brain maturation at term appears similar to that of preterm infants, as shown by the frequency of white matter injury (WMI) and white matter maturational delays.[19,20] Several theories have been proposed to explain this interesting feature of infants with CHD, with particular attention paid to blood flow measurements and brain oxygenation. In a study comparing fetal MRIs of confirmed CHD fetuses with controls, CHD fetuses had reduced arterial oxygen saturation (Sao_2) in the aorta without difference in cerebral blood flow.[21] This was found to be associated in a reduced cerebral oxygen consumption of 32% and a 13% overall reduction in brain volume.[21] Fetuses with single-ventricle physiology had a greater reduction in Sao_2 than those with biventricular physiology. Reductions in head circumference in fetuses with CHD were observed with lower cerebral-to-placental resistance ratios as measured by Doppler ultrasound, suggesting that fetuses with CHD have potentially decreased cerebrovascular resistance compared with controls.[22,23] This appears to have a global effect on brain growth, with total brain volumes, gray matter, and subcortical brain volumes all being affected.[24,25] These effects are most notable in the third trimester of the growing fetus with slower brain volume growth and lower N-acetylaspartate (NAA)-to-choline ratios on MR spectroscopy reflecting a white matter maturation delay.[20] Routine ultrasonography of fetuses with CHD can identify brain volume and abdominal circumference growth abnormalities that are independent indicators of delayed brain growth and development.[26,27] Identification of reduced cerebral fissure depths in fetuses with CHD has been shown to be correlated with lower neurodevelopmental scores at 6 months of age.[28] Fetuses with hypoplastic left heart syndrome (HLHS), transposition of the great arteries (TGA), hypoplastic aortic arch, and other congenital abnormalities resulting in lower placental blood delivery to the brain are at greatest risk of decreased brain maturation and growth delays evident on fetal MRI.[29,30]

Fetal MRI investigation of the fetus with CHD has revealed that subsequent brain abnormalities are commonly found (Table 15.1), whether as a result of underlying genetic syndromes, in utero events, or a result of volume loss from chronic hypoxia.[31] The most common brain abnormality on fetal MRI is abnormal width of the cerebrospinal fluid spaces identified in 43% of affected patients, followed by malformations in 33%, and acquired lesions in 24%.[31] These findings support the significance of the multifactorial determinants of development of the brain in the fetus with CHD and the role of fetal MR in assessing the neurodevelopmental prognosis preoperatively. The investigation of the fetus with CHD with MRI and Doppler ultrasound is of particular importance to the cardiologist in determining the ideal early hemodynamic and surgical approach, yet is equally important to the neonatologist and pediatrician in optimizing brain development.

Prenatal Diagnosis

Rates of prenatal detection of major CHD vary considerably across centers.[32] The best quoted European rate is 47%.[33] However, better training in fetal echocardiography may help improve clinicians' diagnostic skills.[32] Prenatal diagnosis of TGA and HLHS is associated with decreased perioperative morbidity and mortality.[34,35] This positive impact on the development of the brain likely is a result of earlier prostaglandin treatment and earlier monitoring of the hemodynamic state of newborns with CHD.[36] Prenatally diagnosed infants are more likely to be transported while receiving prostaglandin E_1, will have a more physiologic pH on admission to a tertiary care center, and have a lower early mortality.[37] Prenatal diagnosis also results in less WMI and/or stroke and allows for better white and grey matter maturation as evidenced by advanced MRI techniques.[36] There is also a reduced likelihood of seizures following prenatal diagnosis.[38] These observations support the importance of prenatal CHD screening and early prostaglandin treatment in the care of the newborn with CHD.

Postnatal Diagnosis

Delayed or missed diagnosis of critical CHD accounts for 0.4 to 2.0 deaths per 10,000 live births in a U.K. series.[39] These infants typically present with serious

Table 15.1 SUMMARY OF STUDIES INVESTIGATING FETAL BRAIN ABNORMALITIES

Study: Author (Year)	Study Design	Neuroimaging Modality	Brain Abnormalities
Ruiz et al. (2017)	Prospective cohort CHD (n = 119)	Fetal ultrasound	Smaller biparietal diameter z score (-1.32) and head circumference z-score (-0.79), which remained small throughout gestation
Sun et al. (2015)	Case-control CHD (30/60)	Fetal MRI	Smaller total brain volume ($P < .001$) with reduced cerebral oxygen consumption ($P < .001$)
Zeng et al. (2015)	Case-control CHD (73/241)	3D Fetal ultrasound	Smaller total brain volumes in CHD from 28 weeks onwards ($P < .05$), largest in the frontal lobes. The differences were largest in the HLHS, aortic hypoplasia, and TGA populations.
Andescavage et al. (2015)	Case-control fetal CHD (41/135)	Fetal MRI	Smaller total brain and cerebral volumes in CHD group ($P < .001$), with larger brainstem volumes ($P < .001$).
Schellen et al. (2015)	Case-control tetralogy of Fallot (24/48)	Fetal MRI	Smaller total brain ($P < .001$), gray matter ($P = .003$), and subcortical brain ($P = 0.001$) volumes with increased external CSF spaces ($P < .001$) in TOF cases
Masoller et al. (2016)	Case-control CHD (58/116)	Fetal MRI, MRSI, and fetoplacental Doppler ultrasound	Lower biparietal diameter, head circumference and cerebral blood flow (all $P < .05$). Lower NAA/choline values in basal ganglia and frontal lobe ($P < .05$) Lower brain volumes in CHD infants ($P < .05$)
Brossard-Racine et al. (2014)	Case-control fetal CHD (144/338)	Fetal MRI	Higher risk of brain abnormalities (23% vs. 1.5% in controls, $P < .001$). Unilateral ventriculomegaly and increased extraaxial spaces most common abnormalities.
Al-Nafasi et al. (2013)	Case-control fetal CHD (22/34)	Fetal MRI	Lower ventricular output in CHD fetuses ($P < .01$). CHD fetuses had lower brain weights.
Mlczoch et al. (2013)	Prospective cohort CHD (n = 53)	Fetal MRI	Congenital brain disease 39%
Clouchoux et al. (2012)	Case-control fetal HLHS (18/48)	Fetal MRI	Progressively lower subcortical gray ($P < .05$) and white matter ($P < .001$) volumes in third trimester. Delays in cortical gyrification ($P < .001$)
Berman et al. (2011)	Case-control fetal CHD (3/31)	Fetal MRI, DWI	ADC values were higher in CHD fetuses in the thalamus ($P < .05$) with strong trend in the parietal white matter ($P = .071$)
Limperopoulos et al. (2010)	Case-control CHD (55/105)	Fetal MRI, MRSI	Total brain volumes lower ($P < .001$) NAA/choline lower in CHD infants ($P < .001$)

3D, Three-dimensional; *ADC,* apparent diffusion coefficient; *CHD,* congenital heart disease; *DWI,* diffusion-weighted image; *HLHS,* hypoplastic left heart syndrome; *MRI,* magnetic resonance imaging; *MRSI,* magnetic resonance spectroscopic imaging; *NAA,* N-acetylaspartate; *TGA,* transposition of the great arteries; *TOF,* tetralogy of Fallot.

and life-threatening symptoms, such as cyanosis, tachycardia, pulmonary edema, and cardiogenic shock.[5] The timing of presentation depends on the type of cardiac malformation and its dependence on a patent ductus arteriosus to maintain oxygenated circulation to the brain and other major organs. Before pulse oximetry screening was standard practice in neonatology, 30% of infants with CHD were undiagnosed at the time of discharge from the nursery,[40] especially if they appeared normal physically during their first few days of life.[5] In these undiagnosed newborns, the risk of mortality reaches 30%.[41–43]

Malformation Grouping

Severe congenital cardiac malformations are typically categorized as either single-ventricle or biventricular lesions, which can be associated with or without aortic arch obstructions such as coarctation, atresia, or stenosis. Any of these lesions can be further complicated by intracardiac (e.g., atrial septal defect or ventricular septal defect) or extracardiac shunts (e.g., patent ductus arteriosus). The presence of shunts, malformed valves, or obstructed blood flow may cause reduced oxygen delivery owing to the mixing of venous and arterial blood. Two common forms of CHD, accounting for more than 80% of surgeries required during the first week of life, are TGA and HLHS.[44]

CHD can be caused by a number of factors, ranging from inherited or spontaneous genetic mutations to environmental factors.[45,46] The most common genetic syndromes associated with CHD include Down syndrome (trisomy 21), Edward syndrome (trisomy 18), Patau syndrome (trisomy 13), DiGeorge syndrome (22q11.2 deletion), Williams syndrome, and Turner syndrome. Antenatal exposure to certain infections (e.g., rubella), teratogens (e.g., retinoic acid, phenytoin, lithium), maternal diseases (e.g., diabetes mellitus, systemic lupus erythematosus, phenylketonuria), and air pollution are also considered significant contributors.

Transposition of Great Vessels

TGA (Fig. 15.1) results from a ventriculoarterial discordance when the aorta arises from the right ventricle and the pulmonary artery from the left ventricle. Dextro-looped TGA (D-TGA) is the most common type and is characterized by the right ventricle being positioned to the right of the left ventricle and the origin of the aorta being anterior and rightward to the origin of the pulmonary artery. This malformation leads to two parallel circulatory systems and causes the affected infant to be cyanotic. One of these systems carries deoxygenated venous blood from the body to the right atrium and then returns it to the systemic circulation through the right ventricle and aorta. The other system brings oxygenated venous blood from the lungs to the left atrium and sends it back to the lungs via the left ventricle and pulmonary artery. D-TGA can be associated with other cardiac abnormalities, such as ventricular septal defects, left ventricular outflow tract obstruction, mitral and tricuspid valve abnormalities, and coronary artery variations.[47,48] In this situation, the TGA defect is said to be complex. D-TGA can be difficult to diagnose antenatally with ultrasound. Postnatally, affected infants can present with cyanosis, tachypnea, heart murmurs, and diminished femoral pulses. The severity of symptoms is inversely related to the degree of mixing between the two parallel circulations and the presence of other cardiac anomalies.

The initial management of D-TGA is to stabilize the infant's condition until the corrective surgery is performed. This stabilization first consists of a continuous intravenous prostaglandin E_1 infusion to maintain the patency of the ductus arteriosus to optimize the intercirculatory mixing between the two systems.[49] Another procedure that is used to promote mixing of the two parallel circulations is balloon atrial septostomy (BAS). In this intervention, during cardiac catheterization a balloon is pulled vigorously across the atrial septum through the foramen ovale or an existing defect, leading to increased atrial mixing. This procedure dramatically improves the survival of infants with D-TGA and has recently been performed in a series of fetuses.[50,51] The arterial switch, optimally done during the first week of life, is now the standard corrective procedure.[52] An alternative surgical approach, called the Rastelli procedure, is preferred in neonates with significant pulmonary stenosis.[53]

Levo-looped TGA (L-TGA) is much rarer, accounting for less than 1% of CHD.[54] L-TGA is best described as congenitally corrected transposition of great arteries (CCTGA) in which there are discordant atrioventricular and ventriculo-arterial connections. It is due to abnormal leftward looping of the primitive heart. In this cardiac malformation, the heart is physiologically corrected such that the systemic deoxygenated venous blood returns to the pulmonary circulation and oxgenated pulmonary venous blood returns to the systemic circulation. In more than 90% of cases, L-TGA

Normal Heart

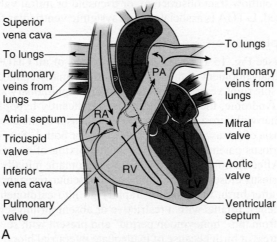

Superior vena cava

To lungs

Pulmonary veins from lungs

Atrial septum

Tricuspid valve

Inferior vena cava

Pulmonary valve

AO

PA

RA

RV

To lungs

Pulmonary veins from lungs

Mitral valve

Aortic valve

LA

LV

Ventricular septum

A

Transposition of Great Arteries

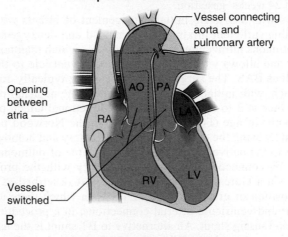

Vessel connecting aorta and pulmonary artery

Opening between atria

AO   PA

RA

RV

LA

LV

Vessels switched

B

Hypoplastic Left Heart Syndrome

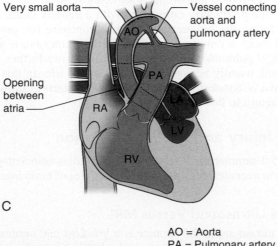

Very small aorta

AO

Opening between atria

RA

PA

RV

Vessel connecting aorta and pulmonary artery

LA

LV

C

AO = Aorta
PA = Pulmonary artery
LA = Left atrium
RA = Right atrium
LV = Left ventricle
RV = Right ventricle

☐ Oxygen-rich blood
☐ Mixed blood
☐ Oxygen-poor blood

Fig. 15.1 Anatomic images of a (A) normal heart, (B) transposition of the great arteries, and (C) hypoplastic left heart syndrome.

is associated with other cardiac abnormalities such as ventricular septal defect, pulmonary outflow tract obstruction, or tricuspid or mitral valve abnormalities.[55] Even if isolated, L-TGA is associated with systemic ventricular failure in the long term.[56]

Hypoplastic Left Heart Syndrome

HLHS (see Fig. 15.1) accounts for 2% to 3% of all CHD[3] and is characterized by an underdevelopment of the left heart with normally connected great vessels,[57] leaving the sole right ventricle to perfuse both the pulmonary and systemic circulations. In this syndrome, the left ventricle is significantly hypoplastic and can be associated either with atresia, stenosis, and hypoplasia of the aortic or mitral valves; with hypoplasia of the ascending aorta and arch; or both.[57] Survival is dependent on ductus arteriosus patency to ensure adequate mixing of oxygenated and deoxygenated blood. Affected infants are relatively asymptomatic initially; however, when the ductus arteriosus closes and the pulmonary vascular resistances decrease, as expected shortly after birth, these infants rapidly go into cardiogenic shock and respiratory insufficiency. Infants with a restrictive or absent atrium septal defect at birth do not benefit from this "honeymoon period" and present with severe cyanosis and respiratory distress at birth because of inadequate interatrial blood mixing. Fortunately, prenatal diagnosis with routine obstetrical ultrasound is often possible, usually between 18 and 24 weeks' gestation.

As with TGA, the initial management of infants with HLHS is focused on providing sufficient mixing of oxygenated and deoxygenated blood with the use of continuous intravenous prostaglandin E_1, which maintains the ductus arteriosus patent and allows vital flow from the right ventricle to the systemic circulation, as well as BAS. The surgical palliative repair typically consists of a three-staged approach, with initial surgery performed in the neonatal period (Norwood procedure), then at 3 to 6 months of age (bidirectional Glenn procedure), and at 18 to 30 months of age (Fontan procedure). In the Norwood procedure, a neoaorta is created by using the proximal pulmonary artery and homograft material, then connected to the native ascending aorta. A source of pulmonary blood flow is established by connecting the innominate artery with the proximal right pulmonary artery via a Gore-Tex shunt L-TGA is best described as congenitally corrected transposition of great arteries (CCTGA) in which there are discordant atrioventricular and ventriculo-arterial connections, in a procedure known as a modified Blalock-Taussig shunt. An alternative to BT shunt is the use of a right ventricle to pulmonary artery shunt. When the child reaches 3 to 6 months of age, pulmonary vascular resistance has dropped sufficiently to allow substitution of the arterial shunt to the pulmonary circulation with a venous shunt, thus unloading the ventricle. During the bidirectional Glenn procedure (or cavopulmonary shunt), the original shunt is removed and the superior vena cava is anastomosed end-to-side to the right pulmonary artery. As the child grows further, the Fontan procedure is performed, usually between 2 and 3 years of life. In this third stage, the inferior vena cava is connected to the pulmonary arteries, allowing the entire systemic venous return to flow passively to the lungs.

Brain Injury and Brain Maturation

Table 15.2 summarizes a selected list of studies associating CHD and brain abnormalities in neonates. Fig. 15.2 shows examples of brain injuries found in infants with CHD.

Cranial Ultrasound Versus MRI

Cranial ultrasound in the neonate is a low-cost and noninvasive bedside procedure that provides an assessment of cerebral volumes and ventricle size and can often identify large hemorrhages, infarcts, and cystic WMI. Advanced ultrasound with Doppler measurements is also informative of the flow in the largest venous sinuses. Unfortunately, the reliability of cranial ultrasound for the detection of ischemic lesions is poor, with up to one-third of infarcts being missed.[58] MRI is increasingly

Table 15.2 SUMMARY OF STUDIES ASSOCIATING CONGENITAL HEART DISEASE AND BRAIN ABNORMALITIES IN NEONATES

Study: First Author (Year)	Study Design	Neuroimaging Modality	Risk Factors	Brain Abnormalities
Fogel et al. (2017)	Prospective cohort SVP (n = 168)	MRI	Presurgical, bidirectional Glenn (BDG), Fontan procedures	WMI and PVL most common in BDG group; more WMI and brain atrophy seen postoperatively than preoperatively
Knirsch et al. (2016)	Prospective cross-sectional SVP (n = 47)	MRI	Fontan procedure	Abnormal MRI in 36% Enlarged CSF spaces, small gray, and white matter injuries were seen; half of the individuals had combined lesions.
Birca et al. (2016)	Prospective cohort CHD (n = 33)	MRI, DTI cEEG	—	WMI and stroke in 25% Brain injury and dysmaturation were both associated with increased high-frequency EEG connectivity and greater discontinuity
Peyvandi et al. (2016)	Prospective cohort TGA and SVP (n = 153)	MRI, DTI	Postnatal diagnosis of CHD	Brain injury rates higher in postnatal diagnosis ($P = .003$) Faster white matter ($P = .04$) and gray matter development ($P = .02$) in infants with prenatal diagnosis of CHD
Knirsch et al. (2016)	Prospective cohort SVP (n = 47)	MRI	—	Abnormal MRI in 36%
Von Rhein et al. (2015)	Case-control Surgical CHD (19/38)	MRI	—	Reduced regional (8%-28%) and total (21%) brain volumes ($P < .001$)
Naim et al. (2015)	Retrospective cohort Surgical CHD patients (n = 161)	cEEG	—	Electrographic seizures in 8% (85% subclinical), beginning at a median of 20 hours after return to ICU. Higher mortality in those with seizures ($P < .001$)
Kelly et al. (2014)	Prospective cohort Surgical CHD (n = 152)	MRI	—	Subdural hemorrhage 43%
Bertholdt et al. (2014)	Case-control Surgical CHD with CPB (30/50)	MRI	—	WMI and stroke 23% vs. 0% in controls Neuromotor scores 15 days postoperatively median 2.5 (95% CI 0–7)
Glass et al. (2011)	Prospective cohort Surgical CHD	MRI	Acquired infection (23/127)	No significant increase in WMI was seen with acquired infection
Block et al. (2010)	Prospective cohort TGA and SVP (n = 92)	MRI	BAS ($P = .003$) Lowest arterial oxygen saturation ($P = .007$)	WMI and stroke (preoperative) 43%
Ter Horst et al. (2010)	Prospective cohort Cyanotic and acyanotic CHD post-PGE (n = 62)	aEEG	—	Abnormal background in 45% of infants, severe in 14%. Electrographic seizure activity in 19%, more commonly in acyanotic CHD ($P = .039$)

Continued

15

Table 15.2 SUMMARY OF STUDIES ASSOCIATING CONGENITAL HEART DISEASE AND BRAIN ABNORMALITIES IN NEONATES—CONT'D

Study: First Author (Year)	Study Design	Neuroimaging Modality	Risk Factors	Brain Abnormalities
Shadeed et al. (2011)	Case-control Cyanotic CHD (38/76)	MRSI, DTI	—	Poor brain development on MRSI ($P < .001$) and DTI ($P < .001$)
Andropoulos et al. (2010)	Prospective cohort Surgical CHD with CPB	MRI	Single-ventricle physiology (32/68)	Increased WMI and stroke postoperatively Single-ventricle ($P = .02$)
Beca et al. (2009)	Prospective cohort TGA	MRI	BAS (33/44)	WMI and stroke Both NS
Miller et al. (2007)	Case-control TGA and SVP (41/57)	MRI, DTI, MRSI	—	WMI and stroke (32% CHD vs. 0% controls) Poor brain development on MRSI ($P < .001$), DTI ($P < .001$)
McQuillen et al. (2006)	Prospective cohort TGA	MRI	BAS (19/29)	WMI, stroke, and IVH $P = .001$ (41%–85% risk difference)
Gaynor et al. (2005)	Prospective cohort Surgical CHD patients (n = 178)	cEEG	Duration of DHCA	Seizures were identified in 11%, with higher likelihood in increased duration of DHCA ($P = .001$)
Tavani et al. (2003)	Prospective cohort Surgical CHD (n = 24)	MRI	—	Intracranial hemorrhage Preoperatively 62%; postoperatively 88% with increased size in 43%
Mahle et al. (2002)	Prospective cohort Surgical CHD (n = 24)	MRI, MRSI	—	WMI and stroke: 24% preoperatively; 67% new lesions postoperatively Elevated lactate preoperatively 53% ($P < .02$) Atrophy late post-operatively 12%

BAS, Balloon atrial septostomy; *cEEG*, continuous EEG; *CHD*, congenital heart disease; *CI*, confidence interval; *CSF*, cerebrospinal fluid; *DHCA*, deep hypothermic circulatory arrest; *DTI*, diffusion tensor imaging; *EEG*, electroencephalography; *MRI*, magnetic resonance imaging; *MRSI*, magnetic resonance spectroscopic imaging; *NS*, not significant; *PGE*, prostaglandin; *PVL*, periventricular leukomalacia; *TGA*, transposition of the great arteries; *SVP*, single ventricle physiology; *WMI*, white matter injury.

recognized as an important addition to the early investigation of neonates with CHD, given the high burden of radiation associated with computed tomography (CT) and the poor reliability of cranial ultrasound. In the investigation of the infant with CHD, it is important to recognize that the majority of injuries are clinically silent and can be present in well-appearing infants.[59,60] MR diffusion-weighted imaging (DWI), in combination with T1- and T2-weighted imaging, is an early and sensitive test for brain ischemia and acute injury. Owing to the postinjury pseudonormalization of the DWI signal beyond 5 to 7 days in the neonate, MR DWI is best performed within the first week of life to assess for silent infarcts. Appropriate investigation of the neonate with CHD is necessary to aid determine the medical treatments, neurodevelopmental prognosis, and subsequent follow-up procedures for those at greatest risk of developmental deficits.

Cerebral Ischemia and Stroke

Up to 40% of infants with CHD will have preoperative brain injuries, with an acute cerebral infarct or stroke the most predominant early injury types.[44] Neonates with cyanotic CHD have been shown to have ischemic lesions in up to 60% of cases.[38] In the preoperative period, low oxygen saturation is associated with increased risk of stroke and WMI.[60,61] Several groups have speculated that BAS is a cause of acute infarcts and WMI in TGA, showing an increased incidence of embolic strokes in

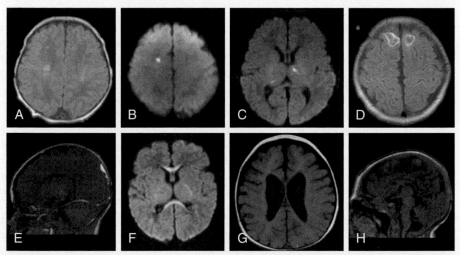

Fig. 15.2 Magnetic resonance imaging of brain injury in congenital heart disease. (A) White matter injury: T1-weighted axial preoperative image of a 2-week-old neonate with pulmonary atresia. Multiple, bilateral punctate white matter lesions are seen in the frontal and parietal white matter. (B) Acute infarct: axial diffusion-weighted image of a 2-day-old with transposition of the great arteries with an intact ventricular septum done following a balloon atrial septostomy. A right frontal white matter infarct is seen with acute diffusion restriction. (C) Multiple acute infarcts: axial diffusion-weighted image of an 8-day-old with tetralogy of Fallot and pulmonary atresia done following a cardiac arrest. Multiple areas of acute diffusion restriction are seen in the left basal ganglia and right thalamus. (D) Cerebrosinovenous thrombosis: axial T1-weighted image of a 5-day-old with tricuspid atresia done preoperatively. Bilateral frontal parasagittal hemorrhages with surrounding edema are seen suggestive of cerebral sinovenous thrombosis. (E) Subdural hemorrhage: sagittal T1-weighted image of a 10-week-old with single ventricle physiology showing a right posterior parasagittal, posterior convexity of the tentorium and right inferior cerebellar subdural hemorrhage. (F) Wallerian degeneration secondary to an acute infarct: a diffusion-weighted image of a 4-week-old neonate with a hypoplastic right ventricle and pulmonary stenosis showing diffusion-weighted image changes in the right posterior limb of the internal capsule and corpus callosum bilaterally indicative of acute pre-Wallerian degeneration of white matter fibers. (G) White matter volume loss: an axial T1-weighted image of a 10-week-old infant with tetralogy of Fallot and pulmonary atresia showing significant white matter volume loss with increased anterior extraaxial spaces and ventriculomegaly. (H) Congenital brain malformation: a sagittal T1-weighted image of a 5-week-old infant with hypoplastic left heart syndrome and multiple congenital brain malformations. The brainstem is small with an abnormally formed medulla and small cerebellum. In addition, there is suspected fusion of the left caudate and lentiform nucleus.

patients treated with BAS; however, this remains controversial.[60,62,63] As clinically silent infarcts and WMI are common in CHD and have a low risk of progressing with surgery, in most cases medically necessary surgical procedures should not be delayed in the event of brain injury findings.[60]

White Matter Injury

WMI, the predominant injury of the premature neonate, is a well-recognized complication of CHD in the term neonate.[19] Infants with CHD are particularly prone to WMI as a result of fluctuations in the cerebral blood flow both preoperatively and postoperatively.[64,65] Although stroke is the most common preoperative complication, WMI is the most common lesion acquired after surgery, with the greatest risk in neonates with single-ventricle physiology and aortic arch obstruction.[44,59] Intraoperatively, during bidirectional Glenn and Fontan procedures it has been shown that higher levels of cerebral blood flow are associated with reduced risk of WMI, suggesting the ischemic nature of this complication.[66] The timing of the injury appears most frequently in the neonatal period, as 1- to 3-month-old infants have a significantly reduced risk of postoperative WMI (4% compared with 54% in neonates).[64] This may reflect the relative immaturity of the cerebral autoregulation systems in the brain of the infant with CHD, much like that of the preterm neonate. In those neonates with known preoperative WMI, worsening of white matter lesions was identified in 19%, with new lesions occurring in 48%.[67] In neonates with follow-up beyond 3 months, MRI scans will reveal that many of the existing lesions have resolved though nearly 30% of patients show new lesions.[59] Similar

15

to cohorts of preterm infants, the incidence of WMI in neonates with CHD appears influenced by nosocomial infections the incidence of WMI in neonates with CHD appears influenced by nosocomial infections.[68] In the assessment of WMI and stroke it is important to remember that their pathophysiologies and subsequent outcomes are shared, and optimizing oxygenation and hemodynamic monitoring provides the best neuroprotection.

Cerebral Sinovenous Thrombosis

Cerebral sinovenous thrombosis (CSVT), a serious hemostatic complication in the ill neonate, is a common finding in autopsies of infants with cyanotic CHD.[69] Yet in a study of several European pediatric registries, patients with CHD represented only 4% of the cases with confirmed CSVT.[70] In an adult study, a greater incidence of thrombosis and bleeding was found in subjects with hypoxemia compared with a nonhypoxemic group (12% vs. 2% and 14% vs. 2%, respectively).[71] The etiology of these abnormalities in hemostasis remains incompletely understood, although chronic endothelial damage, increased blood volume and viscosity, low pulmonary artery velocity, biventricular dysfunction, and chronic right-to-left shunting all likely contribute.[71] The investigation for suspected CSVT should include either unenhanced CT and/or MRI T1- and T2-weighted imaging, in addition to venography (CT venography or MR venography) in investigating for clots within the venous sinuses as well as parenchymal injury with infarction or hemorrhage.[72] An experienced neuroradiologist familiar with neonatal vascular imaging should be involved because of the difficult interpretation of the imaging. In a study comparing CSVT and arterial infarct presentation, parietal involvement and lack of caudate infarction were more suggestive of CSVT.[70]

Subdural Hemorrhage

Serial MRI assessments of neurologically asymptomatic infants with CHD both preoperatively and postoperatively revealed that 43% had subdural hemorrhage (SDH) on at least a single scan, with many infants having more than one focus of hemorrhage.[73] Infants with CHD born by vaginal delivery had a higher incidence compared with those delivered by cesarean section (50% vs. 27%, respectively).[73] These rates are altogether higher than in infants without CHD, normally ranging from 6% to 26% and are highest with assisted vaginal delivery.[74,75] In neonates with CHD, 61% of SDH were small (≤2 mm deep), and only 10% were 5 mm or more deep; the locations were supratentorial in 43% and infratentorial in 57%.[73] There was no significant difference in the location of the hemorrhages between infants with CHD and those without CHD.[30–32] In monitoring SDH lesions over time, 24% of foci resolved within the first 2 to 4 weeks and 95% resolved by 3 months of age, with persistent hemorrhages generally observed in the posterior fossa.[30] Postoperatively 9% of infants with CHD showed new foci of hemorrhage; increased size of SDH was observed in 48% in one study.[73,76] The prevalence of recent preoperative SDH in neonates with chronic hypoxia did not differ significantly from nonhypoxic neonates.[73] Although SDH appears to occur more frequently at birth and postoperatively in infants with CHD, SDHs are generally asymptomatic and resolve over time without treatment. The impact of SDH on the neurodevelopmental outcome of the infant with CHD remains unknown.

Brain Dysmaturation

Brain development during the fetal period requires a high energy supply from the placenta. Failure to meet these demands may disrupt brain growth and maturation, especially in fetuses in whom CHD determines decreased cerebral blood flow and hypoxemia. In infants with HLHS, for example, more than half have microcephaly (<10th percentile) at birth.[77] The head growth seems to be directly linked to the degree of ascending aortic flow.[77] Brain maturation delay and cortical malformations are frequently seen on brain MRI[78] and autopsy.[79] Other prospective studies performed antenatally or postnatally in newborns with CHD demonstrate impairment of brain growth and metabolism in the third trimester,[20] decreased pyramidal tract maturation,[80] or widespread metabolic and microstructural brain abnormalities preoperatively,[19] similar to preterm infants. Together, these studies support the concept that brain dysmaturation in CHD originates in utero.

Brain injury in neonates with CHD shares mechanisms common to preterm infants. WMI in neonates with CHD is linked to ischemia (e.g., hypotension) and inflammation.[68,81,82] Based on experimental data,[83] Buser et al. described how the primary mechanism of myelination failure in the human preterm neonate involves dysmaturation rather than cell loss, through a disrupted cellular response whereby pre-oligodendrocytes fail to differentiate into mature oligodendrocytes (i.e., oligodendrocyte progenitor maturation arrest).[84] Similar findings were recently confirmed in a rodent model of CHD-related WMI.[85] During the third trimester of gestation, early lineage oligodendroglia are vulnerable to insults that do not affect mature myelinating oligodendroglia. This results in a preponderance of WMI in neonates born before term, rather than the gray matter vulnerability seen in term neonates.[86] Surprisingly, WMI is the characteristic brain injury pattern in term neonates with CHD and is indistinguishable from that seen in preterm neonates.[81,82,87–89] Thus brain vulnerability in CHD appears to be a consequence of dysmaturation.

In human newborns, recent works have led to the recognition of abnormal brain maturation in utero and the importance of impaired brain maturation as a substrate for postnatal injury.[19,81] In similar studies of neonates born preterm term, brain dysmaturation, rather than brain injury, is the major driver of adverse neurodevelopment.[90,91] As the primary issue appears to be brain maturation arrest rather than cell loss, these data highlight the potential for brain recovery from injury.

Neuromonitoring

Intraoperative Monitoring

The modern surgical approach to the most complex cardiac lesions includes cardiopulmonary bypass (CPB) and deep hypothermic circulatory arrest (DHCA). Both procedures carry a risk of injury for the neonatal brain and are frequently associated with postoperative lesions. Infants 3 months of age or younger who undergo CHD surgery are at greater risk of transient cerebral ischemia from hypotension than older children, likely as a result of reduced cerebral autoregulation.[64,92] As neuromonitor usage has increased in recent decades, improvements in neurodevelopmental outcomes of the infant with CHD have similarly been seen. Transcranial Doppler ultrasound is one method that has shown effectiveness in determining adequate cerebral perfusion and arterial saturation in real time during the low-flow CPB period.[93,94] Similarly, somatosensory evoked potentials used intraoperatively are very specific and sensitive for neurological complications from hemodynamic disturbances.[95] A study using multimodal intraoperative neuromonitoring combining electroencephalography (EEG), transcranial Doppler ultrasound, and near-infrared spectroscopy (NIRS) identified alterations in brain perfusion in 70% of patients,[30] allowing corrective interventions in 74%.[96] Such interventions were shown to improve neurologic outcomes (6% complication rate vs. 26% in the no-intervention group) and resulted in a decreased hospital length of stay.[96] With the continued focus on improving neurodevelopmental outcomes in infants with CHD, intraoperative monitoring will continue to be an important tool in maximizing intraoperative cerebral protection.

Near-Infrared Spectroscopy

NIRS is a noninvasive bedside monitor that uses nonpulsatile oximetry to monitor hemoglobin oxygen saturation in a localized tissue bed. When used on the head, NIRS provides real-time information on the cerebral cortex oxygenation.[97] NIRS has been shown to correlate well with superior vena cava oxygen saturation, highlighting its utility as a cerebral monitor.[98] NIRS appears useful in both cyanotic and acyanotic heart disease, with optimal correlation at superior vena cava oxygenation concentrations of 40% to 60%, a point at which it is critical to intervene and improve oxygenation to protect brain function and homeostasis.[98] As an intraoperative neuromonitoring system, NIRS has been shown to be a valuable tool in the assessment of hypocarbia and hypoxia and can alarm the surgical team to low cerebral perfusion.[99]

15

Whether or not intraoperative NIRS results in measurable improvements in neurodevelopmental outcomes remains uncertain; one study suggested that the only measurable negative outcome correlated with the NIRS intraoperative nadir was receptive language delay.[100] Another report showed that neonates with values 20% to 40% below baseline during CHD surgery had increased neurologic dysfunction 12 months after surgery.[101] NIRS as a marker of cerebral functioning is well supported by the literature, with its use in multimodal neuromonitoring providing significant benefit to both the infant with CHD as well as the surgical and clinical care teams.

Amplitude-Integrated Electroencephalography

As a marker of cerebral activity, amplitude-integrated EEG (aEEG) provides clinicians with valuable bedside information about the background electrical activity and can identify abnormal activity consistent with seizures. In a study of neonates with cyanotic and acyanotic CHD, aEEG patterns before and after the initiation of prostaglandin treatment showed abnormal voltage patterns in 60% of neonates at some point in the first 72 hours versus only 13% that continued to be abnormal at 72 hours after administration of prostaglandin.[38] Severely abnormal patterns of burst suppression, continuous low voltage, or flat tracings were identified in 15% of neonates with no difference between the acyanotic and cyanotic groups.[38] Abnormal aEEG patterns directly correlated with preoperative brain MRI injury scores; infants with severely abnormal aEEGs had the highest MRI injury scores.[102] Severely abnormal aEEG background activity was associated with brain atrophy in 80% of cases with fewer numbers of focal infarcts and/or WMI.[102] Sleep-wake cycling was present in up to 60% of neonates in the first 72 hours and was not associated with brain injury, although those with brain atrophy were less likely to have sleep-wake cycling present.[38,102] Electrical seizures were identified in 19% of neonates; 11 of 12 were characterized as having acyanotic CHD.[38] Clinical seizures strongly correlated with aEEG, with subclinical seizures identified in 2 of 12 neonates with seizures.[38] Three neonates with suspected clinical seizures and aEEG patterns not consistent with a seizure were identified on conventional EEG to have focal electrographic seizure activity.[38] This reflects a difficulty of aEEG as it has poor sensitivity for focal seizures not localized near the electrodes and showcases the importance of conventional EEG for further characterization of suspected seizures.

Continuous Electroencephalography

Neonates with CHD are at risk of seizures in both the preoperative and postoperative periods.[38,103] The American Clinical Neurophysiology Society guideline on neonatal EEG monitoring in infants with CHD recommends consideration for continuous EEG (cEEG) monitoring during the postoperative period where seizure rates are 5% to 20%.[104–106] HLHS has been shown to carry a greater risk of seizures in the postoperative period with 18% having seizures, compared with 4% in tetralogy of Fallot (TOF), 8% in TGA, and 12% with other biventricular defects.[107] In a study of cEEG in the postoperative period at a single center, 8% of all infants with CHD had electrographic seizures with a median onset time at 20 hours (interquartile range 15–34 hours) after return to the cardiac intensive care unit.[108] Clinical seizures with an electrographic correlate occurred in 15% of patients, with 85% of seizures occurring subclinically and identified purely on the basis of cEEG changes.[108] Status epilepticus, classified as a single seizure lasting more than 30 minutes or recurrent seizures lasting for at least 30 minutes in a 60-minute period, occurred in 62% of those with seizures or 5% of all infants with CHD.[108] Younger age at surgery, longer CPB and DHCA times, single-ventricle physiology and arch obstruction, delayed sternal closure, postoperative cardiac arrest, and extracorporeal membrane oxygenation were all factors that increased the likelihood of seizures.[108] For every 10-minute increase in DHCA time, the odds ratio of developing seizures was 1.47, indicating an association with increased surgical time and subsequent brain dysfunction and injury.[108] All infants with seizures were identified on neuroimaging as having either diffuse or multifocal lesions on either head ultrasound or brain MRI.[108] Electrical seizure activity itself was associated with a 14-fold increase in the likelihood of an abnormal MRI scan.[38] Given the strong association between seizures and CHD, cEEG should be considered in all neonates with CHD, particularly in the postoperative period, to better identify seizures, allowing for timely treatment, and assist in the identification of underlying brain injury.

Advanced Magnetic Resonance Imaging Techniques in Congenital Heart Disease

Identifying the mechanisms of impaired brain maturation in neonates with CHD is hampered by a relative lack of appropriate animal models, and until now, by a lack of ways to noninvasively measure fetal hemodynamics. Advanced brain imaging tools enable quantification of brain maturation with MRI. As shown by several studies, brain injury is common before and after heart surgery.[44,62,67] Yet, the extent of these injuries does not account for global neurodevelopmental impairments seen in childhood. Observations with advanced MR techniques indicate that WMI contributes to impaired brain maturation in areas that appear normal on conventional (T1 and T2) MRI.[19,89,109,110] Using these advanced MR techniques, recent studies suggest that brain dysmaturation is apparent even in the fetal period and may affect subsequent development of the newborn's brain.[19,81,111]

MR Diffusion Tensor Imaging

MR diffusion is calculated based on the measurement of the three-dimensional movement of water molecules within a region, with *isotropic* molecules free to move in any direction. *Anisotropic* molecules are restricted in their movement by the presence of cellular architecture. In the normal development of the neonatal brain, significant increases in the degree of white matter maturation and neuronal development results in decreasing average diffusivity (AD) and increasing mean fractional anisotropy (FA), a measure of anisotropic variance.[110] FA is a composite based on measures of radial and axial diffusivity that reflect myelination, axonal, and cortical maturation. Delays in the maturation are considered to reflect brain maturation through mechanisms of the developing brain are signified by increased AD and decreased FA, robust markers of microstructural brain development. In the assessment of infants with CHD, measurable delays in both preoperative and postoperative AD and FA, particularly within white matter regions, were seen independent of preoperative brain injury.[19] Diffusion tensor imaging provides a sensitive measure of regional microstructural maturity and connectivity in preterm newborns.[112] Prenatal diagnosis has similarly been shown to result in a greater improvement in brain maturation compared with postnatally diagnosed infants, likely as a result of early treatment with prostaglandin.[36]

Magnetic Resonance Spectroscopy

A further measure of brain maturation with MR includes ratios of substrates of regional brain biochemistry with magnetic resonance spectroscopy: lactate, NAA, choline, and creatine. Of these compounds, NAA and lactate are the most useful for assessing brain maturation and injury; abnormal levels of metabolites are predictive of neurodevelopmental outcome following neonatal brain injury.[89,91,113–117] NAA is an acetylated amino acid found at high levels in neurons of the central nervous system. NAA increases with advancing cerebral maturity[113] and decreases with cerebral injury.[19,87,89,115–117] High lactate reflects an ongoing disturbance in cerebral energy substrate delivery and oxidative metabolism (e.g., secondary to hypoxia-ischemia).[19,87,89,115–117] In preoperative neonates with CHD, compared with normal controls, a measurable delay with lower mean NAA-to-choline ratio of 10% and increased lactate-to-choline ratio of 28% were demonstrated in both white and gray matter.[19] Similarly, postoperative increases in the lactate-to-choline ratio were associated with increases in AD, highlighting magnetic resonance spectroscopy as a marker of microstructural brain development.[81]

Functional MRI

To date, functional resting state MRI (fMRI) has not been reported in the neonatal population in infants with CHD. In a recent study of fMRI in neonates, the adoption of an optimized preprocessing pipeline enhanced the detection of functional networks, overcoming many of the complexities of the T2-weighted imaging related to the greater water content within the neonatal brain.[118] A study of adolescents with a history of surgically treated CHD found differences with less task-induced deactivation during working memory tasks compared with controls.[119] Deactivation of prefrontal networks in adolescents with CHD correlated with improved working memory task performance.[119] Further research is needed to better understand the connectivity of the brain in the neonate with CHD and how injury to the brain may alter these functional networks.

Other Techniques

With the continued development of advanced neuroimaging techniques in neonates with CHD, clinicians and researchers alike are able to gain further insight into the neurodevelopment of sick neonates. One such test quantifies cortical folding measurements using postprocessing MR and calculates a *gyrification index,* a ratio of cortical surface to overall cortical hull that provides information about the gyral folding of the neonatal brain, a marker of brain development.[120] In neonates with CHD a decreased gyrification index was found in preoperative neonates compared with healthy controls.[120] Postoperative MR also showed a lower index in infants with single-ventricle physiology compared with both infants with TGA and controls.[120,121] Measures of brain volume, surface area, and folding patterns can be obtained using advanced segmentation and deformation-based morphometry of high-resolution MR images.[122–124] Specifically, deformation-based morphometry can be used to assess local changes in brain volume, both as a three-dimensional map and as volumes of individual brain structures (e.g., white matter, basal ganglia, thalamus, hippocampi, cerebellum). Other novel techniques using optics-based devices with diffuse optical metabolism and diffuse correlation spectroscopy have been used in CHD and are able to noninvasively measure microvascular tissue oxygenation, microvascular cerebral blood flow, and global oxygen metabolism.[125] In a comparison study with MRI measurements there was close correlation across all measures, highlighting a potential future for the increased use of optics in CHD.[125]

Neurodevelopment of the Infant With CHD

Predictors of Outcomes

Children with CHD exhibit deficits in multiple developmental domains that are not necessarily explained by focal injuries identified before and after cardiac surgery[44,60,64,67]: visuospatial skills, memory, executive function, language, and motor function (Table 15.3).[126] In a cohort of children with neonatal cyanotic CHD, the level of memory impairment correlated with the amount of hippocampal atrophy.[127] Despite only a modest decrease in intelligence quotient (IQ) scores, many children have behavioral problems, and up to half receive remedial academic services.[128] In many ways, the neurodevelopmental outcome of children with CHD parallels that of children born prematurely. Long-term outcome data from cohorts of very low-birth-weight infants followed to adulthood indicate that even mild developmental impairment at the time of school entry can translate into significantly impaired functional outcomes with lower rates of educational achievement, independent living, and employment.[129] Based on estimates of lifetime earning potential and the prevalence of CHD survivors, even modest 5-point decreases in IQ translate into losses to society of tens of billions of dollars.[130]

As the survival of infants and children with CHD improves, increasingly more adults are living with CHD. Children with complex CHD have been shown to have suboptimal outcomes at school age with attentional, behavioral, executive functioning, handwriting, and school performance issues.[131] Several large cohort studies have confirmed that infants with CHD have overall lower IQs than the general population, although their values still place them within the normal range.[132,133] Deficits in fine motor and cognition, including higher-order language skills, are evident at 8 years of age in children with TGA corrected surgically in the neonatal period.[132] The

Table 15.3 SUMMARY OF STUDIES INVESTIGATING NEURODEVELOPMENTAL OUTCOMES IN CHILDREN WITH CONGENITAL HEART DISEASE

Study: First Author (Year)	Study Design	Assessment Modality	Neurodevelopmental Abnormalities
Aly et al. (2017)	Prospective cohort Complex CHD (n = 75)	6, 15, and 21 months BSID-II	BSID were abnormal in 46% of survivors; poorer outcomes were associated with lower mean cerebral tissue oxygenation index, higher lactate, and ionotrope use postoperatively
Brosig et al. (2017)	Prospective cohort Complex CHD (n = 102)	4–5 years Neuropsychological testing (WPPSI-III, ABAS-II)	Neurodevelopmental scores were lower than norms on fine motor and adaptive motor skills, but within 1 SD of norms; patients with genetic disorders scored worse on most measures
Knirsch et al. (2017)	Prospective cohort SVP (n = 47)	2 years BSID-III	Lower language composite scores ($P = .040$), with motor and cognitive scores within reference range CSF space enlargement was associated with poorer performance on all subscores (all $P < .02$)
Peng et al. (2016)	Case-control CHD (45/90)	6 months BSID-II	Lower PDI and MDI scores (both $P < .001$); greatest correlation was seen with sylvian fissure depth ($P < .001$)
Hansen et al. (2016)	Prospective cohort HLHS (n = 43)	4.5 years WPPSI	Mean IQ scores were in the lower-normal range Mean preoperative oxygenation was lower in patients scoring below average on full-scale IQ scores
Bergemann et al. (2015)	Case-control HLHS	7–10 years Kaufman assessment battery for children	Lower nonverbal intelligence ($P < .001$), long-term memory ($P = .035$), and processing speed ($P = .012$)
Gaynor et al. (2015)	Retrospective cohort CHD (n = 1770)	6–30 months BSID-I or BSID-II	Lower PDI and MDI than normative means ($P < .001$)
Williams et al. (2015)	Case-control fetal CHD (68/109)	18 month BSID-III	Lower cognitive ($P = .002$), motor and language scores (both $P < .001$) in CHD infants
Hahn et al. (2016)	Prospective cohort SVP (n = 82)	14 months BSID-II	Lower MCA pulsatility index at initial ultrasound predicted higher PDI in CHD infants ($P = .03$); lower abdominal circumference z-scores in the third trimester predicted lower MDI ($P < .05$) with 24- to 29-week z-scores predicting PDI ($P = .04$)
Williams et al. (2013)	Prospective cohort SVP (n = 72)	14 months BSID-II	Mean MDI and PDI were lower in infants than normative means ($P < .001$) Middle cerebral artery pulsatility index z-score negatively correlated with PDI ($P = .03$)
Brosig et al. (2013)	Prospective cohort HLHS (n = 37)	4–6 years Neuropsychological testing	Lower visual-motor integration, fine motor skills, memory, and word structure ($P < .005$). All others were nonsignificant Higher attentional problems ($P < .005$)

ABAS, Adaptive Behavior Assessment System; *BSID,* Bailey Scales of Infant Development; *CSF,* cerebrospinal fluid; *CHD,* congenital heart disease; *HLHS,* hypoplastic left heart syndrome; *IQ,* intelligence quotient; *MCA,* middle cerebral artery; *MDI,* mental development index; *PDI,* psychomotor development index; *SD,* standard deviation; *SVP,* single ventricle physiology; *WPPSI,* Wechsler Preschool and Primary Scale of Intelligence.

15

incidence of disabilities in newborns with HLHS is greater than 60%.[134,135] These impairments result in significant detriment to the child, family, and society.[136,137]

Despite this situation, follow-up studies of infants with CHD report rates of developmental impairments between 27% and 40% and neurologic examination abnormalities in 30%.[138–140] In dividing the factors contributing to poor outcomes into time frames of maximal vulnerability, clinicians and surgeons alike are able to identify various risk periods across the care pathway and implement specific neuro-protection techniques. Previous studies of brain injury in newborns with CHD have focused largely on surgical and CBP-related factors, yet a significant number of children are found to have cognitive impairments, regardless of CBP strategy.[132,141,142]

Preoperative Factors

It is well known that many common genetic disorders with various complexities of CHD (e.g., trisomy 21, DiGeorge, Noonan syndromes) are associated with neurodevelopmental impairments independent of CHD.[143] It has been hypothesized that impacts on neurodevelopment may be equally determined by the underlying genetic abnormalities and injuries to the developing brain.[143] This can be seen in the increasing severity of developmental abnormalities in children with CHD who have chromosomal abnormalities, most of whom have moderate to severe impairments.[131] Injuries to the developing brain in the form of WMI, ischemic infarcts, and microstructural alterations detected on neuroimaging all are determinants of significance in the neurologic outcomes of infants with CHD.[19,36,81] Prenatal diagnosis also appears to be associated with improved brain development and likely reflects the significance of early hypotension and perfusion abnormalities, as demonstrated by the positive effect of prostaglandins on the neurologic outcome in the prenatally diagnosed population.[36] Moreover, recommendations for preoperative management of infants with CHD include ensuring adequate brain perfusion and oxygenation with close monitoring of hematocrit, blood saturation, and hemodynamic circulation in reducing the likelihood of injury. At present, the optimal timing for many CHD surgical repairs in maximizing neurodevelopment and protection remains unknown.

Intraoperative Factors

In the most complex forms of CHD, DHCA and CPB are used during the surgical cardiac repair to minimize the movement of the heart and improve the surgical field. Both DHCA and CPB times have been shown to directly correlate with risk of greater neurologic deficit and mortality, with CPB times longer than 40 to 60 minutes resulting in a greater likelihood of injury.[105,108,139] Pulsatile CPB with close monitoring of pH through a strategy termed the "pH-stat" strategy, was shown to result in improved developmental outcomes.[144] In a randomized clinical trial, intraoperative hematocrit levels above 30% have similarly been correlated with improved neurodevelopment at 1 year after surgery compared with levels less than 20%.[145] Steroids used intraoperatively, shown in animal models to improve outcomes, result in a reduction of circulating inflammatory interleukins, although a measureable short-term clinical benefit was not seen.[146] With the development of newer surgical techniques and increasing use of perfusion and oxygenation monitors, we are seeing improvements in outcomes, although we will need to monitor their development closely to determine which factors are associated with improved long-term outcomes.

Postoperative Factors

Immediately following the surgical repair of the infant with CHD, several significant changes occur in the transition from the intraoperative to postoperative period during which the brain may be injured. Temperature control remains a critical component to postoperative management, where mild hyperthermia is shown to exacerbate injury in animal models.[147] Neurologic dysfunction evident with seizures has been shown to be associated with poor long-term outcomes as a marker of brain injury.[148] Postoperative extracorporeal membrane oxygenation is associated with high rates of mortality, highest in those with postoperative cardiac arrest, with nearly half of survivors having long-term neurologic deficits.[149]

New Interventions and Neuroprotection

Through the 1990s and early 2000s several large initiatives, such as the Boston Circulatory Arrest Trial, focused on optimizing CPB for the surgical management of CHD.[105] Aspects of bypass were further refined over this period (e.g., pH strategy,[150] optimal hemodilution,[145] allopurinol[151]), and there was a concurrent reduction of overt postoperative neurologic dysfunction of 25% in 1990 to 2% in 2002.[152,153] However, we have since learned that at school age, neurodevelopmental outcomes do not differ by bypass strategy used but that the entire cohorts are performing below expectations.[132,141] Most recently, erythropoietin was evaluated for neuroprotection in neonatal cardiac surgery; in a large pilot study neurodevelopmental outcomes were not improved by erythropoietin.[154] The failed attempts to improve neurodevelopmental outcomes through modifications of CPB necessitate a paradigm shift in focus toward fetal, preoperative, and postoperative opportunities to improve the brain health of neonates with CHD. Failed trials of brain protection in neonates with CHD have historically focused on acute protection rather than on promoting brain recovery.[151] By determining how a limitation in brain oxygen delivery that persists after birth impedes brain recovery, clinical strategies to promote brain maturation and optimal neurodevelopmental outcomes should be identified. For example, modifications in the use of atrial septostomy, a technique designed to improve systemic oxygen delivery before surgery but itself associated with stroke,[62] the timing of definitive surgery in newborns with TGA, and optimal postoperative hemodynamic targets could improve brain health.

Antenatally, maternal hyperoxygenation may be a potential treatment for cardiac ventricular hypoplasia. The feasibility of this approach has been demonstrated in fetuses with impaired ventricular growth.[155,156]

Gaps in Knowledge

The care of a child with CHD must manage multiple potential complications in a continuum that begins in the fetus and continues into adulthood. Several gaps continue to exist in the understanding of the ideal management of the ill infant, and there are multiple areas of potential improvement. In the developing fetus we still struggle to fully appreciate the cause for the majority of infants with nonsyndromic CHD, nor do genetics allow us a perfect correlation with anatomic variants. The developing fetus with CHD has been shown to have a maturational delay in the brain similar to preterm infants and infants of diabetic mothers. With the growth of fetal medicine in this field, we have gained significant insight into many potential mechanisms, yet we fail to have any treatments for these fetuses, or their mothers, that may help to advance brain maturation during this period of vulnerability. Surgical advancements have made huge strides in the survival of infants with CHD, and the current treatments with DHCA and CPB can be performed safely and without major injury to the infant brain in the majority of cases. What remains relatively unknown is the ideal time during which surgical treatment maximizes brain development while continually improving survival rates. As the neurodevelopmental profile of the CHD infant continues to be explored, there continues to be a greater gap in the needs of the infant beyond the acute surgical periods to that of community care with physiotherapy, occupational therapy and speech and language therapy, among others. What remains clear is that infants with CHD will continue to improve their survival and neurodevelopmental outcomes as research in the field remains important to the surgeons, clinicians, researchers, parents, and the general public.

Acknowledgment

We thank Dr. Steven P. Miller for his support and mentorship.

REFERENCES

1. Ferencz C, Rubin JD, McCarter RJ, et al. Congenital heart disease: prevalence at livebirth. The Baltimore-Washington Infant Study. *Am J Epidemiol.* 1985;121(1):31–36.
2. Tanner K, Sabrine N, Wren C. Cardiovascular malformations among preterm infants. *Pediatrics.* 2005;116(6):e833–e838.
3. Reller MD, Strickland MJ, Riehle-Colarusso T, Mahle WT, Correa A. Prevalence of congenital heart defects in metropolitan Atlanta, 1998–2005. *J Pediatr.* 2008;153(6):807–813.

4. Ishikawa T, Iwashima S, Ohishi A, Nakagawa Y, Ohzeki T. Prevalence of congenital heart disease assessed by echocardiography in 2067 consecutive newborns. *Acta Paediatr.* 2011;100(8):e55–e60.
5. Khoshnood B, Lelong N, Houyel L, et al. Prevalence, timing of diagnosis and mortality of newborns with congenital heart defects: a population-based study. *Heart.* 2012;98(22):1667–1673.
6. Bernier PL, Stefanescu A, Samoukovic G, Tchervenkov CI. The challenge of congenital heart disease worldwide: epidemiologic and demographic facts. *Semin Thorac Cardiovasc Surg Pediatr Card Surg Annu.* 2010;13(1):26–34.
7. Hoffman JI, Kaplan S. The incidence of congenital heart disease. *J Am Coll Cardiol.* 2002;39(12):1890–1900.
8. van der Linde D, Konings EE, Slager MA, et al. Birth prevalence of congenital heart disease worldwide: a systematic review and meta-analysis. *J Am Coll Cardiol.* 2011;58(21):2241–2247.
9. Romano-Zelekha O, Hirsh R, Blieden L, Green M, Shohat T. The risk for congenital heart defects in offspring of individuals with congenital heart defects. *Clin Genet.* 2001;59(5):325–329.
10. Oyen N, Poulsen G, Boyd HA, Wohlfahrt J, Jensen PK, Melbye M. Recurrence of congenital heart defects in families. *Circulation.* 2009;120(4):295–301.
11. Liu S, Joseph KS, Lisonkova S, et al. Association between maternal chronic conditions and congenital heart defects: a population-based cohort study. *Circulation.* 2013;128(6):583–589.
12. Oyen N, Diaz LJ, Leirgul E, et al. Prepregnancy diabetes and offspring risk of congenital heart disease: a nationwide cohort study. *Circulation.* 2016;133(23):2243–2253.
13. Cohen LS, Friedman JM, Jefferson JW, Johnson EM, Weiner ML. A reevaluation of risk of in utero exposure to lithium. *JAMA.* 1994;271(2):146–150.
14. Loser H, Majewski F. Type and frequency of cardiac defects in embryofetal alcohol syndrome. Report of 16 cases. *Br Heart J.* 1977;39(12):1374–1379.
15. Alverson CJ, Strickland MJ, Gilboa SM, Correa A. Maternal smoking and congenital heart defects in the Baltimore-Washington Infant Study. *Pediatrics.* 2011;127(3):e647–e653.
16. Sullivan PM, Dervan LA, Reiger S, Buddhe S, Schwartz SM. Risk of congenital heart defects in the offspring of smoking mothers: a population-based study. *J Pediatr.* 2015;166(4):978–984.e972.
17. Oster ME, Riehle-Colarusso T, Alverson CJ, Correa A. Associations between maternal fever and influenza and congenital heart defects. *J Pediatr.* 2011;158(6):990–995.
18. Castaneda ARJR, Mayer JE, Hanley FL. *Cardiac Surgery of the Neonate and Infant.* Philadelphia: WB Saunders; 1994.
19. Miller SP, McQuillen PS, Hamrick S, et al. Abnormal brain development in newborns with congenital heart disease. *N Engl J Med.* 2007;357(19):1928–1938.
20. Limperopoulos C, Tworetzky W, McElhinney DB, et al. Brain volume and metabolism in fetuses with congenital heart disease: evaluation with quantitative magnetic resonance imaging and spectroscopy. *Circulation.* 2010;121(1):26–33.
21. Sun L, Macgowan CK, Sled JG, et al. Reduced fetal cerebral oxygen consumption is associated with smaller brain size in fetuses with congenital heart disease. *Circulation.* 2015;131(15):1313–1323.
22. Donofrio MT, Bremer YA, Schieken RM, et al. Autoregulation of cerebral blood flow in fetuses with congenital heart disease: the brain sparing effect. *Pediatr Cardiol.* 2003;24(5):436–443.
23. Ruiz A, Cruz-Lemini M, Masoller N, et al. Longitudinal changes in fetal biometry and cerebroplacental hemodynamics in fetuses with congenital heart disease. *Ultrasound Obstet Gynecol.* 2017;49(3):379–386.
23a. Adescavege, et al. 3-D volumetric MRI evaluation of the placenta in fetuses with complex congenital heart disease. *Placenta.* 2015;36:1024–1030.
24. Schellen C, Ernst S, Gruber GM, et al. Fetal MRI detects early alterations of brain development in tetralogy of Fallot. *Am J Obstet Gynecol.* 2015;213(3):392.e391–392.e397.
25. Von Rhein M, Buchmann A, Hagmann C, et al. Brain volumes predict neurodevelopment in adolescents after surgery for congenital heart disease. *Brain.* 2014;137(1):268–276.
26. Zeng S, Zhou C, Zhou W, Li M, Long C, Peng Q. Volume of intracranial structures on three-dimensional ultrasound in fetuses with congenital heart disease. *Ultrasound Obstet Gynecol.* 2015;46:174–181.
27. Masoller N, Sanz-Cortes M, Crispi F, et al. Mid-gestation brain Doppler and head biometry in fetuses with congenital heart disease predict abnormal brain development at birth. *Ultrasound Obstet Gynecol.* 2016;47:65–73.
28. Peng Q, Zhou Q, Zang M, et al. Reduced fetal brain fissures depth in fetuses with congenital heart diseases. *Prenatal Diagnosis.* 2016;36:1047–1053.
29. Masoller N, Sanz-Cortes M, Crispi F, et al. Severity of fetal brain abnormalities in congenital heart disease in relation to the main expected pattern of in utero brain blood supply. *Fetal Diagn Ther.* 2016;39(4):269–278.
30. Sakazaki S, Masutani S, Sugimoto M, et al. Oxygen supply to the fetal cerebral circulation in hypoplastic left heart syndrome: a simulation study based on the theoretical models of fetal circulation. *Pediatr Cardiol.* 2015;36:677–684.
31. Mlczoch E, Brugger P, Ulm B, et al. Structural congenital brain disease in congenital heart disease: results from a fetal MRI program. *Europ J Paediatr Neurol.* 2013;17:153–160.
31a. Al-Nafasi, et al. Fetal circulation in left-sided congenital heart disease measured by cardiovascular magnetic resonance: a case-control study. *J Cardiovasc Magn Reson.* 2013;15:65.
31b. Clouchoux, et al. Delayed cortical development in fetuses with complex congenital heart disease. *Cereb Cortex.* 2013;23:2932–2943.
31c. Berman, et al. Diffusion-weighted imaging in fetuses with severe congenital heart defects. *AJNR Am J Neuroradiol.* 2012;32:E21–E22.

15

32. McGovern E, Sands AJ. Perinatal management of major congenital heart disease. *Ulster Med J.* 2014;83(3):135–139.
33. Khoshnood B, De Vigan C, Vodovar V, et al. Trends in prenatal diagnosis, pregnancy termination, and perinatal mortality of newborns with congenital heart disease in France, 1983–2000: a population-based evaluation. *Pediatrics.* 2005;115(1):95–101.
34. Bonnet D, Coltri A, Butera G, et al. Detection of transposition of the great arteries in fetuses reduces neonatal morbidity and mortality. *Circulation.* 1999;99(7):916–918.
35. Tworetzky W, McElhinney DB, Reddy VM, Brook MM, Hanley FL, Silverman NH. Improved surgical outcome after fetal diagnosis of hypoplastic left heart syndrome. *Circulation.* 2001;103(9): 1269–1273.
36. Peyvandi S, De Santiago V, Chakkarapani E, et al. Association of prenatal diagnosis of critical congenital heart disease with postnatal brain development and the risk of brain injury. *JAMA Pediatrics.* 2016;170(4).
37. Colaco SM, Karande T, Bobhate PR, Jiyani R, Rao SG, Kulkarni S. Neonates with critical congenital heart defects: impact of fetal diagnosis on immediate and short-term outcomes. *Ann Pediatr Cardiol.* 2017;10(2):126–130.
38. Ter Horst HJ, Mud M, Roofthooft MTR, Bos AF. Amplitude integrated electroencephalographic activity in infants with congenital heart disease before surgery. *Early Hum Dev.* 2010;86(12):759–764.
39. Mahle WT, Newburger JW, Matherne GP, et al. Role of pulse oximetry in examining newborns for congenital heart disease: a scientific statement from the American Heart Association and American Academy of Pediatrics. *Circulation.* 2009;120(5):447–458.
40. Hoffman JI. It is time for routine neonatal screening by pulse oximetry. *Neonatology.* 2011;99(1):1–9.
41. Kuehl KS, Loffredo CA, Ferencz C. Failure to diagnose congenital heart disease in infancy. *Pediatrics.* 1999;103(4 Pt 1):743–747.
42. Chang RK, Gurvitz M, Rodriguez S. Missed diagnosis of critical congenital heart disease. *Arch Pediatr Adolesc Med.* 2008;162(10):969–974.
43. Eckersley L, Sadler L, Parry E, Finucane K, Gentles TL. Timing of diagnosis affects mortality in critical congenital heart disease. *Arch Dis Child.* 2016;101(6):516–520.
44. McQuillen PS, Barkovich AJ, Hamrick SE, et al. Temporal and anatomic risk profile of brain injury with neonatal repair of congenital heart defects. *Stroke.* 2007;38(suppl 2):736–741.
45. Pierpont ME, Basson CT, Benson DW Jr, et al. Genetic basis for congenital heart defects: current knowledge: a scientific statement from the American Heart Association Congenital Cardiac Defects Committee, Council on Cardiovascular Disease in the Young: endorsed by the American Academy of Pediatrics. *Circulation.* 2007;115(23):3015–3038.
46. Lage K, Greenway SC, Rosenfeld JA, et al. Genetic and environmental risk factors in congenital heart disease functionally converge in protein networks driving heart development. *Proc Natl Acad Sci U S A.* 2012;109(35):14035–14040.
47. Moene RJ, Oppenheimer-Dekker A, Bartelings MM. Anatomic obstruction of the right ventricular outflow tract in transposition of the great arteries. *Am J Cardiol.* 1983;51(10):1701–1704.
48. Deal BJ, Chin AJ, Sanders SP, Norwood WI, Castaneda AR. Subxiphoid two-dimensional echocardiographic identification of tricuspid valve abnormalities in transposition of the great arteries with ventricular septal defect. *Am J Cardiol.* 1985;55(9):1146–1151.
49. Freed MD, Heymann MA, Lewis AB, Roehl SL, Kensey RC. Prostaglandin E1 infants with ductus arteriosus-dependent congenital heart disease. *Circulation.* 1981;64(5):899–905.
50. Rashkind WJ, Miller WW. Creation of an atrial septal defect without thoracotomy. A palliative approach to complete transposition of the great arteries. *JAMA.* 1966;196(11):991–992.
51. Marshall AC, Levine J, Morash D, et al. Results of in utero atrial septoplasty in fetuses with hypoplastic left heart syndrome. *Prenat Diagn.* 2008;28(11):1023–1028.
52. Jatene AD, Fontes VF, Paulista PP, et al. Anatomic correction of transposition of the great vessels. *J Thorac Cardiovasc Surg.* 1976;72(3):364–370.
53. Emani SM, Beroukhim R, Zurakowski D, et al. Outcomes after anatomic repair for D-transposition of the great arteries with left ventricular outflow tract obstruction. *Circulation.* 2009;120(suppl 11):S53–S58.
54. Samanek M, Voriskova M. Congenital heart disease among 815,569 children born between 1980 and 1990 and their 15-year survival: a prospective Bohemia survival study. *Pediatr Cardiol.* 1999;20(6):411–417.
55. Graham TP Jr, Bernard YD, Mellen BG, et al. Long-term outcome in congenitally corrected transposition of the great arteries: a multi-institutional study. *J Am Coll Cardiol.* 2000;36(1):255–261.
56. Hornung TS, Bernard EJ, Celermajer DS, et al. Right ventricular dysfunction in congenitally corrected transposition of the great arteries. *Am J Cardiol.* 1999;84(9):1116–1119. A1110.
57. Tchervenkov CI, Jacobs ML, Tahta SA. Congenital heart surgery nomenclature and database project: hypoplastic left heart syndrome. *Ann Thorac Surg.* 2000;69(suppl 4):S170–S179.
57a. Knirsch, et al. Structural cerebral abnormalities and neurodevelopmental status in single ventricle congenital heart disease before Fontan procedure. *Eur J Cardiothorac Surg.* 2016:1–7.
57b. Birca, et al. Interplay of brain structure and function in neonatal congenital heart disease. *Ann Clin Transl Neurolo.* 2016;3(9):708–722.
57c. Shadeed, Elfaytouri. Brain maturity and brain injury in newborns with cyanotic congenital heart disease. *Pediatr Cardiol.* 2011;32:47–54.
57d. Von Rhein, et al. Severe congenital heart defects are associated with global reduction of neonatal brain volumes. *J Pediatr.* 2015;167:1259–1263.

58. Cowan F, Mercuri E, Groenendaal F, et al. Does cranial ultrasound imaging identify arterial cerebral infarction in term neonates. *Arch Dis Child Fetal Neonatal Ed.* 2005;90:F252–F256.
59. Andropoulos DB, Hunter JV, Nelson DP, et al. Brain immaturity is associated with brain injury before and after neonatal cardiac surgery with high-flow bypass and cerebral oxygenation monitoring. *J Thorac Cardiovasc Surg.* 2010;139(3):543–556.
60. Block AJ, McQuillen PS, Chau V, et al. Clinically silent preoperative brain injuries do not worsen with surgery in neonates with congenital heart disease. *J Thorac Cardiovasc Surg.* 2010;140(3):550–557.
61. Bertholdt S, Latal B, Liamlahi R, et al. Cerebral lesions on magnetic resonance imaging correlate with preoperative neurological status in neonates undergoing cardiopulmonary bypass surgery. *Europ J Cardio-Thoracic Surg.* 2014;45:625–632.
62. McQuillen PS, Hamrick SE, Perez MJ, et al. Balloon atrial septostomy is associated with preoperative stroke in neonates with transposition of the great arteries. *Circulation.* 2006;113(2):280–285.
63. Beca J, Gunn J, Coleman L, et al. Pre-operative brain injury in newborn infants with transposition of the great arteries occurs at rates similar to other complex congenital heart disease and is not related to balloon atrial septostomy. *J Am Coll Cardiol.* 2009;53:1807–1811.
64. Galli KK, Zimmerman RA, Jarvik GP, et al. Periventricular leukomalacia is common after neonatal cardiac surgery. *J Thorac Cardiovasc Surg.* 2004;127(3):692–704.
65. Kinney HC, Panigrahy A, Newburger JW, Jonas RA, Sleeper LA. Hypoxic-ischemic brain injury in infants with congenital heart disease dying after cardiac surgery. *Acta Neuropathol (Berl).* 2005;110(6):563–578.
66. Fogel MA, Li C, Elci OU, et al. Neurological injury and cerebral blood flow in single ventricles throughout staged surgical reconstruction. *Circulation.* 2017;135(7):671–682.
67. Mahle WT, Tavani F, Zimmerman RA, et al. An MRI study of neurological injury before and after congenital heart surgery. *Circulation.* 2002;106(12 suppl 1):I109–I114.
68. Glass HC, Bowman C, Chau V, et al. Infection and white matter injury in infants with congenital cardiac disease. *Cardiol Young.* 2011;21(5):562–571.
69. Cottrill C, Kaplan S. Cerebral vascular accident in cyanotic congenital heart disease. *Ann J Dis Child.* 1973;125:484–487.
70. Sebire G, Tabarki B, Saunders E, et al. Cerebral venous sinus thrombosis in children: risk factors, presentation, diagnosis and outcome. *Brain.* 2005;128:477–489.
71. Martinez-Quintana E, Rodriguez-Gonzalez F. Thrombocytopenia in congenital heart disease patients. *Platelets.* 2015;26(5):432–436.
72. Dlamini N, Billinghurst L, Kirkham F. Cerebral venous sinus (sinovenous) thrombosis in children. *Neurosurg Clin N Am.* 2010;21:511–527.
73. Kelly P, Hayman R, Shekerdemian L, et al. Subdural hemorrhage and hypoxia in infants with congenital heart disease. *Pediatrics.* 2014;134:773–781.
74. Looney C, Smith J, Merck L, et al. Intracranial hemorrhage in asymptomatic neonates: prevalence on MR images and relationship to obstetric and neonatal risk factors. *Radiology.* 2007;242(2):535–541.
75. Whitby E, Griffiths P, Rutter S, et al. Frequency and natural history of subdural haemorrhages in babies and relation to obstetric factors. *Lancet.* 2004;363(9412):846–851.
76. Tavani F, Zimmerman R, Clancy R, Licht D, Mahle W. Incidental intracranial hemorrhage after uncomplicated birth: MRI before and after neonatal heart surgery. *Neuroradiology.* 2003;45:253–258.
77. Hinton RB, Andelfinger G, Sekar P, et al. Prenatal head growth and white matter injury in hypoplastic left heart syndrome. *Pediatr Res.* 2008;64(4):364–369.
78. Licht DJ, Shera DM, Clancy RR, et al. Brain maturation is delayed in infants with complex congenital heart defects. *J Thorac Cardiovasc Surg.* 2009;137(3):529–536, discussion 536–527.
79. Glauser TA, Rorke LB, Weinberg PM, Clancy RR. Congenital brain anomalies associated with the hypoplastic left heart syndrome. *Pediatrics.* 1990;85(6):984–990.
80. Partridge SC, Vigneron DB, Charlton NN, et al. Pyramidal tract maturation after brain injury in newborns with heart disease. *Ann Neurol.* 2006;59(4):640–651.
81. Dimitropoulos A, McQuillen PS, Sethi V, et al. Brain injury and development in newborns with critical congenital heart disease. *Neurology.* 2013;81(3):241–248.
82. Miller SP, McQuillen PS. Neurology of congenital heart disease: insight from brain imaging. *Arch Dis Child Fetal Neonatal Ed.* 2007;92(6):F435–F437.
83. Segovia KN, McClure M, Moravec M, et al. Arrested oligodendrocyte lineage maturation in chronic perinatal white matter injury. *Ann Neurol.* 2008;63(4):520–530.
84. Buser JR, Maire J, Riddle A, et al. Arrested preoligodendrocyte maturation contributes to myelination failure in premature infants. *Ann Neurol.* 2012;71(1):93–109.
85. Agematsu K, Korotcova L, Scafidi J, Gallo V, Jonas RA, Ishibashi N. Effects of preoperative hypoxia on white matter injury associated with cardiopulmonary bypass in a rodent hypoxic and brain slice model. *Pediatr Res.* 2014;75(5):618–625.
86. Miller SP, Ferriero DM. From selective vulnerability to connectivity: insights from newborn brain imaging. *Trends Neurosci.* 2009;32(9):496–505.
87. McQuillen PS, Miller SP. Congenital heart disease and brain development. *Ann N Y Acad Sci.* 2010;1184:68–86.
88. Miller SP, Ferriero DM, Leonard C, et al. Early brain injury in premature newborns detected with magnetic resonance imaging is associated with adverse early neurodevelopmental outcome. *J Pediatr.* 2005;147(5):609–616.

89. Chau V, Poskitt KJ, McFadden DE, et al. Effect of chorioamnionitis on brain development and injury in premature newborns. *Ann Neurol*. 2009;66(2):155–164.

90. Vinall J, Grunau RE, Brant R, et al. Slower postnatal growth is associated with delayed cerebral cortical maturation in preterm newborns. *Sci Transl Med*. 2013;5(168):168ra8.

91. Chau V, Synnes A, Grunau RE, Poskitt KJ, Brant R, Miller SP. Abnormal brain maturation in preterm neonates associated with adverse developmental outcomes. *Neurology*. 2013. In press.

92. Hayashida M, Kin N, Tomioka T, et al. Cerebral ischaemia during cardiac surgery in children detected by combined monitoring of BIS and near-infrared spectroscopy. *BrJ Anaesth*. 2004;92(5):662–669.

93. Zimmerman A, Burrows F, Jonas R, Hickey P. The limits of detectable cerebral perfusion by transcranial Doppler sonography in neonates undergoing deep hypothermic low-flow cardiopulmonary bypass. *J Thorac Cardiovasc Surg*. 1997;114:594–600.

94. Hoffman G, Ghanayem N. Perioperative neuromonitoring in pediatric cardiac surgery: techniques and targets. *Prog Pediatr Cardiol*. 2010;29:123–130.

95. Ghariani S, Spaey J, Liard L, et al. Sensitivity, specificity and impact on preoperative neuromonitoring of surgical strategy by somatosensory evoked potentials in vascular surgery performed in deep hypothermic circulatory arrest. *Clin Neurophysiol*. 1998;28(4):335–341.

96. Austin E, Edmonds H, Auden S, et al. Benefit of neurophysiologic monitoring for pediatric cardiac surgery. *J Thorac Cardiovasc Surg*. 1997;114:707–717.

97. Hirsch J, Charpie J, Ohye R, Gurney J. Near infrared spectroscopy (NIRS) should not be standard of care for postoperative management. *Semin Thorac Cardiovasc Surg Pediatr Card Surg Ann*. 2010;13:51–54.

98. Ricci Z, Garisto C, Favia I, et al. Cerebral NIRS as a marker of superior vena cava oxygen saturation in neonates with congenital heart disease. *Pediatr Anesth*. 2010;20:1040–1045.

99. Quarti A, Nardone S, Manfrini F, et al. Effect of the adjunct of carbon dioxide during cardiopulmonary bypass on cerebral oxygenation. *Perfusion*. 2012;28(2):152–155.

100. Simons J, Sood E, Derby C, Pizarro C. Predictive value of near-infrared spectroscopy on neurodevelopmental outcome after surgery for congenital heart disease in infancy. *J Thorac Cardiovasc Surg*. 2012;143:118–125.

101. Sanchez-de-Toledo J, Chrysostomou C, Munoz R, et al. Cerebral regional oxygen saturation and serum neuromarkers for the prediction of adverse neurologic outcome in pediatric cardiac surgery. *Neurocrit Care*. 2014;21:133–139.

102. Mulkey SB, Yap VL, Bai S, et al. Amplitude-integrated EEG in newborns with critical congenital heart disease predicts preoperative brain magnetic resonance imaging findings. *Pediatr Neurol*. 2015;52(6):599–605.

103. Clancy RR, McGaurn SA, Wernovsky G, et al. Risk of seizures in survivors of newborn heart surgery using deep hypothermic circulatory arrest. *Pediatrics*. 2003;111(3):592–601.

104. Shellhaas R, Chang T, Tsuchida T, et al. The American Clinical Neurophysiology Society's guideline on continuous electroencephalography monitoring in neonates. *J Clin Neurophysiol*. 2011;28:611–617.

105. Newburger JW, Jonas RA, Wernovsky G, et al. A comparison of the perioperative neurologic effects of hypothermic circulatory arrest versus low-flow cardiopulmonary bypass in infant heart surgery. *N Engl J Med*. 1993;329(15):1057–1064.

106. du Plessis AJ, Jonas RA, Wypij D, et al. Perioperative effects of alpha-stat versus pH-stat strategies for deep hypothermic cardiopulmonary bypass in infants. *J Thorac Cardiovasc Surg*. 1997;114(6):991–1000, discussion 1000–1001.

107. Gaynor J, Nicolson S, Jarvik G, et al. Increasing duration of deep hypothermic circulatory arrest is associated with an increased incidence of postoperative electroencephalographic seizures. *J Thorac Cardiovasc Surg*. 2005;130:1278–1286.

108. Naim M, Gaynor J, Chen J, et al. Subclinical seizures identified by postoperative electroencephalographic monitoring are common after neonatal cardiac surgery. *J Thorac Cardiovasc Surg*. 2015;150:169–180.

109. Adams E, Chau V, Poskitt KJ, Grunau RE, Synnes A, Miller SP. Tractography-based quantitation of corticospinal tract development in premature newborns. *J Pediatr*. 2010;156(6):882–888.

110. Miller SP, Vigneron DB, Henry RG, et al. Serial quantitative diffusion tensor MRI of the premature brain: development in newborns with and without injury. *J Magn Reson Imaging*. 2002;16(6):621–632.

111. Brossard-Racine M, du Plessis AJ, Vezina G, et al. Prevalence and spectrum of in utero structural brain abnormalities in fetuses with complex congenital heart disease. *AJNR Am J Neuroradiol*. 2014;35(8):1593–1599.

112. Nossin-Manor R, Card D, Morris D, et al. Quantitative MRI in the very preterm brain: assessing tissue organization and myelination using magnetization transfer, diffusion tensor and T(1) imaging. *Neuroimage*. 2013;64:505–516.

113. Kreis R, Hofmann L, Kuhlmann B, Boesch C, Bossi E, Huppi PS. Brain metabolite composition during early human brain development as measured by quantitative in vivo ¹H magnetic resonance spectroscopy. *Magn Reson Med*. 2002;48(6):949–958.

114. Vigneron DB. Magnetic resonance spectroscopic imaging of human brain development. *Neuroimaging Clin N Am*. 2006;16(1):75–85. viii.

115. Miller SP, Newton N, Ferriero DM, et al. Predictors of 30-month outcome after perinatal depression: role of proton MRS and socioeconomic factors. *Pediatr Res*. 2002;52(1):71–77.

116. Thayyil S, Chandrasekaran M, Taylor A, et al. Cerebral magnetic resonance biomarkers in neonatal encephalopathy: a meta-analysis. *Pediatrics*. 2010;125(2):e382–e395.

117. Card D, Nossin-Manor R, Moore AM, Raybaud C, Sled JG, Taylor MJ. Brain metabolite concentrations are associated with illness severity scores and white matter abnormalities in very preterm infants. *Pediatr Res.* 2013;74(1):75–81.

118. Smith-Collins A, Luyt K, Heep A, Kauppinen R. High frequency functional brain networks in neonates revealed by rapid acquisition resting state fMRI. *Hum Brain Mapp.* 2015;36:2483–2494.

119. King T, Smith K, Burns T, et al. fMRI investigation of working memory in adolescents with surgically treated congenital heart disease. *Appl Neuropsychol Child.* 2016.

120. Ortinau C, Alexopoulos D, Dierker D, Essen DV, Beca J, Inder T. Cortical folding is altered before surgery in infants with congenital heart disease. *J Pediatr.* 2013;163(5):1507–1510.

121. Claessens N, Moeskops P, Buchmann A, et al. Delayed cortical gray matter development in neonates with severe congenital heart disease. *Pediatr Res.* 2016;80(5):668–674.

122. Nossin-Manor R, Chung AD, Whyte HE, Shroff MM, Taylor MJ, Sled JG. Deep gray matter maturation in very preterm neonates: regional variations and pathology-related age-dependent changes in magnetization transfer ratio. *Radiology.* 2012;263(2):510–517.

123. Nossin-Manor R, Chung AD, Morris D, et al. Optimized T1- and T2-weighted volumetric brain imaging as a diagnostic tool in very preterm neonates. *Pediatr Radiol.* 2011;41(6):702–710.

124. Chakravarty MM, Steadman P, van Eede MC, et al. Performing label-fusion-based segmentation using multiple automatically generated templates. *Hum Brain Mapp.* 2013;34(10):2635–2654.

125. Jain V, Buckley EM, Licht DJ, et al. Cerebral oxygen metabolism in neonates with congenital heart disease quantified by MRI and optics. *J Cereb Blood Flow Metabol.* 2014;34(3):380–388.

126. Majnemer A, Limperopoulos C, Shevell MI, Rohlicek C, Rosenblatt B, Tchervenkov C. A new look at outcomes of infants with congenital heart disease. *Pediatr Neurol.* 2009;40(3):197–204.

126a. Aly, et al. Cerebral tissue oxygenation index and lactate at 24 hours postoperative predict survival and neurodevelopmental outcome after neonatal cardiac surgery. *Congenital Heart Disease.* 2017;12:188–195.

126b. Brosig CL, et al. Preschool neurodevelopmental outcomes in children with congenital heart disease. *J Pediatr.* 183, 80–86.e1.

126c. Brosig CL, et al. Neurodevelopmental outcomes for children with hypoplastic left heart syndrome at the age of 5 years. *Pediatr Cardiol.* 2013;34:1597–1604.

126d. Hansen, et al. Neurodevelopmental outcome in hypoplastic left heart syndrome: Impact of perioperative cerebral tissue oxygenation of the Norwood procedure. *J Thorac Cardiovasc Surg.* 2016;151:1358–1366.

126e. Bergemann A, Hansen JH, Rotermann I, et al. Neuropsychological performance of school-aged children after staged surgical palliation of hypoplastic left heart syndrome. *Eur J Cardiothorac Surg.* 2015;47:803–811.

126f. Gaynor, et al. Neurodevelopmental outcomes after cardiac surgery in infancy. *Pediatrics.* 2015;135(5):816–825.

126g. Williams, et al. Fetal growth and neurodevelopmental outcome in congenital heart disease. *Pediatr Cardiol.* 2015;36:1135–1144.

126h. Williams, et al. The association of fetal cerebrovascular resistance with early neurodevelopment in single ventricle congenital heart disease. *Am Heart J.* 2013;165:544–550.e1.

126i. Hahn, et al. Association between fetal growth, cerebral blood flow and neurodevelopmental outcome in univentricular fetuses. *Ultrasound Obstet Gynecol.* 2016;47:460–465.

127. Munoz-Lopez M, Hoskote A, Chadwick MJ, et al. Hippocampal damage and memory impairment in congenital cyanotic heart disease. *Hippocampus.* 2017;27(4):417–424.

128. Majnemer A, Mazer B, Lecker E, et al. Patterns of use of educational and rehabilitation services at school age for children with congenitally malformed hearts. *Cardiol Young.* 2008;18(3):288–296.

129. Hack M. Adult outcomes of preterm children. *J Dev Behav Pediatr.* 2009;30(5):460–470.

130. Grosse SD, Matte TD, Schwartz J, Jackson RJ. Economic gains resulting from the reduction in children's exposure to lead in the United States. *Environ Health Perspect.* 2002;110(6):563–569.

131. Wernovsky G. Current insights regarding neurological and developmental abnormalities in children and young adults with complex congenital cardiac disease. *Cardiol Young.* 2006;16(suppl 1):92–104.

132. Bellinger DC, Wypij D, Duplessis AJ, et al. Neurodevelopmental status at eight years in children with dextro-transposition of the great arteries: the Boston Circulatory Arrest Trial. *J Thorac Cardiovasc Surg.* 2003;126(5):1385–1396.

133. Bellinger DC, Wypij D, Kuban KC, et al. Developmental and neurological status of children at 4 years of age after heart surgery with hypothermic circulatory arrest or low-flow cardiopulmonary bypass. *Circulation.* 1999;100(5):526–532.

134. Miller G, Tesman JR, Ramer JC, Baylen BG, Myers JL. Outcome after open-heart surgery in infants and children. *J Child Neurol.* 1996;11(1):49–53.

135. Rogers BT, Msall ME, Buck GM, et al. Neurodevelopmental outcome of infants with hypoplastic left heart syndrome. *J Pediatr.* 1995;126(3):496–498.

136. Majnemer A, Limperopoulos C, Shevell M, Rohlicek C, Rosenblatt B, Tchervenkov C. Health and well-being of children with congenital cardiac malformations, and their families, following open-heart surgery. *Cardiol Young.* 2006;16(2):157–164.

137. Majnemer A, Limperopoulos C, Shevell M, Rohlicek C, Rosenblatt B, Tchervenkov C. Developmental and functional outcomes at school entry in children with congenital heart defects. *J Pediatr.* 2008;153(1):55–60.

138. Dittrich H, Buhrer C, Grimmer I, Dittrich S, Abdul-Khaliq H, Lange PE. Neurodevelopment at 1 year of age in infants with congenital heart disease. *Heart.* 2003;89(4):436–441.

139. Limperopoulos C, Majnemer A, Shevell MI, et al. Predictors of developmental disabilities after open heart surgery in young children with congenital heart defects. *J Pediatr*. 2002;141(1):51–58.
140. Limperopoulos C, Majnemer A, Shevell MI, et al. Functional limitations in young children with congenital heart defects after cardiac surgery. *Pediatrics*. 2001;108(6):1325–1331.
141. Karl TR, Hall S, Ford G, et al. Arterial switch with full-flow cardiopulmonary bypass and limited circulatory arrest: neurodevelopmental outcome. *J Thorac Cardiovasc Surg*. 2004;127(1):213–222.
142. Bellinger DC, Jonas RA, Rappaport LA, et al. Developmental and neurologic status of children after heart surgery with hypothermic circulatory arrest or low-flow cardiopulmonary bypass. *N Eng J Med*. 1995;332(9):549–555.
143. McQuillen PS, Goff DA, Licht DJ. Effects of congenital heart disease on brain development. *Prog Pediat Cardiol*. 2010;29(2):79–85.
144. Murkin J, Martzke J, Buchan A, Bentley C, Wong C. A randomized study of the influence of perfusion technique and pH management strategy in 316 patients undergoing coronary artery bypass surgery. *J Thorac Cardiovasc Surg*. 1995;110:340–348.
145. Jonas RA, Wypij D, Roth SJ, et al. The influence of hemodilution on outcome after hypothermic cardiopulmonary bypass: results of a randomized trial in infants. *J Thorac Cardiovasc Surg*. 2003;126(6):1765–1774.
146. Amanullah M, Hamid M, Hanif H, et al. Effect of steroids on inflammatory markers and clinical parameters in congenital open heart surgery: a randomised controlled trial. *Cardiol Young*. 2016;26(3):506–510.
147. Shum-Tim D, Nagashima M, Shinoka T, et al. Postischemic hyperthermia exacerbates neurologic injury after deep hypothermic circulatory arrest. *Cardiovasc Surg*. 1998;116:780–792.
148. Rappaport LA, Wypij D, Bellinger DC, et al. Relation of seizures after cardiac surgery in early infancy to neurodevelopmental outcome. Boston Circulatory Arrest Study Group. *Circulation*. 1998;97(8):773–779.
149. Chow G, Koirala B, Armstrong D, et al. Predictors of mortality and neurological morbidity in children undergoing extracorporeal life support for cardiac disease. *Europ J Cardio-Thoracic Surg*. 2004;26(1):38–43.
150. Bellinger DC, Wypij D, du Plessis AJ, et al. Developmental and neurologic effects of alpha-stat versus pH-stat strategies for deep hypothermic cardiopulmonary bypass in infants. *J Thorac Cardiovasc Surg*. 2001;121(2):374–383.
151. Clancy RR, McGaurn SA, Goin JE, et al. Allopurinol neurocardiac protection trial in infants undergoing heart surgery using deep hypothermic circulatory arrest. *Pediatrics*. 2001;108(1):61–70.
152. Ferry PC. Neurologic sequelae of open-heart surgery in children. An 'irritating question'. *Am J Dis Child*. 1990;144(3):369–373.
153. Menache CC, du Plessis AJ, Wessel DL, Jonas RA, Newburger JW. Current incidence of acute neurologic complications after open-heart operations in children. *Ann Thorac Surg*. 2002;73(6):1752–1758.
154. Andropoulos DB, Brady K, Easley RB, et al. Erythropoietin neuroprotection in neonatal cardiac surgery: a phase I/II safety and efficacy trial. *J Thorac Cardiovasc Surg*. 2013;146(1):124–131.
155. Borik S, Macgowan CK, Seed M. Maternal hyperoxygenation and foetal cardiac MRI in the assessment of the borderline left ventricle. *Cardiol Young*. 2015;25(6):1214–1217.
156. Say L, Gulmezoglu AM, Hofmeyr GJ. Maternal oxygen administration for suspected impaired fetal growth. *Cochrane Database Syst Rev*. 2003;(1):CD000137.

15

CHAPTER 16

Long-Term Follow-Up of the Very Preterm Graduate

Neil Marlow

- Very preterm graduates may develop complex and subtle deficits of neuropsychological function that have implications for health and well-being across childhood.

- Major neurosensory deficits, such as cerebral palsy or vision and hearing impairment, are decreasing in frequency among survivors, but medical services need to remain alert to their presentation and need for support.

- Recognition and support over infancy may be effective in ensuring optimal outcomes.

- Very preterm children at school are at risk of key executive function deficits that may lead to poor performance in the classroom and in behavior.

- These issues have importance for attainment and wealth as adults.

The continuum of perinatal casualty extends to adverse neuropsychological outcomes after very preterm (VPT) birth, which consist of an important spectrum of impairments that has become more apparent with increasing academic study over the past 20 years. Increasing survival without severe impairment at extremely low gestational ages[1] has fueled increasing intervention in the perinatal period and a recognition that "less" intervention may be "more" in terms of outcomes. Birth at extremely low gestations is nonetheless attended with a high risk of neurologic injury and complex sequelae. Outcome evaluation has resulted in an explosion of interest in this area that has contributed to our current understanding of the problems faced by VPT children through infancy to adolescence and into adult life. This chapter focuses on the child and the support necessary to ensure optimal outcomes as a result of our perinatal investment.

Most follow-up services are associated with individual neonatal programs and fulfill two roles: first, as individual family-infant support and detection of atypical neurodevelopment so that families can receive appropriate services, and second, collecting information for quality assurance and research. Support may be most intensive over the first year as the child develops and anxiety is highest for families. Most serious impairment should be detected during this time, including cerebral palsy (CP), and significant developmental delay, and issues with feeding, regulation, and growth should be addressed. As the infant develops, respiratory function improves, and supplemental oxygen and feeding support can be withdrawn. Over the second year the intensity of support required lessens, and most services now carry out a formal assessment at 18 to 24 months to categorize outcome for quality assurance purposes. Services then may transfer children to the care of their family medical support team or continue to monitor progress intermittently. As will be noted, continuing support helps to support families in decision-making—for example, about education—and can provide advice and direction when new problems arise. Research into the neuropsychological impairments found in middle childhood is important in helping us to understand the educational and wider support needs of VPT children.

The Major Sequelae of Very Preterm Birth

Key neurosensory adverse outcomes found among VPT survivors include:

- CP
- Cognitive impairment
- Visual impairment
- Hearing loss
- Behavioral problems

These outcomes are inversely related to gestational age at birth, best exemplified by the exponential rise of educational special needs with increasing immaturity[2] and the similar relationship between mean intelligence quotient (IQ) of studies and gestational age.[3,4]

Cerebral Palsy

Classically, CP following VPT birth is described as bilateral spastic in type, tending to be worse in the lower limbs and associated with periventricular leukomalacia (spastic diplegia). However, with increasing immaturity, the pattern of CP is complex and more mixed in distribution among more modern cohorts. Among infants with birth weights between 1000 and 1500 g, there is some evidence that CP rates are falling in Europe and a suggestion that rates for infants weighting less than 1000 at birth are following the trend.[5] There is also evidence in multiple studies that less severe motor problems are more common among VPT survivors. Strong prognostic risk factors for CP and motor problems are intraventricular hemorrhage and periventricular leukomalacia, together with use of postnatal or nonuse of antenatal steroids for CP. Male sex and lower gestational age are also related to the prevalence of CP, but in studies with restricted study size or gestational range this may not be as clear.[6]

The definition of CP varies from physician to physician. Various classification systems are in place, such as that from the Surveillance of Cerebral Palsy in Europe group (SCPE; www.scpenetwork.eu). Their simple classification tree provides for consistent classification into spastic (bilateral, unilateral), dyskinetic (dystonic, choreoathetoid), ataxic, or other. Functional outcome in children with CP is increasingly important. Simple classifications, such as the Gross Motor Function Classification System (GMFCS)[7] and Manual Ability Classification System (MACS),[8] are valuable schemes to maintain some consistency between reports and are often used in published studies. However, functional outcome extends beyond motor outcomes to other aspects of daily living and societal integration, as described by Bax and colleagues in their extended definition of CP.[9]

Early detection of CP is challenging before discharge. Critical imaging findings may indicate high risk but distribution and severity are hard to predict. Most nonambulatory CP can be identified using sequential cranial ultrasound, supplemented by assessment of the posterior limb of the internal capsule on magnetic resonance imaging (MRI).[10] All VPT infants should have a formal structured neurologic examination before discharge.[11,12] Many services, particularly in Europe, find a video recording of general movements, classified as suggested by Prechtl,[13] to be valuable. Most predictive of later problems is a repeat video at 3 months postterm, in particular evaluating for the normal presence or absence of fidgety movements. Classic persistence of primitive reflexes and ongoing neurologic abnormalities raise suspicion. When there is anxiety about evolving neurologic signs, early referral to neurodisability services is important to provide enhanced surveillance and monitoring, with intervention as indicated.

During follow-up in infancy, VPT children may display what are considered abnormal patterns of neurologic development, mainly related to persisting trunk extension and shoulder retraction. Such a pattern is not associated with the typical evolving pattern of spastic CP; on occasions it may masquerade as such when it is severe. Such transient dystonias or transient neurologic abnormalities are well described and they tend to resolve over the second year; hence distinguishing them from evolving CP may be of great importance. First described by Drillien,[14] such findings may be associated with persisting periventricular echodensities on sequential neonatal ultrasound[15] and may signal children at risk of later educational challenges.[14] Recognition should nonetheless initiate support from neurodisability services to encourage optimal posture and facilitate development.

Cognitive Impairment in Infancy

Developmental progress should be monitored as part of routine follow-up. Repeated formal assessments may provide a suitable framework on which to counsel parents, but are not strictly necessary. Most follow-up programs will develop key assessment points. National recommendations in the United Kingdom are to make a single formal assessment point at 24 months of age corrected for preterm birth. At this age, there are a range of screening and assessment tools available.[16] Choice of tools will depend on resources. In the United Kingdom, there is a proposal to use a parental questionnaire (Parent Report of Children's Abilities-Revised [PRCA-R][17]) at 2 years but to supplement this by a formal general cognitive score in the preschool period. Other schemes include assessment using formal comprehensive assessments, such as the Bayley Scales of Toddler and Infant Development (Bayley-III). Formally assessed developmental scores underpin much outcome research activity. There is some evidence that the second edition of the Bayley Scales has a high predictive value for IQ over childhood to 19 years, emphasizing the importance of accurate and well-conducted assessments in the third postnatal year.[18] It is too early to review the predictive value of the third edition, but concerns have been raised over the rather higher-than-anticipated scores,[19,20] possibly because of overscoring of performance at lower scores.[21]

Children who are causing developmental concern or who score poorly on screening or developmental testing should be referred to early intervention services, which can provide longitudinal monitoring and support. Early intervention programs may show early benefit through to the preschool period, but there is little evidence the effects persist into childhood from current studies.[22] Parental support and reassurance are equally important in the early months when uncertainty and anxiety may compromise maternal-infant interaction but are rarely assessed.

Sensory Outcomes

Neonatal screening for hearing impairment and vision screening will identify those children with severe or profound impairment; formal testing where good population screening and intervention services exist is not necessary. Because the increased prevalence of acquired hearing loss and milder degrees of visual impairment are very common in VPT children, in the absence of specialized screening programs formal assessment is an important part of follow-up services for this group.

Behavior

Assessing behavior at 2 years of age is fraught with problems. Most disability classifications (see later text) at around 2 years of age do not include behavioral criteria.

However, there is little doubt that the prevalence of autistic symptoms is increased after very preterm birth and detection before 2 years may help with intervention, if it is deemed necessary. Screening is recommended by the American Academy of Pediatrics at 18 months followed by referral. Screening for autistic symptoms is frequently undertaken in many follow-up programs, but the screening tools available, designed to identify at-risk children in the general population, are confounded by their reliance on developmental questions[23] and the obligatory telephone follow-up and clinical assessment are rarely reported.[24] Very high rates of positive screening results have been reported[23,25,26] but the necessary screening is not followed by diagnostic testing. Later follow-up indicates that the proportion with a diagnosis of autism may be considerably less than these estimates.[27] Screening tools should be used with caution and follow-up diagnostic assessments undertaken before disclosure. Some of the newer screening tools may be better in this respect,[28] but further work is required in the preterm population to define their performance.

Classification of Impairment

For the purposes of research and audit, several classification systems are in use. The most common reports include children with what are called "moderate or severe impairments" or "neurodevelopmental impairment." Such data are frequently used to support counseling without real reference to their predictive validity. Other systems use a more graded approach, separating severe and moderately disabling impairments.[29] The prevalence of "severe impairment" in some situations is a useful construct, such as delivery room decisions about active care and decisions concerning palliative care, and forms part of the widely used the U.K. National Institute for Health Research (NIHR) prognostic calculator.[30] In contrast, most individuals with "moderate impairment" at 2 years will achieve independent living. Although on an individual basis the categorization of impairment at 2 to 3 years is a relatively poor predictor of childhood status, on a population basis it provides a good estimate of risk throughout childhood; children with borderline results frequently move between categories in both directions.

CASE 1   ABIGAIL

Abigail was born to a 33-year-old primigravid Afro-Caribbean mother following spontaneous preterm labor at 26 weeks. Her mother presented with 6-cm dilatation and proceeded to deliver without steroids. Abigail was ventilated for 2 weeks and then received continuous positive airway pressure/supplemental oxygen until 32 weeks of postmenstrual age (PMA). Her course was complicated by feeding difficulties and several episodes of neonatal sepsis (*Staphylococcus epimermidis*). She was discharged home at 38 weeks PMA. Results of neurologic examination were normal, and ultrasound revealed mild ventriculomegaly (+2 standard deviations bilaterally). No brain MRI scanning was performed.

Prechtl video assessment at 3 months corrected age (CA) (i.e., postterm) was inconclusive as to the presence of fidgety movements; neurologic and developmental examinations were unremarkable. Feeding was slow and weight gain borderline. Working with the speech and language team, solids foods were introduced but no developmental interventions were planned.

At 6 months CA Abigail was just starting to roll over, with tendency to go into extension, but limb tone and reflexes were unremarkable. The parents were resistant to intervention at this stage, so early review was planned but this appointment was missed.

Abigail was evaluated again at 12 months CA when generalized hypertonia was evident. She was not sitting and reflexes were generally brisk. Hand function was poor without pincer grasp. She was bright and communicative, with three clear words. Assessment by physiotherapy confirmed the hypertonia, and referral was made to the community disability team, who confirmed our findings and organized support with physiotherapy as the lead professional team. Formal disclosure of a diagnosis of CP was made, which the parents denied.

Over the next 6 months Abigail made rapid progress and was walking at 18 months CA. When seen formally at 24 months CA, her motor developmental score was 95 and her cognitive score 106. Neurologic assessment demonstrated a resolution of her hypertonia, and her overall classification was unimpaired.

Learning Points

The early clinical course included the evolution of mild bronchopulmonary dysplasia (BPD), sepsis, and the absence of treatment with antenatal steroid—all risk factors for poor outcomes. Despite normal neurologic examination results at discharge, two factors point to the need for close surveillance: the presence of ventriculomegaly and subsequently the lack of convincing fidgety movements at 3 months CA. Interestingly Abigail appears to have developed transient dystonia, a condition well described in very preterm children. Important clues that this might not be severe CP at 6 months were the lack of tonal changes in the lower limbs (one might expect severe CP to demonstrate hypertonicity in ankle flexion and abduction, with hyperreflexia, upgoing plantar responses, and perhaps even clonus). However, by 12 months this had progressed to cause widespread professional concern that this was indeed CP. The rapid resolution over the second year is typical of transient dystonia and indeed at 24 months CA she was classed as unimpaired. In view of the history, however, the team considered it prudent to continue observation.

Transition to School

VPT children are increasingly followed up through to school age. In the transitional preschool period, there is a focusing of cognitive development into recognizable patterns of executive processing, and accessing general cognitive function (IQ) becomes more reliable. Over this period children frequently attend nursery education in preparation for learning in the school environment. Behavior changes alongside this, as the relative overactivity of the 2-year-old is replaced by the emerging internalized phenotype seen across school age and into adult life. Language and socialization develop rapidly at this time.

Starting School

In some settings, school readiness is assessed to help determine when children appear ready to go to school. Such structured assessments can inform follow-up programs. In other settings, neonatal follow-up services may provide support over this transition. When school entry is age dependent, there is controversy whether former VPT children should be held back to be allowed to catch up, particularly if their birthday and due date would place them in different school intakes (e.g., see the Bliss website at www.bliss.org.uk/starting-school). There is little evidence either way. In the EPICure study, children born before 26 weeks' gestation who were in school in the correct year by due date had attainment similar to that of children who had gone to school in an earlier intake, but the children received more special needs support to do so.[31] Decisions may be better made considering the social development of the child, bearing in mind that keeping a child back a year will not necessarily improve this.

Emerging Impairments at Early School Age

Over the period of transition to school, difficulties in learning, behavior, and motor function may evolve or appear de novo. It is important that such issues are detected early, so that strategies can be put in place to support and optimize learning. Formal assessments by follow-up teams may be structured to assist in this and to inform educational teams.

Cognitive Function

General cognitive scores for very preterm children are, on average, lower than those of children whose pregnancies deliver at full term. As gestation decreases below around 32 weeks, mean scores at each gestational week are progressively lower.[4,32] Traditionally the scores for school age children are calculated on chronological age, rather than age corrected for prematurity, for two reasons—firstly, the school age child is compared to their peers in the school year and, secondly, proportionately the correction is less. More recently this has been challenged with the suggestion that correction should continue,[33] but there appears to be little consensus.

General cognitive scores are the product of a range of executive processes, which themselves may be impaired. The size of the discrepancy, compared with individuals born at term, depends on the process and the postnatal and gestational age of the child.[34] Some executive functions will catch up during childhood—for example, selective or sustained attention—whereas others may diverge—for example, planning or phonemic fluency. Hence the pattern of cognitive problems changes as the children grow through school. At 8 to 10 years of age, key functions such as working memory or information-processing speed appear to underpin the cognitive,[35] learning,[36] and behavioral problems[37] seen in VPT children, which point to foci that may provide opportunity for intervention.

School Attainment

Very preterm children at school are more frequently reported to have special needs, with increasing proportions as gestation decreases.[2] At 24 weeks' gestation around 50% of children will have some special needs in the classroom,[2] varying from 1:1 or small group teaching, to support from therapists. In the EPICure study 13% of children born at less than 26 weeks were in non-mainstream schools because of special needs. Attainment is lower across all educational domains but seems particularly problematic with mathematics, scores in which are depressed more than in other domains. Mathematics difficulties may have a different origin in the VPT child compared with children born at term; more often the problem is related more frequently to underlying executive and working memory problems rather than number estimation, which is most often the cause for children born at term.[38] Key strategies to optimize learning in VPT children may be the presentation of sequential information (i.e., breaking tasks down into smaller steps) and careful monitoring of attention in the classroom.

Behavior

Over the past 20 years there has been increasing recognition of common behavioral and psychiatric morbidity in cohorts of VPT and extremely preterm children.[39–41] Current estimates suggest that VPT 7-year-olds have 3 times the odds of being assigned a psychiatric diagnosis.[42] The most frequent diagnosis is attention deficit disorder, which is most commonly of the inattentive subtype, consistent with the working memory and processing deficits observed. Autism is currently of interest and has been recognized for some time in association with prematurity. Eight percent of an extremely preterm cohort was assigned a diagnosis of autism using a standardized assessment protocol.[43] The literature on preterm infants is somewhat confusing because making a formal diagnosis and scoring high on screening tests are different things. Indeed, symptoms of attention deficit (as scored using the DuPaul RS4 Rating Scale [RS-IV][44]) or of autistic traits (Social Communication Questionnaire,[45] Social Responsiveness Scale[46]) are much more frequently found in VPT children compared with diagnoses. Comorbid with symptoms of anxiety in early adolescence, this excess of symptoms has led to the definition of a preterm behavioral phenotype consisting of internalized individuals with common symptoms within the domains of anxiety, inattention, and social communication.[40] There is some evidence that this may be exacerbated by bullying, which is reported more frequently in preterm populations.[47] It is important that teachers and follow-up teams are aware of these risks if they are to be detected early and support provided to minimize the impact they have on the child and family.

Motor Problems

CP aside, VPT children are frequently reported to have impairments of motor function, referred to variously in the literature. The commonest assessment tool is the Movement Assessment Battery for Children, which is a test of motor impairment as opposed to a motor performance test. Rates of scores above the 5th or 15th percentiles (higher scores reflect more impairment) are significantly higher in VPT populations. In a recent study 28% of VPT children scored at or above the 5th percentile at 8 years, which was a similar proportion to their findings at 4 years.[48] The proportion scoring above these thresholds has not changed appreciably for some time[49] and seems to be related to both perinatal risk and comorbid cognitive scores. These impairments may need assessment and support from physical or occupational therapists. When assessed alongside a detailed neurologic examination—for example, as described by Touwen[50]—motor problems also may be comorbid with a range of soft neurologic signs and seem to reflect a less well-organized motor system.

Changes Over Time for Individual Children

Assessments in infancy are often considered relatively poor predictors of school age outcomes. Particularly when categorical outcomes are used, children may shift between categories. Within the EPICure study at 6 years, only 65% of children classified as having a severe disability at 30 months were still classified as such. In other categories movement was greater. Hence it can be difficult to be certain from even earlier assessments of the likely outcomes if emphasis is placed on categorization. There is often uncertainty about population scores catching up over school age, but such data are very challenging to interpret as the tests will have changed and may measure slightly different mixtures of functions. Generally, in our cohorts mean cognitive scores have remained the same and, although scores in individual children may rise, in others they fall.[51] Cognitive scores in particular appear to be conserved over childhood and adolescence, particularly in those with impairments.[18]

CASE 2   JOSEPH

Joseph was born at 25 weeks' gestation by cesarean section following maternal preeclampsia; his weight was 720 g 48 hours after a course of antenatal steroid treatment. His mother was single and supported by her family. Magnesium sulfate was administered before delivery as a neuroprotective agent. He developed severe respiratory disease and was ventilated for 14 days, with supplemental oxygen remaining to 38 weeks postmenstrual age. Cranial ultrasound results were unremarkable but head growth to discharge home at 39 weeks remained at the 10th percentile. Neurologic examination at discharge was unremarkable and at 3 months he demonstrated fidgety movements. Early development was delayed, and at 12 months of age corrected for prematurity he scored between 86 and 93 for the three composite scales on the Bayley-III. He was referred to the early intervention team because of low developmental scores and social disadvantage. He began nursery school at 2 years of age. Progress over the next 2 years was good and assessment at 4 years of age revealed no neuromotor problems and an IQ score of 104 using the Wechsler Preschool and Primary Scale of Intelligence-Fourth Edition (WPPSI-IV). He remained small but had thrived at nursery school and was well adjusted. Language skills were good. His major problem was in terms of somatic growth and he remained at the 9th percentile for height and weight, with head circumference on the 25th percentile. His mother presented to the clinic at 4 years with a request that he be held back from going to school for a year because he had been born in July and his expected date of delivery was in September and she was concerned about his small size. We discussed his good progress and his behavior in his current social group—which was well adjusted—and discussed this with his nursery. After some further thought we agreed he should be placed in school with his current social group. Over the next 2 years it became clear he was inattentive in the classroom but managing well with his schoolwork, and with some classroom support was achieving performance in the middle of that of his peer group. There were no significant cognitive or behavior problems.

Learning Points

There were several points to the request for him to be kept back a year. First was the potential disadvantage from his age considering his expected date of delivery. Second, his mother considered that he might be bullied because of his small size. And third, there was pressure from within her family to hold him back to protect him so he could be more mature when he went to school. In fact, discussing the situation with the nursery school personnel showed he had a good range of friends in his year at school, he interacted well with staff and the other children, and was certainly holding his own. It was considered not to be to his advantage to take him out of his stable peer group and thus he progressed with his friends.

Transition to Young Adult Life

Studies that span the adolescent period are few in number. The period of adolescence is associated with different demands on individuals compared with early school ages, alongside emerging social competences and independence. Emphasis on physical performance may be less marked, for example, and motor problems appear to be less evident as issues with VPT adolescents, even though differences in scores remain.

Cognitive processes seem relatively conserved over adolescence in terms of general cognitive scores,[18][51] but despite improvements in attention span and attentional problems over adolescence,[52] executive processing problems persist.[53] Relatively poor cognitive performance reduces attainment at school. For example, compared with term-born controls, young people of former preterm very low-birth-weight born in Liverpool, United Kingdom, were more likely to attain vocational qualifications (odd ratios [OR] 4.11 [2.01–8.36]) and fewer achieved university degrees (OR 0.21; 95% confidence interval [CI] [00.11–0.44]).[54] Similar findings have been reported across a range of studies from longitudinal cohorts and database association studies over multiple countries as summarized in detail by Hack.[55] Lower educational attainment reduces employment opportunities, which may be further reduced by poor health outcomes, as evidenced by increased sickness and disability payments with decreasing gestational age at birth.

Of major neurologic concern is the continuity of behavioral and psychiatric problems into adult life recently reviewed.[56] There is evidence for persistence of the preterm behavioral phenotype, consisting of internalizing symptoms of inattention, anxiety, and depression, into adult life, but despite database associations between psychotic disorders such as schizophrenia and preterm birth,[57] for example, none of the longitudinal studies have confirmed this as yet. Such disorders commonly present during the third decade and most longitudinal studies have not yet followed up with populations to the fourth decade.

The social associates of these outcomes are of interest. The lower prevalences of risk-taking, sexual experience, and criminality reported among VPT adults[58,59] may reflect the internalized phenotype and a restricted peer group. Health-related quality of life, as measured using the Health Utilities Index (HUI-3), remains less optimal in extremely low-birth-weight survivors through to the fourth decade, particularly in those with neurosensory impairments, although there is no evidence that the gap with term-born controls is increasing.[60] In the fourth decade, despite reasonable adaptation at 20 years,[61] adults who were of extremely low birth weight were less likely to be employed, overall or full-time, more likely to require social assistance, and on average earned Can$20,000 less than controls. Fewer were married, had sexual intercourse, or had children. Poor health contributed to these differences and after exclusion of chronic health conditions differences were no longer significant.[59]

CASE 3   MARTIN

Martin was born at 24 weeks' gestation following a pregnancy complicated by preterm rupture of membranes. Spontaneous delivery occurred 24 hours after a course of steroids, but the infant was in good condition and admitted in minimal supplemental oxygen but was ventilated to the neonatal unit. His early cardiorespiratory course over the first few days was stormy and, by day 10, cranial ultrasound revealed a left-sided hemorrhagic infarction. This progressed to porencephaly with mild ventriculomegaly on the contralateral side. Neurologic assessment indicated asymmetry at term and over the first 6 months he developed signs of unilateral CP. General development was in keeping with his age but motor milestones were delayed. He received support from the community disability team, receiving regular physiotherapy. At 2 years CA he was categorized

16

CASE 3   MARTIN—cont'd

with moderate impairment; he was not yet ambulant and had clear signs of CP. The Bayley Mental Development Index score was 90 and the Psychomotor Development Index score was 65. Over the preschool years Martin acquired good ambulation with an aid and had surgery for tendon releases at 6 and 12 years of age to maintain ambulation with a crutch. Physiotherapy continued until he moved to senior school at 11 years, when it ceased except around the episode of surgery. At school he remained introverted and shy but teacher reports suggested good learning. He started to play the cello and passed his early examinations easily despite his disability. He graduated with good grades and was offered a place in college studying computer science. At 20 years, he undertook a range of charitable events to raise money for his local neonatal intensive care unit and started a small company to market software. Clinical evaluation at 20 years confirmed a monoplegia involving the right leg, with spasticity and requiring aids to walk but excellent upper limb function.

Learning Points

Despite major ultrasound evidence of brain injury and adverse disability grading at 2 years of age, Martin demonstrated good learning and drive to overcome his physical limitations and entered college with all prospects of a good degree. Early adversity does not necessarily indicate poor outcome, although nominally his health-related quality of life was reduced because of his physical disability. Prediction of outcome from early examinations is never precise and good outcomes are not infrequent.

Components of a Follow-Up Program

Neonatal follow-up programs have evolved that are often based around research and audit. For such programs to be of value to the family, it is important that they provide support and information to help the family provide for and understand their choices for their child.

Over the first year, services need to be available to reassure and provide advice over a range of issues that, while mundane to the professional, are of great importance to families: feeding, vaccination, developmental milestones, growth monitoring, and for those children with ongoing morbidity after their neonatal stay, specific support— for example, for children with bronchopulmonary dysplasia. Regular visits and availability are important, and access to multidisciplinary support is highly valued by parents because advice from professionals not versed in the problems of the preterm may be contradictory. Such follow-up services need to be well connected to community services and early referral for support is critical when issues that require intervention arise.

Over the second year, face-to-face visits are less frequent. At around 2 years of age (corrected for prematurity) a formal assessment of development and outcome is generally undertaken. This should cover the key neurologic domains, hearing and vision, a formal assessment of development, and other clinical systems. Standardized reporting is recommended at 2 years as part of most service activity for audit purposes, using standardized definitions—for example, as part of the British Association of Perinatal Medicine program.[62]

Over the third and subsequent years, we usually undertake annual assessments for those who are of concern, usually those with gestational ages less than 27 weeks at birth, or those for whom there are concerns, and carry out a formal cognitive assessment in the third or fourth year to identify children who may need special needs services early in their educational career.

Each service will identify those who need further follow-up, but research-oriented services will provide intermittent assessments throughout childhood as part of their areas of interest. These data are critically important in educating the profession as to the import of the long-term impairments within this group of vulnerable individuals.

16

Gaps in Knowledge

1. Accurate biomarkers in infancy of later cognitive problems need to be developed so that these can be identified early, leading to earlier intervention and also to act as short-term outcomes to reduce the time required to study their prevention.
2. Identification of the optimal developmental intervention timing and strategy to prevent later neuropsychological problems is required.
3. Identification of family and biologic factors that promote robustness over child-hood would be helpful in targeting interventions.
4. Early childhood markers of adolescent and adult outcomes would be of value in demonstrating improvement, or lack of it, in long-term outcomes.
5. Better neonatal neuroprotective strategies are required.

Conclusions

Neonatal care is continually changing. There is some evidence that these advances work together to produce incremental improvements in outcome, promoting survival of children without serious impairment. Recognition of the pervasive effects of prematurity on brain, and therefore, functional development over childhood, has led to increased research activity in the field, but effective strategies to ameliorate some of the developmental disadvantage in a significant proportion of very preterm children remain elusive. The effects of core neurologic functions, such as slower processing speed and working memory, compared with term-born children, have wide-ranging effects on neurologic function and behavior that may affect socialization and integration for some children, adolescents, and adults. Recognition and support remain critically important functions for follow-up services in the foreseeable future.

REFERENCES

1. Moore T, Hennessy EM, Myles J, et al. Neurological and developmental outcome in extremely preterm children born in England in 1995 and 2006: the EPICure studies. *BMJ*. 2012;345:e7961.
2. MacKay DF, Smith GC, Dobbie R, et al. Gestational age at delivery and special educational need: retrospective cohort study of 407,503 schoolchildren. *PLoS Med*. 2010;7(6):e1000289.
3. Marlow N. Outcome following preterm birth. In: Rennie JM, ed. *Roberton's Textbook of Neonatology*. London: Churchill Livingstone; 2005.
4. Kerr-Wilson CO, Mackay DF, Smith GC, et al. Meta-analysis of the association between preterm delivery and intelligence. *J Public Health*. 2012;34(2):209–216.
5. Sellier E, Platt MJ, Andersen GL, et al. Decreasing prevalence in cerebral palsy: a multi-site European population-based study, 1980 to 2003. *Dev Med Child Neurol*. 2016;58(1):85–92.
6. Linsell L, Malouf R, Morris J, et al. Prognostic factors for cerebral palsy and motor impairment in children born very preterm or very low birthweight: a systematic review. *Dev Med Child Neurol*. 2016;58(6):554–569.
7. Palisano RJ, Hanna SE, Rosenbaum PL, et al. Validation of a model of gross motor function for children with cerebral palsy. *Phys Ther*. 2000;80(10):974–985.
8. Eliasson AC, Krumlinde-Sundholm L, Rosblad B, et al. The Manual Ability Classification System (MACS) for children with cerebral palsy: scale development and evidence of validity and reliability. *Dev Med Child Neurol*. 2006;48(7):549–554.
9. Bax M, Goldstein M, Rosenbaum P, et al. Proposed definition and classification of cerebral palsy, April 2005. *Dev Med Child Neurol*. 2005;47(8):571–576.
10. de Vries LS, van Haastert IC, Benders MJ, et al. Myth: cerebral palsy cannot be predicted by neonatal brain imaging. *Semin Fetal Neonatal Med*. 2011;16(5):279–287.
11. Gosselin J, Gahagan S, Amiel-Tison C. The Amiel-Tison neurological assessment at term: conceptual and methodological continuity in the course of follow-up. *Ment Retard Dev Disabil Res Rev*. 2005;11(1):34–51.
12. Dubowitz L, Ricciw D, Mercuri E. The Dubowitz neurological examination of the full-term newborn. *Ment Retard Dev Disabil Res Rev*. 2005;11(1):52–60.
13. Einspieler C, Prechtl HFR. Prechtl's assessment of general movements: a diagnostic tool for the functional assessment of the young nervous system. *Ment Retard Dev Disabil Res Rev*. 2005;11(1):61–67.
14. Drillien CM. Low-birthweight children at early school-age: a longitudinal study. *Develop Med Child Neurol*. 1980;22:26–47.
15. De Vries LS, Regev R, Pennock JM, et al. Ultrasound evolution and later outcome of infants with periventricular densities. *Early Hum Dev*. 1988;16(2–3):225–233.
16. Johnson SJ, Marlow N. Assessment of the development of high risk infants in the first two years. In: Cioni G, Mercuri E, eds. *Clinics in Developmental Medicine*. London: McKeith Press; 2007.

17. Johnson S, Wolke D, Marlow N. Developmental assessment of preterm infants at 2 years: validity of parent reports. *Dev Med Child Neurol.* 2008;50(1):58–62.
18. Breeman LD, Jaekel J, Baumann N, et al. Preterm cognitive function into adulthood. *Pediatrics.* 2015;136(3):415–423.
19. Anderson PJ, De Luca CR, Hutchinson E, et al. Underestimation of developmental delay by the new bayley-III scale. *Arch Pediatr Adolesc Med.* 2010;164(4):352–356.
20. Vohr BR, Stephens BE, Higgins RD, et al. Are outcomes of extremely preterm infants improving? Impact of Bayley assessment on outcomes. *J Pediatr.* 2012;161(2):222–228.e3.
21. Moore T, Johnson S, Haider S, et al. Relationship between test scores using the second and third editions of the bayley scales in extremely preterm children. *J Pediatr.* 2012;160(4):553–558.
22. Spittle A, Orton J, Anderson PJ, et al. Early developmental intervention programmes provided post hospital discharge to prevent motor and cognitive impairment in preterm infants. *Cochrane Database Syst Rev.* 2015;(11):CD005495.
23. Moore T, Johnson S, Hennessy E, et al. Screening for autism in extremely preterm infants: problems in interpretation. *Dev Med Child Neurol.* 2012;54(6):514–520.
24. Guy A, Seaton SE, Boyle EM, et al. Infants born late/moderately preterm are at increased risk for a positive autism screen at 2 years of age. *J Pediatr.* 2015;166(2):269–275.e3.
25. Limperopoulos C. Autism spectrum disorders in survivors of extreme prematurity. *Clin Perinatol.* 2009;36(4):791–805.
26. Kuban KC, O'Shea TM, Allred EN, et al. Positive screening on the Modified Checklist for Autism in Toddlers (M-CHAT) in extremely low gestational age newborns. *J Pediatr.* 2009;154(4):535–540.e1.
27. Kim SH, Joseph RM, Frazier JA, et al. Predictive validity of the Modified Checklist for Autism in Toddlers (M-CHAT) born very preterm. *J Pediatr.* 2016;178:101–107.e2.
28. Wong HS, Huertas-Ceballos A, Cowan FM, et al. Evaluation of early childhood social-communication difficulties in children born preterm using the quantitative checklist for autism in toddlers. *J Pediatr.* 2014;164(1):26–33.e1.
29. Marlow N. Is survival and neurodevelopmental impairment at 2 years of age the gold standard outcome for neonatal studies? *Arch Dis Child Fetal Neonatal Ed.* 2015;100(1):F82–F84.
30. Tyson JE, Parikh NA, Langer J, et al. Intensive care for extreme prematurity—moving beyond gestational age. *N Engl J Med.* 2008;358(16):1672–1681.
31. Johnson S, Hennessy E, Smith R, et al. Academic attainment and special educational needs in extremely preterm children at 11 years of age: the EPICure study. *Arch Dis Child Fetal Neonatal Ed.* 2009;94(4):F283–F289.
32. Marlow N. Chapter 3: outcome following preterm birth. In: Rennie J, ed. *Robertson's Textbook of Neonatology.* Edinburgh: Churchill Livingstone; 2005.
33. Wilson-Ching M, Pascoe L, Doyle LW, et al. Effects of correcting for prematurity on cognitive test scores in childhood. *J Paediatr Child Health.* 2014;50(3):182–188.
34. Mulder H, Pitchford NJ, Hagger MS, et al. Development of executive function and attention in preterm children: a systematic review. *Dev Neuropsychol.* 2009;34(4):393–421.
35. Mulder H, Pitchford NJ, Marlow N. Processing speed mediates executive function difficulties in very preterm children in middle childhood. *J Int Neuropsychol Soc.* 2011:1–10.
36. Mulder H, Pitchford NJ, Marlow N. Processing speed and working memory underlie academic attainment in very preterm children. *Arch Dis Child Fetal Neonatal Ed.* 2010;95(4):F267–F272.
37. Mulder H, Pitchford NJ, Marlow N. Inattentive behaviour is associated with poor working memory and slow processing speed in very pre-term children in middle childhood. *Br J Educ Psychol.* 2011;81(Pt 1):147–160.
38. Simms V, Gilmore C, Cragg L, et al. Nature and origins of mathematics difficulties in very preterm children: a different etiology than developmental dyscalculia. *Pediatr Res.* 2015;77(2):389–395.
39. Johnson S, Wolke D. Behavioural outcomes and psychopathology during adolescence. *Early Hum Dev.* 2013;89(4):199–207.
40. Johnson S, Marlow N. Preterm birth and childhood psychiatric disorders. *Ped Res.* 2011;69(5 Pt 2):11R–18R.
41. Hille ET, den Ouden AL, Saigal S, et al. Behavioural problems in children who weigh 1000 g or less at birth in four countries. *Lancet.* 2001;357(9269):1641–1643.
42. Treyvaud K, Ure A, Doyle LW, et al. Psychiatric outcomes at age seven for very preterm children: rates and predictors. *J Child Psychol Psychiatry.* 2013;54(7):772–779.
43. Johnson S, Hollis C, Kochhar P, et al. Autism spectrum disorders in extremely preterm children. *J Pediatr.* 2010;156(4):525–531.e2.
44. Brogan E, Cragg L, Gilmore C, et al. Inattention in very preterm children: implications for screening and detection. *Arch Dis Child.* 2014;99(9):834–839.
45. Johnson S, Hollis C, Hennessy E, et al. Screening for autism in preterm children: diagnostic utility of the social communication questionnaire. *Arch Dis Child.* 2011;96(1):73–77.
46. Padilla N, Eklof E, Martensson GE, et al. Poor brain growth in extremely preterm neonates long before the onset of autism spectrum disorder symptoms. *Cereb Cortex.* 2015.
47. Wolke D, Baumann N, Strauss V, et al. Bullying of preterm children and emotional problems at school age: cross-culturally invariant effects. *J Pediatr.* 2015;166(6):1417–1422.
48. Griffiths A, Morgan P, Anderson PJ, et al. Predictive value of the movement assessment battery for children—second edition at 4 years, for motor impairment at 8 years in children born preterm. *Dev Med Child Neurol.* 2017.
49. Marlow N, Roberts B, Cooke R. Motor skills in extremely low birthweight children at the age of 6 years. *Arch Dis Child.* 1989;64(6):839–847.

16

50. Touwen B. Examination of the child with minor neurological dysfunction. *Clin Dev Med.* 1984.
51. *Cognitive Outcomes Following Extremely Preterm Birth to 19 Years of Age: The EPICure Study.* Baltimore: Pediatric Academic Societies (PAS); 2016.
52. Breeman LD, Jaekel J, Baumann N, et al. Attention problems in very preterm children from childhood to adulthood: the bavarian longitudinal study. *J Child Psychol Psychiatry.* 2016;57(2):132–140.
53. Nosarti C, Giouroukou E, Micali N, et al. Impaired executive functioning in young adults born very preterm. *J Int Neuropsychol Soc.* 2007;13:571–581.
54. Cooke RW. Health, lifestyle, and quality of life for young adults born very preterm. *Arch Dis Child.* 2004;89(3):201–206.
55. Hack M. Adult outcomes of preterm children. *J Dev Behav Pediatr.* 2009;30(5):460–470.
56. Johnson S, Marlow N. Growing up after extremely preterm birth: lifespan mental health outcomes. *Semin Fetal Neonatal Med.* 2014;19(2):97–104.
57. Moster D, Lie RT, Markestad T. Long-term medical and social consequences of preterm birth. *N Engl J Med.* 2008;359(3):262–273.
58. Hack M, Flannery DJ, Schluchter M, et al. Outcomes in young adulthood for very-low-birth-weight infants. *N Engl J Med.* 2002;346(3):149–157.
59. Saigal S, Day KL, Van Lieshout RJ, et al. Health, wealth, social integration, and sexuality of extremely low-birth-weight prematurely born adults in the fourth decade of life. *JAMA Pediatr.* 2016;170(7):678–686.
60. Saigal S, Ferro MA, Van Lieshout RJ, et al. Health-related quality of life trajectories of extremely low birth weight survivors into adulthood. *J Pediatr.* 2016;179:68–73.e1.
61. Saigal S, Stoskopf B, Streiner D, et al. Transition of extremely low-birth-weight infants from adolescence to young adulthood: comparison with normal birth-weight controls. *JAMA.* 2006;295(6):667–675.
62. Report of a BAPM/RCPCH working group. *Classification of Health Status at 2 Years as a Perinatal Outcome.* London: BAPM; 2008.

Index

Note: Page numbers followed by "f" refer to illustrations; page numbers followed by "t" refer to tables; page numbers followed by "b" refer to boxes.

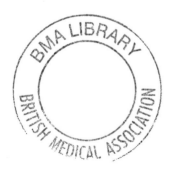